Governing Systems

BERKELEY SERIES IN BRITISH STUDIES

Edited by Mark Bevir and James Vernon

Governing Systems

*Modernity and the Making of Public
Health in England, 1830–1910*

Tom Crook

UNIVERSITY OF CALIFORNIA PRESS

University of California Press, one of the most
distinguished university presses in the United States,
enriches lives around the world by advancing scholarship
in the humanities, social sciences, and natural sciences.
Its activities are supported by the UC Press Foundation
and by philanthropic contributions from individuals and
institutions. For more information, visit www.ucpress.edu.

University of California Press
Oakland, California

© 2016 by The Regents of the University of California

Library of Congress Cataloging-in-Publication Data

Names: Crook, Tom, 1977–author.
Title: Governing systems : modernity and the making of
    public health in England, 1830-1910 / Tom Crook.
Other titles: Berkeley series in British studies ; 11.
Description: Oakland, California : University of
    California Press, [2016] | "2016 | Series: Berkeley
    series in British studies ; 11 | Includes bibliographical
    references and index.
Identifiers: LCCN 2015045708| ISBN 9780520290341
    (cloth : alk. paper) | ISBN 9780520290358 (pbk. : alk.
    paper)
Subjects: LCSH: Public health—England—History—19th
century. | Public health—England—History—20th
century. | Medical policy—England—History—19th
century. | Medical policy—England—History—20th
century.
Classification: LCC RA487 .C735 2016 | DDC
    362.10941—dc23
LC record available at http://lccn.loc.gov/2015045708

Manufactured in the United States of America

25 24 23 22 21 20 19 18 17 16
10 9 8 7 6 5 4 3 2 1

In keeping with a commitment to support
environmentally responsible and sustainable printing
practices, UC Press has printed this book on Natures
Natural, a fiber that contains 30% post-consumer waste
and meets the minimum requirements of ANSI/NISO
Z39.48-1992 (R 1997) (*Permanence of Paper*).

For Holly

Contents

Illustrations

Acknowledgments

All books take time. This one has taken ages. It began life at the University of Manchester in 2001 as an ESRC-funded doctoral project. This book bears only a passing resemblance to my Ph.D.; but it is here where my thanks begin. Most of all, I would like to thank Patrick Joyce, who was my supervisor back then, and who first stirred my interest in "systems." Bertrand Taithe and Ian Burney also provided support and guidance, which at times was much needed. I am delighted to say that I'm still friends with my fellow Ph.D.-ers in that great city of Manchester, Francis Dodsworth, Chris Otter, and Gavin Rand. Of late, as this book staggered toward completion, it has been the friendship of James Vernon that I have cherished and benefited from most. His patience has been immense, his advice brilliant and generous.

My colleagues at Oxford Brookes, where I began working in 2005, have kept me going over the years: supportive, collegiate, and incredibly good humored all at once. Special thanks to Carol Beadle, Joanne Begiato, Virginia Crossman, Anne-Marie Kilday, Donal Lowry, Angela McShane, David Nash, Viviane Quirke, Andrew Spicer, Marius Turda, Cassie Watson, and Jane Stevens Crawshaw. Still more special thanks must go to Glen O'Hara, with whom I've had countless productive discussions about why governing is such a messy process—and enjoyed many laughs and beers along the way. But good company has never been in short supply in Oxford, and for that I must thank Simon Baalham, Markus Butler, Stephen Byrne, Ady Davey, Mike Esbester,

Matthew Feldman, Stefan Fisher-Høyrem, and Pete Mills. The next round is on me.

All this pales in comparison to the support I have received from my family—or rather, happily enough, various families these days, from the Crook and the Wright to the Hiscox and the Peace. And Jo, you are simply the best; Malcolm, the one who keeps on keeping on, always—inspirations both. And this pales again in relation to the support of the one who matters the most. This book is for you, Holly, though I shall spare you any extended words of thanks. They could never be enough, ever.

Abbreviations

AMSES	Association of Municipal and Sanitary Engineers and Surveyors
ARLGB	*Annual Report of the Local Government Board*
ARRG(s)	*Annual Report(s) of the Registrar-General*
BMA	British Medical Association
BMJ	*British Medical Journal*
CBH	Central Board of Health
CDAs	Contagious Diseases Acts
CLH(s)	common lodging house(s)
GBH	General Board of Health
GRO	General Register Office
HMSO	Her/His Majesty's Stationery Office
ICD	International List of Causes of Death
ICE	Institution of Civil Engineers
ISC(s)	International Sanitary Conference(s)
JSSL	*Journal of the Statistical Society of London*
LCC	London County Council
LGAO	Local Government Act Office
LGB	Local Government Board
LMA	London Metropolitan Archives

LPDA	Liberty and Property Defence Association
LSA	Ladies' National Association for the Diffusion of Sanitary Knowledge
MAB	Metropolitan Asylums Board
MALSC	Manchester Archives and Local Studies Centre
MBW	Metropolitan Board of Works
MCS	Metropolitan Commission of Sewers
MDPC	Medical Department of the Privy Council
MO(s)H	medical officer(s) of health
MSSA	Manchester and Salford Sanitary Association
NALGO	National Association of Local Government Officers
NAPSS	National Association for the Promotion of Social Science
OHC	Oxfordshire History Centre
PAMSES	*Proceedings of the Association of Municipal and Sanitary Engineers and Surveyors*
PLMOs	poor law medical officers
PSA(s)	port sanitary authority(ies)
RSI	Royal Sanitary Institute
SIGB	Sanitary Institute of Great Britain
SSL	Statistical Society of London
TNA	The National Archives
TNAPSS	*Transactions of the National Association for the Promotion of Social Science*

CHAPTER I

In Search of Hygeia

Systems, Modernity, and Public Health

In October 1875, it fell to the physician and sanitary reformer Benjamin Ward Richardson to deliver the presidential address of the health section of the National Association for the Promotion of Social Science (NAPSS). The occasion was the NAPSS's annual congress, which was taking place that year in Brighton, on England's south coast. Since its establishment in 1857, the NAPSS had brought together thousands of ministers, MPs, councillors, local and central officials, professionals, and voluntary activists in order to advance the cause of more rational ways of governing, both at home and in the British Empire. Other sections dealt with education, legal reform, and finance and trade. Richardson later wrote that he had considered giving a lecture entitled "The Statistics of Death Rates." Instead, having been advised that delegates were "worn out with statistics," he decided "to plunge into the imagination" and outline a utopian city of health."[1]

Richardson called this city Hygeia. All houses were furnished with bathrooms and toilets, and were connected to sewerage and water-supply systems. Sewage was channeled to outlying fields, where it was put to use in agriculture. Pedestrians walked tree-lined streets; traffic was directed underground via subways. Sanitary and medical officers worked unhindered. The municipal council was free of political strife. Hospitals were plentiful. All foodstuffs were inspected. And no one smoked or drank alcohol. It was not, he stressed, entirely free of infectious diseases. Scarlet fever, measles, and whooping cough, for instance, would probably persist, even if smallpox, dysentery, cholera, typhoid, and typhus would likely be banished; otherwise, most would die from diseases that arose from "uncontrollable causes," among them cancer and those of a "strong hereditary character." Nonetheless, Hygeia was within reach: Richardson estimated it was only a generation away. The "details" existed in places—the particular technologies, practices, and forms of expertise—and had been "worked out by those pioneers of sanitary science, so many of whom surround me today."[2] It was a question of pulling these elements together to form a coherent and seamless urban system. Like all earthly utopias, it is a vision of wholeness and goodness, and of people and things at their most exemplary, somehow emerging from history at the hands of humans. "Utopia itself is but another word for time," Richardson concluded, having noted that Hygeia contained "nothing whatever but what is at this present moment easily possible."[3]

Richardson's presentation of Hygeia is but a scene within the bigger story that this book seeks to retell: the making of a modern public health system in England, roughly 1830 to 1910. The aim is to rethink the modernity of this system by looking at how it was assembled, reformed and, above all, practiced. We begin with Hygeia because it captures something of the epidemiological priorities of public health in this particular pocket of space and time. In Victorian and Edwardian England, the principal focus of public health efforts was the eradication of infectious diseases of a bacterial and viral sort—diseases that would, mercifully, as part of what demographic historians call an "epidemiological transition," lose their deadly salience in the twentieth century, when more chronic and degenerative conditions became the principal causes of death.[4] It captures, too, the growing administrative capacities of public health. Already more than twenty-five years had passed since the establishment (in 1848) of the General Board of Health (GBH), England's first centralized, specialized public health office. By 1875, it was a bureaucratic function that had passed to the Local Government Board (LGB). Since 1872, local authorities had been obliged to appoint medical officers of health (MOsH) and sanitary inspectors. Large-scale sewerage systems were in the process of being constructed. In fact, the largest of these had been completed just that year: London's Main Drainage Scheme, which carried away the waste of more than three million people. Only months before Richardson spoke, parliament had passed the 1875 Public Health Act, a mammoth piece of legislation that consolidated existing statutes passed during the preceding three decades. Its sprawling scope included regulations relating to the supply of water and the disposal of sewage; the sale of food and the slaughter of animals; the disinfection of insanitary homes and business premises; and the provision of hospitals for those suffering from infectious diseases.

It is easy, then, to understand Richardson's confidence: progress was being made, and might not more be had—significantly more? And yet, quite simply, Hygeia was never realized. In some respects, Richardson's imaginary city is the last place we should begin if we wish to understand, as this book does, the practices and practicalities of governing public health in Victorian and Edwardian England. For a real flavor of what happened we might turn to the papers that followed Richardson's address as part of the deliberations of the health section. For sure, there was no sense of fatalism or powerlessness, but there was frustration and dispute in abundance. Acts had been passed, yet some local authorities, whether out of lethargy or active opposition, had still to implement them; and where they had, the results were disappointing. Any kind of uniformity of practice was wholly absent. At the same time, there was no consensus regarding some basic questions of administration: should water-supply systems, for instance, be publicly or privately owned? Some thought the former, others the latter, invoking as they did so conflicting examples of good practice. Meanwhile, delegates delved into a maddening world of technical intricacies, from those that featured as part of the reform of England's portside quarantine system—an urgent matter, given Britain's global-economic dominance at this point—to those that might strike us as somewhat inconsequential. One paper, for instance, was entitled "Roof Pipes for Ventilating Sewers."

Where, we might ask, is Hygeia in all of this? An editorial in the *Times* was suitably skeptical. It welcomed the ambitions and ideals that informed what it called "Hygeiopolis"; but it was quick to point out that the people of England were just not ready for such a city, given its costs and regulatory burdens. A "model city can never exist," it declared, "until the community intended to inhabit it is educated to render individual freedom subordinate to the public good in a far greater degree than is at present seen to be either useful or necessary by the majority of the people of this country." It went on: "If Hygeiopolis were established tomorrow, before six weeks had passed the Municipal Council would witness a powerful opposition in favour of dirt, freedom and disease."[5] The *Times* was right: governing public health was—and would remain— enmeshed in political struggles and the variable willingness of the public to accept measures designed to improve its health and longevity. To this we might add that reforms were mooted and by turns rejected, adopted, and reworked; that solutions generated new problems; and that administrative anomalies and shortcomings were routinely acknowledged and debated (as in the deliberations of the NAPSS's health section in 1875). So much for Hygeia: not only was England's public health system a work in progress, always in need of reform; its development was unpredictable, confused, and contested.

Yet, as this book argues, this gap between (high, lofty) ideals and (low, practical) realities goes to the heart of the modernity of the public health system that was assembled in England during the period 1830 to 1910. The book develops this argument by exploiting the word *system*. Curiously, given its ubiquity, both past and present, the word has yet to take center stage within histories of public health—or indeed histories of other areas of administration that were (and remain) just as systemic, be they educational, economic, legal, or penal, to name but a few.

Today, as in the past, the term carries two principal meanings.[6] One of these, to quote Johnson's *Dictionary of the English Language* (1755), is "any complexure or combination of many things acting together"; or in the words of a later dictionary, system as an "assemblage of parts adjusted into and working as a whole, being mutually dependent."[7] This, it is argued here, is precisely what the public health system was, *in actu*: a shifting assemblage of interacting parts and practices, people and things, which, crucially, included more specialized systems—or subsystems, as they might be styled—of sanitary inspection, waste disposal, and statistical classification, among many others. The modernity of the system partly resides in its complexity, and in the way it was reflected upon and realized as a series of systems, from the system as a national whole to multiple systems within.

The other meaning is system as method, as a set of practices that are ordered, regular, and uniform; or, as Johnson's *Dictionary* had it, "a scheme which unites many things in order."[8] It is from this meaning that the term *systematic* derives, understood as "methodical, regular," to quote one dictionary published in 1874; or as "methodical, according to a plan, not casual, sporadic, or unintentional," as another later put it in 1914.[9] Let us be clear: England's public health system during the Victorian and Edwardian periods was never systematic—far from it, at all levels, and at each step of the way. And yet, so this book contends, no system, small or large, could have arisen, functioned, or been critiqued without a modicum of desire for, or conception of, systematic systems. To be sure, these conceptions were hugely varied, and at their most extreme they offered visions of total system and administrative perfection; or at least something approaching perfection, as the possibilities were then understood, as in Richardson's Hygeia. Nonetheless, in order to understand what happened and how, the slippage between these two meanings of system should be embraced. It is only by doing so that we can grasp the modern dynamism—the spirit of restless critique and permanent innovation—in which a public health system was put together and practiced in Victorian and Edwardian England. No one was antisystem, even if some were more pragmatic than others. And if there was frustration, then it was frustration born of the assumption of historical progress, and that things might be administered in a more systematic, efficient, and uniform fashion. Modernity is nothing if not a confused, Sisyphean search for cities like Hygeia.

In sum, this is a book about why Hygeia was never built. But it is also a book about modernity, and a culture of governing in which a city such as Hygeia was taken seriously and deemed possible.

FROM THE "HEROIC" TO THE "ANTIHEROIC"

To focus on systems is not the usual way to write the history of modern public health in England. Equally, to seek to refresh and reinvigorate a sense of the modernity of public health in Victorian and Edwardian England is to swim against the tide of the revisionist scholarship that has developed since the 1970s. This is not the place to offer a detailed review of what is now a voluminous literature, characterized by multiple concerns, geographies, arguments, and methodologies; and excellent reviews exist already.[10] Even so, when it comes to thinking about the modernity of Victorian public health—and it is here where the rub lies, in the Victorian period—we might speak of the dissolution of some crucial analytical coordinates; or, to borrow from Dorothy Porter, introducing her comparative collection, *The History of Public Health and the Modern State,* a broad shift from a "heroic" to an "antiheroic" historiography.[11]

The former took shape in the 1950s and 1960s. Whether in a biographical vein or not, accounts of this sort stressed the industry of leading reformers—notably Edwin Chadwick, William Farr, and John Simon—and their allies as they struggled to impose an enlightened, centralized, and science-based program of public administration. Apathetic ministers and parsimonious ratepayers were among the villains, attached as they were to non-interventionism and outmoded traditions of local self-government.[12] Meanwhile, comparative accounts, notably George Rosen's classic study, *A History of Public Health,* situated England firmly in the European van of nations that pioneered modern public health. The "seed-beds" of the "revolution" to come were many, Rosen suggested, not least German conceptions of an all-encompassing "medical police," which emerged in the second half of the eighteenth century. Revolutionary France and industrial England, however, were home to the first public health "movements," he argued, even if the lead quickly passed to the latter during the mid-nineteenth century.[13] It was at this point when towns and cities began building what would become England's most celebrated contribution to the cause of public health: waterborne sewerage systems.

Invariably, this scholarship was of its time. As Richard Price has argued, the 1950s to 1970s were decades when historians took as their starting point the Victorians' own sense of epochal change, while looking backward through the modernizing "lens of the twentieth century."[14] In this case the "lens" offered a vision of a collectivist, social-democratic modernity; or in the case of public health, a future of socialized medicine. In Britain at least, books on public health were thus part of a broader seam of works written on the "origins" of the welfare state, the NHS, and council housing amid the more liberal, laissez-faire modernity of the nineteenth century.[15] It was at this point, in the throes of a society enduring the twin traumas of urbanization and industrialization, when a modern state began to cohere. There was even talk of a Victorian "revolution in government," presaging the more obvious milestones reached by the New Liberalism of the Edwardian period, chief among them the National Insurance Act of 1911.[16]

It would be wrong to caricature this literature. No consensus emerged from these accounts. There was intense debate, for instance, regarding the precise admixture of governing philosophies that presided over the "growth of the state," if indeed they played any role at all. Even so, the welfare state of postwar Britain served as a crucial means of narrative orientation. At the very least it lent the story of Victorian and Edwardian public health a progressive quality, rooted in science and humanitarian sentiments, while amplifying a sense of the modernity and novelty of what happened.

The antiheroic scholarship that began to develop in the 1980s has not dispatched entirely with the conceptual apparatus and terminology of the more heroic historiography, or with some of its claims. "Modern society" and "modern public health" are still invoked. So too is a "modern state" that was at once more centralized, bureaucratic, and information-rich compared to its medieval, early modern, and eighteenth-century predecessors. Comparative accounts still rank England among the homes of modern public health, and still largely for its development of more environmental and sanitary approaches. Every other facet of the scholarship, however, has been significantly modified, even overturned, dissolving any sense of progressive or necessary problem solving, while encouraging a more diminished sense of novelty and change. Crudely, we might distinguish between four lines of revisionist reappraisal.

The first is the most diffuse: the absence of any overarching modernizing trajectory and, accordingly, the constitutive importance of national and local peculiarities. Peter Baldwin's *Contagion and the State in Europe, 1830–1930* is the most striking account in this respect.[17] Baldwin's aim is to contest the correlation, first mooted by Erwin Ackerknecht in 1948, between "politics and prevention," and especially between the styles of regulation pursued in more liberal regimes, such as Britain and France, and those of a more conservative and authoritarian sort, such as Prussia, Austria, and Russia.[18] Instead, examining Britain, France, Germany, and Sweden, Baldwin points to the following in each national case: (a) peculiar and "polymorphous" combinations of prophylactic responses to common pathogenic enemies—in particular cholera, smallpox, and syphilis—ranging from environmental interventions to more person-centered techniques of quarantine, vaccination, and isolation; and (b) a "multiplicity" of explanatory factors, among them political traditions; moral scruples and religious sensibilities; geopolitical interests; and considerations of administrative geography and capability.

The same interpretive attention to detail, however, can now be found in great swaths of scholarship. From within England, at the local level; to Scotland, Wales, and Ireland; to European nations and the United States; and finally, to Britain's empire: in all of these arenas, historians have piled variation upon variation, complexity upon complexity, at all levels, at all moments, and in relation to all manner of diseases and climatic conditions.[19] We would expect as much, perhaps, in accounts of public health in British India, where English innovations were self-consciously "adapted" in the face of "backward" traditions and populations; but it applies just as intensely to accounts of places with a fully developed sense of civilizational kinship, and where English models of innovation were directly emulated, such as the United States and Australia.[20] Ironically, the one quality these multiple sites now have in common is that they were all very different.

The remaining three facets are more or less pronounced in particular works, but all have similarly sapped a sense of linear, modernizing, and even benign state building. One of these is a reappraisal of the role of science, or rather a plurality of sciences, and how each developed in a contested, stumbling fashion. Notably, given the causal role it was once thought to have played, historians point, not to a "bacteriological revolution" in the 1880s and 1890s, but to a series of slowly maturing, disease-specific breakthroughs alongside a methodological eclecticism among professionals.[21] A third aspect is the way historians have recovered the disciplinary and civilizing dimensions of public health reform in England, which were by no means the preserve of imperial endeavors, whether in India or Egypt, Hong Kong or Singapore.[22] Quite the contrary, they were just as pronounced at home, in the "metropole," where they played a role in the realization of a broadly liberal society. In brief, no longer a neutral enterprise driven by science and humanitarian sentiments, public health is now considered part of a wide-ranging attempt to order society according to various norms regarding race, gender, and class, and the moral requirements of respectable citizenship.[23] This is partly based on the work of Michel Foucault, but also on recovering the ways public health was enmeshed in a patriarchal, stratified, and still largely Christian society.

Finally, the causal role once played by the epidemiological pressures created by urbanization and pronounced demographic growth has faded, amid a recovery of the plurality of options that might have been pursued, and the contingency of those that were. No one disputes the enormity of the demographic transformation that took place. The figures speak for themselves. The population of England and Wales rose from roughly 6.5 million in the mid-1750s to roughly 9 million in 1801, before beginning a remarkable course of expansion: by 1851, it had doubled to 18 million, about half of which lived in urban areas; by 1901 it stood at 32.5 million, at which point more than 80 percent lived in towns and cities.[24] The argument is that no necessary solutions followed, even if it was clear to most that something had to be done. Strikingly, the Chadwickian battle against dirt is now viewed as a strategic choice that turned upon a narrow and selective vision of what constituted public health: a vision, that is, that privileged the provision of sewerage systems and water closets over the reform of medical relief, and more holistic conceptions of what caused death and disease.[25] As Christopher Hamlin has emphasized, *public health* was—and remains—a mutable and contested term. Certainly public health understood as an administrative enterprise with particular priorities, forms of expertise, and personnel is a very different thing to the health of the public.[26]

The above is only a sketch. But it will be evident how much the anti-heroic readings have done to undermine any clear sense of the modernity of public health in Victorian England, even if the term *modern* continues to be used (much as it does elsewhere, in relation to various genres of historiography). All that once seemed solidly modern—progress and developmental direction; science and humanitarian endeavor; revolutions and rapid change and innovation—has melted away, amid a suitably skeptical and empirically driven insistence on multifactorial causation and contingent choices; variation at all levels and in all places; and invariably complex mixtures of science and politics, continuity and change, and theories and practices. And this too was, and still is, of its time. At the very least, as Porter has noted, it reflects the broader (even, in her terms, "postmodern," "relativist") skepticism toward grand narratives of historical development that emerged during the 1980s, and a more critical disposition toward science and the modern state as sources of emancipation and betterment.[27]

This book endorses this revisionism. There should be no turning back: no repression of contingencies or variations; no resort to monocausal explanations or sources of change; no reassertions of the origins of a state to come. Yet, the argument of this book is that we can affirm just this—contingency and choice, contestation and variation—while also insisting on the modernity of public health in Victorian and Edwardian England. To do so is to argue that we might find a modern *form* or *structure* in the formation and performance of that which now appears to be without form or structure. Ultimately, to do so is to argue that modernity inheres not in a particular outcome or solution, but in the way in which an administrative problem—in our case, public health—is posed, practiced, and reformed: or, to put it another way, in open-ended processes of modern order*ing*, rather than the attainment of order as such, or movement toward a particular endpoint or telos. The chapter now sets out the key elements of this argument and the understanding of modernity that informs the chapters that follow.

DISPLACING THE STATE

The crucial assumption this book makes is that governing is a matter of discourse and practice: a combination of cultural-intellectual *and* material-logistical forces. In this way, the book works with both the "cultural" and the "material turns," and locates agency and change in shifting amalgams of words and things, meanings and practices, people and technologies.[28] One such historical site is the state. It seems that around 1780, the term *state*—though it was normally capitalized—began to be used in a modern sense to refer to an abstract, singular agent that might act and do things, and so "interfere" and "intervene" in society.[29] This was in contrast to earlier uses, when it referred to social-institutional rituals and exchanges embedded in people's lives, and time-honored hierarchies, as in the "states" or "estates" of society.[30] The Victorians spoke about the state in this functional and impersonal fashion, even if by the end of the century a "skein of states" had emerged, as James Meadowcroft has put it, ranging from the state understood as a legal and political power distinct from society to the state understood as the collective incarnation of the nation's capacity to govern itself.[31] Advocates of public health reform certainly invoked the state, most notably, perhaps, when speaking of "state medicine," a term popularized from the 1850s onwards. Likewise, opponents of reform invoked the state, where it normally meant something quite restricted: legal compulsion of national scope and active central regulation, as distinct from the voluntary efforts of individuals, families, and localities.

But whereas some scholars have argued for "bringing the state back in," this book seeks to displace the state in favor of a focus on systems and governance, and a more diffuse understanding of power and agency.[32] The term *system* captures this (see above), and the term *governance* does much the same. To speak of governance is to focus "less on the state and its institutions and more on social practices and activities," as one introductory has text put it.[33] Historians have used it in just this fashion to describe those practices and processes that organize and enable collective order—or "the ordering of order," as one account has it—but which extend much beyond the state and into civil society, economic markets and commercial agents, local authorities, and even as far as the self.[34] It is not a question of abandoning the state, for it was and remains an important referent and actor. To adopt the minimal definition, laws of national scope were forthcoming on a regular basis, and some of these were of a compulsory sort. And just as crucial were various other practices associated with the modern state that were conceptualized and contested around the early nineteenth century, including center-local relations, statistics, and bureaucracy. All were part of what made governing public health modern in Victorian and Edwardian England.

Why, then, focus on systems, and multiple agents of governance? One reason is that the state itself can be grasped quite empirically in this fashion. As Patrick Joyce and Timothy Mitchell have argued, for all its abstract impersonality, the modern state was, and remains, rooted in intricate systems and the work of the myriad agents that operate and maintain them. Among many other examples, we might note taxation systems (e.g. national income tax), state-owned communication systems (e.g., postal and telegraphic services), and standardized systems of weights and measures.[35] One might even regard the modern state as the *effect*, rather than the cause, of these many systems; but certainly, as we shall see in this book, practices understood in terms of the state, such as the generation of official statistics and the performance of official forms of inspection, were all systemic in that they turned upon the coordination of multiple agents and a medley of technologies and practices. Seemingly innocuous technical details and humble administrative acts were the very stuff of governing, if also of conflict and frustration.

The second key reason is that making decisions about what to do was less a matter of opting for a bigger or a smaller state than it was of adopting, reworking, or choosing between particular systems. Indeed, if there was reference to the state, then reference to systems, of one sort or another, was decidedly more frequent. These included the system as a whole, grasped as a national enterprise, as well as multiple subsystems, from systems of inspection and statistical publicity to domestic toiletry and plumbing systems. Public health was by no means exceptional in this respect. During the early and mid-Victorian period, for instance, the "new poor law system" was contrasted with the "old system"; prison reformers spoke of the "prison system," and discussed the relative merits of "silent" and "separate systems" of incarceration pioneered in the United States; education reformers compared the "monitorial system" of school instruction to the "Glasgow system"; civil engineers building a national "railway system" fought over the practicality of "broad" versus "narrow gauge systems"; and these examples might be multiplied. Put another way, displacing the state in favor of systems and governance enables the historian to grasp contingency not just on various levels and scales—from the system as a whole to systems within—but also in terms of how it was practiced and conceived at the time.

MODERN PROCESSES AND SYSTEMIC DYNAMICS

This is where the book locates the quality of being modern—in the formation and functioning of governing systems—a quality that first became evident, so it is argued here, during the early to mid-Victorian period. This is not to suggest, it should be emphasized, that modernity equates with the existence of systems per se. In fact, another strand of revisionist historiography concerns the recovery of the vibrancy and cogency of public health efforts that predated the nineteenth century, extending as far back as the medieval period.[36] A key feature of this literature has been the desire to avoid the kind of anachronistic readings of a premodern past that began with the Victorians themselves, as Carol Rawcliffe has recently argued, where it is the absence or ill-formed origins of those modern features that were to follow that form the analytical point of departure (e.g., a centralized state or professionalized expertise).[37] Instead, the broad aim has been to understand the past in terms of its own distinctive idioms, administrative customs, and prophylactic rationales. And once we do so, we find not only active assemblages of governance but also a recognized way of doing things.

So what, briefly, of the functioning of the premodern public health systems that preceded the modern systems of this book? Certainly, in some respects, public health was already being posed and practiced as a matter of national governance. Health might be conceived in collective terms via the aggregate notion of "population," a product of the late seventeenth century, and there was occasional reference to the "public health of the nation," as in William Blackstone's *Commentaries on the Laws of England* (1765–69).[38] During the sixteenth century, the Privy Council began issuing national books of orders in times of epidemic emergency, in particular during visitations of bubonic plague, the last of which occurred in 1665–66.[39] From roughly 1700 onward, parliament provided a degree of national mediation, to the extent that it sanctioned acts that applied to specific localities.[40] In 1808, a National Vaccine Establishment was founded to promote smallpox vaccination.

Yet, as the revisionist historiography suggests, this was essentially a localized and hierarchical culture of governance, one where public health measures were embedded in a seam of administrative units designed to secure the "common weal" and the "publick good."[41] Among these units were counties, boroughs, and parishes, whose origins and responsibilities derived from a jumble of ecclesiastical customs, royal charters, Saxon practices, and acts of parliament. There were, however, at least two sources of coherence and system. One was the authority of property and the distribution of offices according to social status. The second was resort to court-based proceedings. In counties, for instance, monthly petty sessions presided over by a duo of gentlemanly magistrates provided the principal means of dealing with a medley of offenses collected under the expansive common law rubric of nuisances.[42] At once judicial and administrative agents, magistrates generally ruled on individual cases "presented" by inhabitants, which might include complaints relating to leaking cesspits and negligent pig keeping.[43] A similar culture of administration prevailed in towns and cities, where corporate mayors and aldermen might act as ex-officio magistrates, or where manorial courts were in place, as in Manchester (up to 1846) and Birmingham (up to 1854).

At the same time, court-based processes were supplemented by the actions of various agents, either paid for or called upon to act in a voluntary capacity. Physicians, apothecaries, and lay healers, for instance, attended to the sick. The neediest might avail themselves of the medicines and food distributed by local overseers, as part of the welfare provisions afforded by a parish-based poor law system. Beyond times of emergency, when tactics of isolation and quarantine were deployed, environmental measures were also implemented, amid an already eclectic sense of the causes and vectors of disease, which ranged from corrupt atmospheres and "fomes" (tiny particles) to rotting flesh and human contact.[44] As early as 1552, the corporation of Norwich established a body of two aldermen and ten freemen, called the Surveyours of the Ryver and Streates, to enforce bylaws relating to the repair and cleanliness of waterways, pavements, and roads.[45] Markets were another site of regulation. During the eighteenth century, Manchester's Court Leet annually appointed a handful of propertied inhabitants to act as Market-Lookers for Fish and Flesh, and Officers for Wholesome Ale and Beer.[46] We can even point to engineering projects, such as the building of artificial "conduits" to channel drinking water to homes, as well as ditches to manage rain and surface water.

Finally, there were significant innovations, even if all served to refine, rather than challenge, established practices and forms of authority. Besides the growing formalization of magisterial powers, the poor laws, as well as common law (as in Blackstone's *Commentaries*), new units of administration developed. Most notably, during the second half of the eighteenth century so-called improvement and police commissions were created in towns to further the work of creating a nuisance-free environment. Empowered by local acts of parliament, and composed of local elites and property owners, these bodies were charged with enhancing the lighting, paving, and sweeping of civic spaces and thoroughfares. Between 1760 and 1799, no fewer than four hundred commissions were established.[47]

More might be said on this front. The point is that the transition to a modern culture of governance does not reside in the existence or invention of systems per se. Premodern systems of governing public health were just that: intricate and active systems, composed of multiple roles and responsibilities, and characterized by a shared sense of order and authority. The differences lie elsewhere. The most obvious of these has been introduced already: the sheer scale and ambition of public health in Victorian and Edwardian England, and its emergence as a differentiated domain of governance. It is not just the functioning and multiplication of bigger, more specialized administrative and technological systems that is distinctively modern; so too is the sense of human possibility that attended their conception and their recurrent critique and refinement. On the one hand, a new order of logistical magnitude and organizational complexity; on the other, a new order of reforming ambition, which extended to totalizing visions of system. We began with Richardson's Hygeia, which might be dismissed as an isolated flourish of enthusiasm. And yet, as we shall see, similarly grandiose schemes of reform were in the mix, competing for attention, setting agendas, and prompting discussion and dissension. Chadwick's sanitary agenda of the 1840s and 1850s is one instance; another, the alternate visions of state medicine that also emerged midcentury. Neither was implemented as initially (and ambitiously) conceived, and for different reasons; but they were not without considerable consequence.

This only partly explains, however, the pervasive struggle to make systems systematic. Certainly another logistical factor was the demographic expansion noted above and the brute fact of more and more human bodies. This made for urgency and impetus, and it clearly shaped a sense of the scale of what needed to be done and how this was articulated; but equally, as the revisionist scholarship suggests, it caused nothing in particular from an administrative point of view (including systems for counting and classifying this very same demographic growth: see chapter 3). To be clear, the account of modernity presented here offers no single sufficient cause. Instead, the book assumes a multiplicity of causes, as inscribed in the development and work of a series of modern dynamics and accompanying dialectical processes. It argues for three of these. None concern particular (contingent) outcomes; rather, the argument is that between them these dynamics lent a modern form or structure to the way "public health" was posed and practiced, contested and frustrated as an ongoing and open administrative problem. Crucially, it is not one or the other that matters most, but their combination and intersection, something which began in the decades after 1830. We begin with levels of governance.

Levels of Governance

Modern public health is routinely associated with the eclipse of localized, personalized means of governing—such as the figure of the magistrate—by the advent of more centralized and distant forms of authority; or, more simply, with the rise of the modern state. This was indeed a defining aspect of the modernity of Victorian and Edwardian public health. The institutional milestones are well known, in particular, as noted above, the establishment of GBH and LGB. Equally, in terms of eclipsing the local and the personal, we might add an international level of governance, given the profusion of conferences that took place during the second half of the century. One list of international meetings contrasts twenty-four entries up to 1851, and only one before 1815, against 1,390 between 1851 and 1899; and some of these concerned sanitary matters.[48]

The emergence of central and international levels of governance was part of what might be termed, after Anthony Giddens, a "disembedding" of public health, and the assumption of a national and global field of reference; or again, a "lifting out" of public health from "local contexts of action," so that innovations and norms of good practice could be discussed and encouraged on a *trans*local basis.[49] As we shall see, the principal frame of reference was the national one, and developments within this frame at the local level, which were subject to increasingly intense and regular forms of scrutiny. But this did not preclude looking beyond England. The assumption, certainly, was that lessons might be learned from abroad, and, conversely, exported there. From the vantage point of the national and the central, governmental gazes were cast both inward and outward.

Yet, the argument here is that this is only half of what happened. For if centralization and internationalization entailed a "lifting out" or "abstraction" of systems of governance, and the promotion of general standards and models of practice, the flipside of this was a *reinvigoration of the local and the personal*. This is not to invert the familiar association of modernity with central, or indeed international, levels of governance, so that the local and the personal are transformed into the crucibles of modern power. Rather, it is to suggest that we need to grasp these levels together, as part of a modern, "multi-scalar" process of mutual elaboration and transformation.[50] Significantly, this is how governing became conceived at the time. It was during the early Victorian period, for instance, when "local self-government" was first opposed to "centralization." Likewise, the Victorians began insisting on a distinction between "public" and "private" realms of hygiene, where the latter referred to the self-governing powers of individuals. And it was also a matter of practice. Public health simply could not have happened without the multiple relations that emerged both between central and local agencies, and *within* the local itself, between officials, councillors, and members of the public. This was partly about meeting a logistical challenge, of course. Ultimately, it was at the local level—in towns, streets, and homes, and in and around human bodies—where policies had to work. But governing on multiple levels was also about wrestling with another modern dynamic: the public of "public health" as both an object and a subject of governance.

Agents of Governance

One development commonly associated with the rise of the modern state in England (and elsewhere) is the increasing power of experts and officials. This too is a key feature of modernity. Bureaucratization and professionalization were hugely complicated processes, of course, not least given the persistence of gentlemanly ideals, especially within the central "civil service" (another novel term, along with *bureaucrat* and *expert*).[51] But both processes were pronounced. What became known as "sanitary science," for instance, found a promotional home in various national and professional bodies, among others the Metropolitan Association of Medical Officers of Health (1856; later, in 1873, the Society of MOsH); the NAPSS; the Sanitary Institute of Great Britain (SIGB, 1876; later, in 1904, the Royal Sanitary Institute); and the British Institute of Public Health (1892; later, in 1897, the Royal Institute of Public Health). To put this into a Foucauldian idiom, bureaucratization and professionalization were means by which the English public was objectified, normalized, and disciplined: which is to say, exposed to inspection and compelled to act in accordance with regulations; counted and classified according to norms of good health; and, ultimately, posited like an *object* governed by scientific laws of health.

Yet, once again, this kind of analysis captures only half of a dynamic and dialectical process. For at the same time, and in multiple ways, this public also featured as a *subject* of governance. As Anne Hardy has suggested, there were a variety of "publics" that made up the public of public health, including those of a more civic and voluntary sort, all part of a flourishing civil society.[52] Equally, there was an active process of public empowerment at work that was just as modern as the rise of expertise and bureaucracy: namely, democratization, and the formation of a parliamentary-political sphere and an extraparliamentary public sphere. The complexities are immense in each case, and not least because of crucial considerations of class and gender. Nonetheless, these developments proceeded more or less in tandem with the rise of professionals and officials. The 1832 Reform Act and the 1835 Municipal Corporations Act marked the beginning of a gradual formalization of the "political nation," and an expansion in the number of those able to vote in local and parliamentary elections. Within and outside parliament, politics became more party-based and organized. A distinction emerged, for instance, between "the Government" and "the Opposition"; and local party groupings were eventually integrated on a mass scale via the formation of national Conservative (1867) and Liberal associations (1877).[53] Meanwhile, "public opinion" became an established point of reference in the 1820s, just as the press began to expand. In 1824, there were 244 local and national newspapers in the United Kingdom; by 1886, there were 2,093—a near ninefold increase.[54]

Theorists of modernity have generated various antinomies to capture the dynamism of this process, among others the dual imperatives of "mastery and autonomy," the twin authorities of "science and liberty," and the interplay of "bureaucracy and democracy."[55] Never a consistent theorist of power, in a lecture he delivered in the mid-1970s Foucault described an analogous antagonism:

> From the nineteenth century until the present day we have then in modern societies, on the one hand, a legislation, a discourse and an organization of public right articulated around the principle of the sovereignty of the social body, and we also have a tight grid of disciplinary coercions that actually guarantees the cohesion of that social body. . . . In modern societies, power is exercised through, on the basis of, and in the very play of the heterogeneity between a public right of sovereignty and a polymorphous mechanics of discipline.[56]

Doubtless the dynamic might be formulated in more than one fashion. The basic point here is that modern governance extends to practices and ideals of popular inclusion and public activism and accountability, as much as to practices and ideals of expert knowledge and bureaucratic administration. Put another way, modernity involves multiplying agents of governance, who form—and indeed are thought of and posited—as both objects and subjects of power.

This is not to deny the advent of increasingly specialist forms of expertise and institutionalized systems of officialdom. Rather, it is to suggest that this needs to be considered as part of a more shared, entangled, and routinely messy process of governing that also relied on the agency of MPs, civic activists, councillors, and members of the public. This certainly made for conflict. If freedom inhered in freedom from disease, and so a whole series of disciplinary and costly interventions, then freedom also inhered in fiscal restraint, domestic privacy, the rights of property, and local self-government. Yet, crucially, this did not preclude cooperation and the formation of coalitions between agents, and at various levels of governance, without which nothing could have been done. It worked both ways. In short, the modernity of England's modern public health system resides in the way it was composed and forged in these multiple relations.

Times of Governance

The final dynamic concerns the temporality of Victorian and Edwardian public health, and the way it assumed and practiced what might be called, after Reinhart Koselleck, modern-historical time: or more specifically, the kind of evolutionary and civilizational time that began to develop during the second half of the eighteenth century, before flourishing in the nineteenth.[57] That the Victorians looked backward as much as forward is well known, making for a "mixed modernity," as Billie Melman has put it, composed of complex accretions of multiple futures and multiple pasts.[58] In terms of the former, we find invocations of progress and immense future possibilities; in terms of the latter, increasingly elaborate recoveries of the past, from the discoveries of geology to new histories and idealizations of the ancient, medieval, and early modern worlds. And what Jerome Buckley once termed the "triumph of time" was also manifest in new practices: among others, the advent of a public culture of museums and exhibitions; organized, professionalized archiving; and the growing popularity of personal autobiography and diary keeping.[59]

All of these developments marked a profound extension of temporal perspective on the present, one that came to underpin all aspects of life and thought. Governing was no exception. As Koselleck argues, from roughly 1800 onward, historical time became central to governmental thought and action, informing the entire "social and political vocabulary": "Since then, there has hardly been a concept of political theory or social programmes which does not contain a coefficient of temporal change, in the absence of which nothing can be recognized, nothing thought or argued, without the loss of conceptual force. Time itself becomes a title of legitimation open to occupation from all sides. Specific legitimating concepts would no longer be possible without temporal perspective."[60] One instance of this, he suggests, is the proliferation of modern "isms" that occurred in the nineteenth century—"conservatism," "liberalism," and "socialism," among them—and how each was tied to particular readings of history.

Yet, as Koselleck and others have argued, this deepening of temporal-historical perspective was only half of a complex dynamic, for it was also bound up with quite the opposite: namely, "time-space *compression*," and the assumption that all spaces, no matter how far apart and whatever it is they contain (particular people and practices, for example, or traditions and customs), inhabit the same clocked, chronological present.[61] Linked to a growth of global connectivity and increased travel, trade, and migration, this temporal dynamic was first developed in the civilizational and proto-anthropological thought of the Enlightenment. Koselleck describes how societies from around the world were increasingly subject to synchronic comparison *and* diachronic ordering, thereby generating ideas of relative "advance" and "backwardness." "From the eighteenth century on," he writes, "it was possible to formulate the postulate of acceleration; or conversely from the point of view of those left behind, the postulate of drawing level or overtaking. This fundamental experience of progress, embodied in a singular concept around 1800 ['Progress'], is rooted in the knowledge of noncontemporaneities which exist at a chronologically uniform time."[62] Not everyone, that is, progressed at the same rate or in the same fashion, even if they inhabited the same ticking, empty chronological present: a given year, month, day, or hour. One might even move backward, regress, and degenerate.

Public health in Victorian and Edwardian England was governed in just this kind of time. Perhaps writers and poets enjoyed epiphanic moments; perhaps Christian evangelicals invoked apocalyptic crises now and then.[63] But when it came to governing public health and figuring out a way forward, it was this form of time that was crucial. Modern-historical time functioned as a kind of operative assumption, and was embedded just as much in the day-to-day work of governing systems, as in the ideals and principles that created and sustained these systems. Crudely, on the one hand, public health was rooted in temporal depth and extension, most of all the simple but crucial assumption of progress and the possibility of leaving behind a filthy, disease-ridden past. Progress was variously defined and the means to secure it were always in dispute. Nonetheless, it formed the principal horizon of thought and action, and was most manifest in the development of a great archive of official "blue book" documentation—central surveys, bureaucratic returns, and the reports of royal commissions, for instance—recovering what had been done and what might be done, and investigating good and bad practices, both at home and abroad. Put another way, it was realized and materialized as an unprecedented investigatory labor into spatial-temporal variations of practice, and existing problems and possible solutions.

On the other hand, however—if also as part of the same dynamic—Victorian and Edwardian public health was rooted in a "shrinking world" of technological infrastructures and administrative systems that assumed the emptiness and homogeneity of time and space, while compressing their interrelations: or more simply, a world of growing speed and acceleration that combined chronological intensity and spatial reach. This process of shrinking is normally associated with the introduction of steam-powered transportation (steam ships and railways), and the advent of imperial news systems and electrical telegraphy, all of which helped to secure increasingly rapid flows of information and people.[64] But it was just as much an administrative and a bureaucratic phenomenon. As we shall see, the governance of public health participated in this kind of compression, most of all in the institutionalization of systems for processing and coordinating change. Notable instances explored here include the development of permanent administrative infrastructures relating to vital statistics, official inspection, and the so-called stamping out of infectious diseases. And yet, just as they performed this function, these same systems also assumed an extended or deeper historical dimension, in that they helped to secure grander narratives of sanitary progress and human possibility. The point, once more, is that we need to grasp the two together, as part of a dynamic, modern process of both temporal extension and compression.

The two elements introduced above—displacing the state, and thinking in terms of modern dynamics, rather than contingent outcomes—might seem like an overly theorized way of seeking to re-engage a basic question: what was modern about modern public health in Victorian and Edwardian England? The book also comes at a time when *modernity* is under immense pressure as a term of historical analysis. As James Vernon has argued, since the 1990s—when the term eclipsed *modernization* as the category of choice—*modernity* has been used to capture so many conditions, processes, peoples, and moments that historians have begun to question its utility.[65] It is no coincidence that the interpretive and periodizing category of "the Victorian" has also come under scrutiny, as historians have weighed up whether some kind of modern transition occurred in the 1830s and 1840s, or in the 1880s and 1890s (the argument here clearly suggests the former).[66] Yet, it is surely worth revisiting the question of the modernity of modern public health, not only in light of extensive revisionist scholarship, but also given how much the term *modern* continues to structure existing narratives regarding the when, how, and extent of historical change. In any case, as an exercise in history, the key test is the empirical one, and whether the argument formulated above can do any useful work in terms of shedding new light on what happened, when and how.

This book makes no claim to comprehensive coverage. It does not pretend to match the scope of works such as F. B. Smith's *The People's Health,* or Anthony Wohl's *Endangered Lives.*[67] Rather, it presents a series of detailed thematic studies that cover some of the core areas and agents of "public health," as it was then defined as an administrative problem. Briefly, the six main chapters explore the following: the organization of public health as a national system of governance composed of local and central parts; the use of statistics to measure the progress of this system; official bureaucracy and the practice of sanitary inspection; the building of sewerage and waste disposal systems; stamping out, and responding to outbreaks of infectious disease; and finally, washing the body and personal cleanliness. Notable absences, then, include smallpox vaccination and the regulation of air, food, and water—if not necessarily, it might be said, the regulation of factories and industrial health, which remained largely a Home Office responsibility, and the medical functions of the poor law (not that this lack of system and integration went unnoticed at the time, as we shall see).

The purpose, however, is not to account in depth for each and every aspect of public health, at each and every level. No account has and no account could—at least not while attending to all of the complex twists and turns of policy formation and implementation. If the book aspires to any sort of comprehensive scope, then this is in two respects. The first is in terms of grasping the multilayered modernity of Victorian and Edwardian public health, and the way it was forged and performed not just through struggles concerning the organization of the system as a national whole, but also in terms of struggles at the local and personal levels. The book thus begins with a chapter on "sanitary centralization," and ends with a chapter on intimate acts of bodily hygiene. The second is in terms of the systemic abundance of public health; which is to say, the sheer diversity of systems that made up public health as a modern field of governance, from those of a more bureaucratic and administrative nature to those of a fully technological and material sort.

Ultimately, this is the kind of history offered here. The book is not a cultural, political, or social history; nor again is it an environmental, administrative, or technological history. Rather, it is a history of systems, and in particular a history of the modern ambitions and frustrations that governed their making and remaking in Victorian and Edwardian England under the mutable rubric of "public health." And in so doing, it argues for the utility of writing history in just this fashion—a point we return to in the concluding chapter.

CHAPTER 2

A Perfect Chaos

Centralization and the Struggle
for National System

Tradition is a modern phenomenon, as various scholars have argued, among them Eric Hobsbawm and J.C.D. Clark.[1] Their point is that tradition, understood as that which is of the past and so opposed to the new, requires a sense of historical development in order to be fully operational and active. Only then can tradition be posited as an object of restoration, preservation, and reform, or even revolutionary abandonment. During the nineteenth century, considerations of this sort became unavoidable, given the ongoing historical change now thought to distinguish "civilized" and "progressive" societies from those judged "backward" and "barbaric." As the Tory leader Benjamin Disraeli declared, during the passage of what would become the 1867 Reform Act: "In a progressive country [Britain] change is constant; and the question is not whether you should resist change which is inevitable, but whether that change should be carried out in due deference to the manners, the customs, the laws and the traditions of the people, or whether it should be carried out in deference to abstract principles, and arbitrary and general doctrines."[2] Counterintuitively perhaps, tradition thrives not before or beyond, but only *within* modern systems of governing, where different readings of the past are embroiled in all kinds of arguments for and against the status quo, and multiple possible futures. As Clark has noted, only during the 1870s did the term *traditionalist* enter the English language, when it began to assume the meaning it still carries today.[3] And we might add that the original meaning of *tradition—*

transmitted orally—became increasingly difficult to sustain, given the intensification of administrative writing practices and "bureaucracy," itself a new concept (see chapter 4).

This is true of the English tradition of local government, long held by historians to be a powerful, if also irksome and anachronistic, ingredient in the making of public health as a national system of governance. This precise formulation—"tradition of local government"—was not much used until the turn of the century, when English local government became the object of increasingly professionalized historical scrutiny.[4] By this point it was commonplace to assert that a strong commitment to local self-government was a long-standing English peculiarity, distinct from most continental practices. "England is pre-eminently the country of local government," declared one primer on the subject, published in 1894.[5] "Central administration" might be traced back to the Norman aristocracy ("French officials") of the twelfth century, but the historical roots of local self-government ran still deeper. "Local administration is at least five hundred years older, and was probably the unconscious adaptation of primeval Teutonic customs to the conditions of new settlement," the primer went on, noting how even recent reforms had remained in the groove of "the old lines." "Nothing more clearly shows the profound conservatism of the English character than this practice," it added.[6]

However, as Joanna Innes has suggested, although projected backward over centuries, this particular English tradition was in fact quite novel, emerging only in the 1830s, when the distinction between "the local" and "the central" first gained currency. In the eighteenth century, the closest distinction was the hierarchical one between "officers of state" or "the Crown," and "inferior officers of government."[7] In the early nineteenth century, as increasingly complex voluntary organizations started to boast "central committees," the term *local government* was applied almost exclusively to institutions in colonial territories, such as India and Australia. Only during the early 1830s did the distinction central/local come to be used in relation to institutions exercising power at home. The short-lived Central Board of Health, set up to combat the cholera epidemic of 1831–32, is one instance (see chapter 6); another, the 1834 Poor Law Amendment Act, which set up a "central" Poor Law Commission to preside over "local" boards of guardians. Similarly, *local self-government* and *centralization* were early Victorian neologisms, and it was precisely at this point when their history started to flourish and deepen. "Barely had the term [local government] been given this domestic application," Innes writes, "than it started to be championed as an age-old principle of the British constitution!"[8]

Clearly this is not to suggest that nothing was happening at the level of boroughs, counties, and parishes prior to the 1830s, still less that established practices somehow ceased to exist. Indeed, the improvement commissions noted in chapter 1 were still part of the nation's administrative landscape as late as the 1870s. The point here is that it attests to the birth of a new and fully modern political-organizational problem: namely, how to secure public health as an integrated national system of governance composed of "local" and "central" parts, whose very institutional being was historical, whether one liked it or not. To be sure, it was sometimes remarked that the English were averse to insisting on total system and uniformity. "Our local institutions, like our political constitution, have developed spontaneously, and both alike bristle with anomalies," stated an introductory text on local government published in 1883. "Englishmen, however, care but little for symmetry," it added. "The fact that an institution is anomalous, or a compromise in administering it illogical, does not disturb them so long as the thing works even tolerably."[9] Yet, in the case of public health, a great many Englishmen did indeed care for just this, quite passionately so. The very text that galvanized Victorian public health reform, Edwin Chadwick's landmark *Sanitary Report* published in 1842, for instance, concluded with a plea for "uniformity in legislation and in the executive machinery, and of doing the same things in the same way, and calling the same officers, proceedings and things by the same names."[10]

Chadwick's report was only the start. Although designed to secure more systematic administration, central institutions such as the GBH and the LGB altogether failed in this regard, as was so often pointed out. In 1886, the Midland branch of the Association of MOsH listened to an address entitled "Our Sanitary System and Its Reorganisation." In terms of administrative boundaries, the speaker pointed to "a perfect chaos." The sanitary district where he resided comprised parts of two counties and two poor law unions. The "present system of sanitary law" was no better: "it consists of something like 700 acts, dating from 1275 to 1885, administered by twenty-three different kinds of authorities, having eighteen different kinds of rates."[11] The same frustrations were still being voiced much later. In 1914, the Liberal MP Christopher Addison delivered an address on "The Health of the People." "No one fairly looking into the organization of our medical and public health services can fail to be struck by the confusion that is presented," he stated. By way of example, he pointed to the agencies that might be called upon should a London worker and his family fall ill: poor law guardians; MOsH and sanitary inspectors of the London County Council (LCC); the Metropolitan Asylums Board; and should he have been injured at work, National Insurance commissioners and the Home Office. Much might be gained, he suggested, "by simplification, and by securing, in an increased degree, a common aim and direction."[12]

Indeed, if anything was systematic—regular, methodical, predictable—it was the struggle for system (understood as systematic), rather than its attainment as such. This goes to the heart of the making of public health as a modern system of governance. Part of the explanation is that it is not enough to speak of the empowerment of professionals and bureaucrats. We also need to attend to the empowerment—just as modern, as chapter 1 detailed—of MPs, civic activists, councillors, and members of the public: all those, in fact, who might be distinguished as "political" or "nonprofessional." Furthermore, as will be argued here, in order to appreciate the contingent and contested nature of this system building, we also need to recognize another element: that is, the way in which the organization of these parts was itself subject to ongoing reformulation, as discussed in terms of the distinction between "the central" and "the local," as well as very different visions of a national administrative framework.

Arguments that simultaneously invoked the past, present, and future of the public health system were not the only means through which it was assembled in a modern-historical fashion. The next two chapters detail the generation of statistics and the production of bureaucratic records, which also served this function, albeit in different ways. But this is where the chronological present of governing was subject to the greatest degree of temporal *extension*, in the sense that reform entailed acknowledging an administrative inheritance that now stretched back over centuries. The trouble was that there was no agreement on what this inheritance amounted to, and whether progress entailed rejecting it, working with it, or even reclaiming it more fully. As we shall see in this chapter, which focuses on the midcentury debate on "sanitary centralization," the politics of public health was made of different readings of the past, as put in the service of different futures. A Whiggish-liberal vision of interactive center-local relations proved dominant, in keeping with the broader ascendancy of liberalism during the period 1830–80; but more technocratic and democratic visions were also in the mix, each offering very different conceptions of the "public" of public health.[13]

The chapter begins with a brief sketch of the dense patchwork of authorities and agents in which arguments of this sort circulated—the same patchwork in fact that these arguments also hoped to reform and reconfigure.

THE PATCHWORK OF LOCAL-CENTRAL GOVERNANCE

The fraught gestation of Victorian and Edwardian public health as a national system of governance has been detailed at length.[14] In towns and cities, especially, public health reforms had to negotiate the battles of councillors and parties, the scrutiny of the local press, and the opposition of pressure groups, including the ratepayer associations that mushroomed during the middle of the century.[15] From the start, the problem of public health was entangled with questions of local finance and fiscal responsibility, and the legal entitlements of individual, commercial, and corporate property holders—all questions with their peculiar, place-specific twists and turns. Equally, the obstruction of public health measures mixed with their active promotion. In some places, they became a matter of civic pride.[16] To note only the best-known examples, this is true of Birmingham in the mid-1870s under the Liberal leadership of Joseph Chamberlain, as well as the LCC during the 1890s and early twentieth century, when it was governed by a Progressive (Liberal-radical) coalition. By this point there were two main tiers of local government: the counties, created in 1888, with the largest cities, the county boroughs, distinct from the administrative counties; and a seam of smaller urban and rural district sanitary authorities, created between 1872 and 1894.

Similarly, we find struggle and conflict—again, both for and against public health measures—in parliament. Though they might receive the advice of professionals urging executive compulsion, ministers had to tread carefully if legislation was to pass at all. Compromise was crucial. During the passage of what would become the 1848 Public Health Act, it was decided that London should be dealt with separately. In late 1847, a Crown-nominated Metropolitan Commission of Sewers (MCS) was formed—of which there would be six in subsequent years—followed in 1855, after much protest and acrimony, by an indirectly elected Metropolitan Board of Works (MBW). More generally, the principal strategy was one of enabling, rather than enforcing, local authorities to undertake public health initiatives; and in any case, there was still the option of pursuing local bills. In the main, legislation was piecemeal and permissive, with local authorities adopting powers set out in general statutes while receiving the advice of a central office based in London: the GBH, followed by the Local Government Act Office (LGAO, 1858, as a subdepartment of the Home Office) and the Medical Department of the Privy Council (MDPC, 1859); and then the LGB (1871), which subsumed both the LGAO and MDPC, as well as the Poor Law Board.

It is difficult to overstate the intricacy and variety with which the public health system developed at the local and central levels. Exceptions, peculiarities, variations: these were the rule, it might be argued, all of which were forged via a confusing patchwork of administrative authorities, among others vestries and councils, and a variety of boards, offices, and commissions. In fact, it could be argued that the notorious patchwork of the seventeenth and eighteenth centuries, famously detailed in the mammoth, multivolume work of the Webbs (published during 1906–29), became *more* and not less confused. Even so, this was a different kind of patchwork, one whose systemic complexity was generated within a different temporality of governance—modern and historical, as understood here—and that was articulated as a matter of the logistical-political relations between central and local authorities. There was certainly a process of centralization at work; but this was accompanied by a process of localization as well, with one informing and complicating the other.

This was so in all sorts of ways, and what is sometimes termed the "autonomy of the local" was never pure, given the oversight of central agencies and the use of general acts of parliament. As David Eastwood has argued, beginning in the 1830s, with royal commissions on the poor laws (1832–34) and municipal corporations (1833–35), local government *itself* became the object of periodic, center-inspired inquiries, all of which sought to collect information from around the country, as well as from abroad.[17] By 1900, few, if any, areas had been left unturned, resulting in a mass of official blue books. The subject of water-supply systems, for instance, attracted over twenty official investigations, variously initiated by the GBH, the LGB, and the Board of Trade. And there were more regular forms of centralized-localized interaction and mutual elaboration. The vital statistics provided by the General Register Office (GRO) might be cited here (see chapter 3); so too the reports of central inspectors and the requirement that bylaws pass through the hands of central officials. Between 1858 and 1871, the LGAO scrutinized roughly fifteen hundred sets of bylaws according to its own model regulations. Similarly, center and locality were intertwined financially. Capital expenditure schemes, for example, required centrally sanctioned loans, normally from the Public Works Loan Commissioners. Relations were also entrenched via a system of district auditing, which began in the 1840s in relation to poor law expenditure. In 1879, by which point it was being applied to almost all areas of local government, the district audit became a fully salaried service under the LGB, giving rise to an annual round of local appeals regarding disallowances and surcharges.[18]

Localization *and* centralization: there was indeed a twofold modern dynamic at work, which included general measures designed by ministers and officials to formalize the status of "the local" as a site of governance. A number of public health acts provided for an expansion of local democracy, however modest given the ongoing attachment to a property-based franchise. A case in point is the 1848 Public Health Act, which besides establishing the GBH also enabled the creation of elected local boards of health in nonincorporated areas, as well as the establishment of sanitary committees of borough councils.[19] To set up a board required the submission to the GBH of a petition signed by 10 percent of the relevant ratepayers. Following a visit by a central inspector, who would assess local conditions and outline what needed to be done, elections to a board would take place, thereby politicizing the otherwise technical question of how a given district might be better mapped and drained (see figure 1). By 1852, the act had been applied in 134 localities, including in a handful of large town and cities, such as Bristol, Derby, Preston, and Hull. But it was rarely a smooth process, as various studies have shown, in places prompting fractious elections and the setting up of ad hoc parties.[20]

At the same time, the political intensification of the local was accompanied by the emergence of new professions, pressure groups, and parties, all of which sought to influence the work of central institutions.[21] Although the intensity of party conflict ebbed and flowed—as indeed did levels of discipline *within* parties—battles between radicals, Whigs, and liberals (or "reformers") on the one hand, and Tories on the other, characterized municipal politics throughout the century. During the 1890s, the political mix was further complicated by the emergence of new parties that sought to build from the local upward. In 1893, the Independent Labour Party entered the fray, espousing a philosophy of so-called municipal socialism. Candidates began to appear in places such as Leeds in the mid-1890s; and though significant advances had to wait until the next century, it did score some gains in the short term: by 1898, the party had taken control of the borough of West Ham in London, and secured a handful of council seats in Bradford and Bristol.[22]

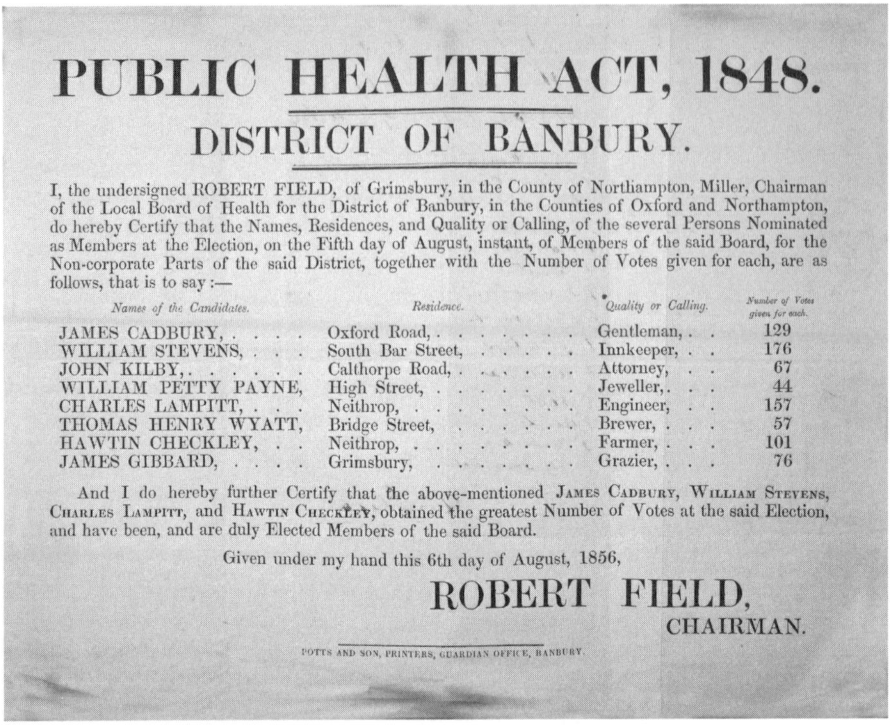

PUBLIC HEALTH ACT, 1848.

DISTRICT OF BANBURY.

I, the undersigned ROBERT FIELD, of Grimsbury, in the County of Northampton, Miller, Chairman of the Local Board of Health for the District of Banbury, in the Counties of Oxford and Northampton, do hereby Certify that the Names, Residences, and Quality or Calling, of the several Persons Nominated as Members at the Election, on the Fifth day of August, instant, of Members of the said Board, for the Non-corporate Parts of the said District, together with the Number of Votes given for each, are as follows, that is to say :—

Names of the Candidates.	Residence.	Quality or Calling.	Number of Votes given for each.
JAMES CADBURY, ...	Oxford Road, ...	Gentleman, . .	129
WILLIAM STEVENS, . . .	South Bar Street, ...	Innkeeper, . .	176
JOHN KILBY, ...	Calthorpe Road, ...	Attorney, . .	67
WILLIAM PETTY PAYNE,	High Street, ...	Jeweller, . . .	44
CHARLES LAMPITT, . . .	Neithrop, ...	Engineer, . .	157
THOMAS HENRY WYATT,	Bridge Street, ...	Brewer, . . .	57
HAWTIN CHECKLEY, . .	Neithrop, ...	Farmer, . . .	101
JAMES GIBBARD, ...	Grimsbury, ...	Grazier, . . .	76

And I do hereby further Certify that the above-mentioned JAMES CADBURY, WILLIAM STEVENS, CHARLES LAMPITT, and HAWTIN CHECKLEY, obtained the greatest Number of Votes at the said Election, and have been, and are duly Elected Members of the said Board.

Given under my hand this 6th day of August, 1856,

ROBERT FIELD,
CHAIRMAN.

POTTS AND SON, PRINTERS, GUARDIAN OFFICE, BANBURY.

FIGURE I. Notice announcing the outcome of the first board of health election in Banbury, Oxfordshire, 1856. Source: Oxfordshire History Centre, H7/A1/4.

Developments of this sort would not have been possible without the gradual expansion of the local franchise, which even included a small class of propertied women by the end of the century; but the public was not the only element subject to empowerment. Crucially, the democratization of a local tier of governance was also accompanied by a process of professionalization and the emergence of multiple associations designed to provide national representation for a growing and localized workforce. Most notably perhaps, the National Association of Local Government Officers (NALGO) was formed in 1905 to represent the interests of white-collar employees; but this particular process of empowerment descended into every nook and cranny of the workforce, including among hands-on roles in public health. The borough engineers examined in chapter 5 formed a national association in 1873; the sanitary inspectors of chapter 4 did the same in 1883. Finally, hybrid associations were formed, containing both professional and political agents. In 1872, an Association of Municipal Corporations was formed, composed of town clerks, mayors, and councillors, which in turn provided the organizational model for the County Councils Association established in 1889.

The frustration noted above regarding the lack of administrative uniformity and system is readily understandable. We might well endorse the views of those professionals who bemoaned the ignorance of MPs and the parsimony of ministers and ratepayers, and who consistently urged more in the way of central compulsion. But this is to overlook the growing complexity of the system, and the commitment to ensuring open and accountable governance. Reforming the system entailed contending with various arguments, from various quarters—local and central; professional, parliamentary, and public—some urging greater uniformity of system, others local exceptions, others still insisting that the system was fine as it was. All of the key legislative building blocks that laid the basis for public health as a national administrative system—notably the 1835 Municipal Corporations Act, and the 1848 and 1872 public health acts—were a product of compromise. Furthermore, as we shall now see, once posited as such, as a national system comprised of "local" and "central" parts, ministers also had to contend with different visions of unity, and how these parts should relate to one another.

VISIONS OF UNITY AND SYSTEM

Public health was not the only system steeped in competing claims about the merits of centralization, a term (*centralisation*) that had originated in revolutionary France in the 1790s.[23] The first sustained struggle in which the term featured prominently surrounded the passage and implementation of the 1834 Poor Law Amendment Act.[24] Indeed, it was not immediately deployed in the context of public health reform. As M. W. Flinn long ago noted, Chadwick's 1842 *Sanitary Report* was "tactfully silent on the question of central supervision," despite being critical of existing arrangements at the local level and calling for national uniformity of administration.[25] It was only with the second report of the Royal Commission on the State of Large Towns and Populous Districts, published in 1845, that national arrangements were broached in any detail. Developing the thrust of Chadwick's report, the commission lamented the absence of any "general law" in relation to the nation's health.[26] Nor were there any means of "comparing, in point of execution and economy," works undertaken in one part of Britain "with those in other parts of the kingdom": the Crown lacked any kind of supervisory powers. Finally, the work undertaken to apply improvement acts was, "in the present system of local government," "frequently placed under the immediate direction of persons, who are seldom qualified by any professional education for the direction of scientific works."[27]

Equally, even after the setting up of the GBH in 1848—by which point, use of the term had become common—centralization was not necessarily defended by professionals. During the early 1850s, Chadwick's attempt to promote the universal introduction of pipe-based systems of sewerage met with fierce resistance among the engineering profession (see chapter 5). Such was the rancor that in 1856 a book appeared entitled *Engineers and Officials,* which staged a scathing attack on centralization and the broader culture of regulation with which it was now associated. The book mocked the capacity of government ministers and officials to pronounce on technical matters of sewerage design; or those it otherwise dubbed the "enthusiastic amateurs of the Chadwickian school."[28] Invoking the "general ignorance of English bureaucrats" and the "system of Blue Books," it lamented the tendency of government "to meddle with everything, object to everything, and finish nothing."[29] "We are all reformers now!" it noted, ironically.[30]

Nonetheless, for all its varied contestation and elaboration, from the start the subject of centralization was enmeshed in a translocal field of reference, which here assumed a pronounced social-historical dimension, in the sense that there was a marked concern with national peculiarities of character, circumstance, and habit. In retrospect, given his subsequent association with the term, it is fitting that Chadwick was among the first—perhaps *the* first—to dwell at length on centralization as a novel means of organizing administrative systems, doing so in 1829 in the *London Review.*[31] His point of departure was a recent work by a Scottish surgeon on French hospitals; and though not uncritical of French practices, Chadwick was especially impressed by the use of a Bureau central d'admission, which oversaw the flow of patients in and out of Parisian hospitals. Dwelling favorably on other organizational facets, he then outlined a series of lessons regarding the benefits of centralization, including a greater division of labor—and so economies of scale—and enhanced institutional flexibility in times of epidemic emergency. In what would become a common defense later in the century, he also noted the greater publicity afforded by centralized institutions: "Further, the great and acknowledged advantages of publicity are increased by the arrangement attendant on centralization, which brings the whole of the [hospital] establishments into view as one system, and enables the public better to compare and appreciate the separate merits of each. Good management in any one department meets with a more speedy, certain and extensive reward or praise; bad management or abuse with more certain blame and discredit." Similarly, clinical innovations in one hospital were quickly communicated to others, thus nurturing the forward march of knowledge as much as administrative efficiency. "It might be proved as the result of this system," exclaimed Chadwick, "that France in medical science is nearly half a century in advance of England."[32]

Generally speaking, as the term gained currency, it assumed two meanings. One was pejorative and carried the charge that centralization was a continental peculiarity, opposed to the English character and England's peculiar constitutional history. In 1836, the MP and diplomat Henry Lytton Bulwer published *The Monarchy of the Middle Classes,* his "social, literary, [and] political" study of contemporary France. Two chapters were dedicated to centralization. One facet of his argument was that, if unchecked, as in the case of France, centralization sapped a nation's capacity for self-reliance. Only if subject to strict limitations might it be suited to England.[33] Equally, given the peculiar conditions of French society, it did have a certain logic: "Looking, then, at the equality among the French people, which prevents the local government of an aristocracy—at the position and divisions of France, which render dangerous the controlled local government of a democracy— centralization, if an evil, is almost an evil of necessity, and cannot be abandoned."[34] Though France remained the paradigmatic case, centralization was also linked to excessive bureaucracy and authoritarian militarism, leading to associations with Prussia, Austria, and Russia. As Bernard Porter has argued, when it came to assessing the progress of England in relation to her continental neighbors, political and institutional considerations were to the fore, rather than racial or religious ones.[35] The "bureaus and barracks" of the European continent were an affront to English traditions of liberty, and the free circulation of people, goods, and ideas.

The other meaning was more neutral and descriptive, to the extent that it evoked the organizational scale of contemporary statecraft, irrespective of its national manifestations and without necessarily suggesting anything malign. This was implicit in the many defenses of centralization that emerged during midcentury, and was subject to elaboration on occasions. In 1847, the Benthamite legal scholar John Austin published an article in the *Edinburgh Review* entitled "Centralization," which sought to inject some nuance into the meaning of this "much extolled and much decried word."[36] Seeking to overcome the negative association with "over-governing," Austin explored its myriad variations in terms of the distributions of power between "supreme" (national, sovereign) and "subordinate" (local) forms of authority, which, he suggested, were common to all types of state, from the monarchical and imperial to the republican and popular. Centralization was neither good nor bad, he argued, surveying Britain, the United States, France, and Germany. It all depended on a variety of "extrinsic causes," not least the political complexion of a given people and its relative state of civilization.

Both meanings are apparent in the midcentury debate on sanitary centralization, which erupted in the wake of the 1848 Public Health Act. At stake was neither laissez-faire nor interventionism; nor, for some at least, the local versus the central, where the two were placed in necessary opposition. Rather, the debate turned on differing visions of unity and system, and how the emerging centralized-localized parts and agents noted above should or should not relate to one another. Three key perspectives might be highlighted: a radical technocratic vision; a radical democratic vision; and a Whiggish-liberal vision. Ultimately, it was variants of the latter that prevailed; but it is only by considering all three together that we can fully appreciate the richness of critique and sense of possibility that flourished at the time.

Technocratic Radicalism

In terms of technocratic visions, the immediate figure that springs to mind is Chadwick. As noted above, he was among the first to reflect on centralization as such, and to promote the virtues of centralized, integrated administrative systems. Moreover, throughout his career the former secretary to Jeremy Bentham demonstrated an aversion toward public opinion and parliament, and he went on to defend centralization across various fields, including the poor law, policing, and public health. "In the present condition and practice of legislation," he informed a meeting of the NAPSS in 1863, "no measure based on administrative principles, partaking of science or system, goes into the House of Commons that, as a general rule, does not come out worse than it went in."[37] He also remained a connoisseur of foreign practices, especially those of France, and a keen advocate of expert input into the public and parliamentary spheres. During the 1850s, he lobbied for the reform of parliamentary information gathering, arguing that all measures subject to debate by MPs should be preceded by the systematic circulation of statements of fact and the testimony of specialist administrators.[38]

There are good reasons, then, why Chadwick provoked the animus that he did, which reached its high point during the late 1840s and early 1850s, following the formation of the MCS and the GBH.[39] But if Chadwick's lifelong loathing of inefficiency was underpinned by strong technocratic impulses, he never advocated bypassing public opinion entirely, only making it better informed and organized. Centralization is a case in point. In the 1830s, he argued that a centralized Poor Law Commission in conjunction with local boards of guardians made for more efficient and accountable governance.[40] Similarly, in one of his last publications, entitled *On the Evils of Disunity in Central and Local Administration* (1885), he argued that centralization was in fact about "decentralization." Central regulation and official guidance did not amount to central control. Rather, it was about securing "superior self-government" for ratepayers: the "best local intelligence under unity in the place of disunity and local ignorance." "The interest of the central administration is really in the most complete and well-organised local self-government, and its smooth unjarring action, which will give it the least trouble."[41] This, he argued, was "centralization for the people."

As we shall see, Chadwick's views bear affinities to the Whiggish-liberal visions of administrative system. More importantly, Chadwick's views competed with other technocratic visions of public health. Beginning in the 1850s, and finding a promotional home in the NAPSS and the organs and associations of the medical profession, "state medicine" emerged as an alternate expert-driven agenda. In general, the term was understood to mean the application of medicine in a collective and preventive—as opposed to individual and curative—fashion, though its adoption was neither smooth nor swift. The term was of German origin and was initially used alongside other terms of continental derivation, such as "medical police" (*medicinal polizei*) and "public hygiène" (*hygiène publique*); and in the case of Britain more generally, it was in Scotland, and more especially Edinburgh, where state medicine had been subject to scrutiny and elaboration.[42] At the same time, state medicine mingled with the environmental idiom of "sanitation" and "sanitary conditions" established by Chadwick and his allies in the 1840s. In 1851, the *Provincial Medical and Surgical Journal* published a paper, "On the Progress of Public Hygiène and Sanitary Legislation in England," which stated: "State medicine, medical police and hygiène are terms which have been used synonymously . . . to express the art or science which has for its object the application of physiological and medical science to securing the well-being and amelioration of society—that is, to improving the sanitary condition of the people, and promoting the health, ease and welfare of the human race, especially that portion of it doomed to live in towns."[43] Even so, the emergence of state medicine as the term of choice occurred only gradually. In an address to the NAPSS in 1869, the MP Sir Stafford Northcote noted that "the phrase State Medicine is absolutely new to many of us," and was "still imperfectly understood by the general public."[44]

These idiomatic complexities should not be overlooked: as Patrick Carroll has argued, the abandonment of the term *medical police* was prompted by an awareness of its un-English connotations.[45] Nonetheless, use of the term *state medicine* was partly an acknowledgment of the growing involvement of the medical profession in the administration of public health, which included various functions that fell under the auspices of boards of guardians, such as the distribution of medical relief and smallpox vaccination. Above all, growing numbers of MOsH were charged with directing activities at the local level. The first MOH was appointed in Liverpool in 1847, and by the mid-1850s there were almost one hundred operating in towns and cities, including forty-eight in London. Medicine also found a home in central government, thanks to the efforts of John Simon.[46] In 1858, the former MOH to the City of London (1848–55) and medical officer of the GBH (1855–58) was made medical officer of the Privy Council; and by 1861 he was in charge of his own department, the MDPC, equipped with its own premises and staff. Though Simon never eschewed Chadwick's concern with filth, he used his position to promote a more medicalized variant of public health. During the 1860s, Simon's medical staff—many of whom were members of the London Epidemiological Society (1850) and the Metropolitan Association of MOsH—produced a series of reports on nutrition, factory work, and infant diarrhea, among other concerns, all of which were incorporated into his annual statements on the health of the nation.[47]

In this respect, state medicine was an evolving reality, complementing, if also complicating, Chadwick's sanitary vision of public health with a new suite of technical facets and features. No doubt doctors had a vested interest in securing a place as paid servants of the public, thus enhancing the prestige of a still insecure and fragmented profession.[48] But state medicine was also an ideal, at once scientific and humanitarian, and something that had yet to be institutionalized in a systematic fashion.

Crucial here were the efforts of the NAPSS and the British Medical Association (BMA), which in 1868 joined forces to form a Joint Committee on State Medicine and the Organization and Administration of the Sanitary Laws. The committee was the product of a tight nexus of leading physicians (such as Henry Acland and Robert Christison) and public health experts (including Chadwick, Simon, and William Farr of the GRO), all with track records in promoting the professionalization of public health, however defined.[49] It bore immediate fruit: just three weeks after its formation, the committee successfully lobbied for the appointment of a royal commission to inquire into the existing state of public health administration with a view to its reform.

What was its vision of reform? It would be wrong to speak of only one vision. State medicine was subject to ongoing deliberation within the NAPSS and the BMA, giving rise to different emphases. But it is possible to isolate "the leading voice," as Simon later put it, the man who, in 1898, was dubbed "the father of State medicine" in Britain: Henry Wyldbore Rumsey, a practicing doctor based in Cheltenham, and a member of the BMA and the NAPSS, as well as of their Joint Committee.[50] Although he already had some publications to his name and had been called upon to give evidence to two select committees on poor law medical relief, Rumsey's key work, *Essays on State Medicine,* was published in 1856.[51] His views have some affinities with those of Chadwick. In particular, Rumsey was keen to defend centralization as a benign feature of any system of government organized on a national scale.[52] He was also scathing about the "sham" that was local self-government, quoting facts and figures attesting to the ignorance and incompetence of "local cabals" and "parochial cliques."[53] Finally, he was concerned with securing unity of administration. "Sanitary reform," he argued, should "be part of ONE large and statesmanlike project," whose various laws and regulations should "fit harmoniously together, like the architectural details of some vast pile, planned at one time though reared at intervals, and when completed, exhibiting its unity of design, and standing in simple grandeur, an object for the admiration of mankind."[54] Rumsey's vision, however, was also unique, offering a particular variant of unity which turned on the preeminence of professionalized science, and especially medicine.

Rumsey was quite explicit about his inspiration in this respect: French and above all German theories and practices. "Germany and France are far in advance of England, as to both legislation and practical administration," he noted in his *Essays.*[55] And he was just as explicit regarding the way his continental research—which had included travels to Belgium and Germany—had enabled him to draw up a normalizing framework by which to judge English efforts.[56] The "sanitary code" which he set forth in the first of his essays, he wrote, "may also serve as a normal project, a theoretical standard, by which to test some of those errors, anomalies and shortcomings of English sanitary legislation and management."[57] In broad terms, the problem with existing arrangements was twofold. On the one hand, the system was infused with ignorance and amateurism, even at its center. In the preface to his *Essays,* Rumsey made reference to the GBH, finding it incredible that "in the last decade of advancing civilization and in a nation boasting of its intellectual and material resources," a "whimsical experiment should have been tried of appointing three non-medical authorities—two Lords [Morpeth, Ashley] and a Barrister [Chadwick]—to preserve the health of the living." The nation did not require a "Central Board of sanitary amateurs"; what it needed was a council, "aided by its [England's] physicians and enlightened by its philosophers," coupled with a two-tier system of local government administered by "a trained and scientific corps of officers."[58]

On the other hand, public health had been construed far too narrowly. In the third of his essays, Rumsey reviewed the evidence presented in the preceding years by the GRO, Chadwick's *Sanitary Report,* the Royal Commission on the Health of Towns, and the GBH. Not only was the evidence incomplete, the conclusions drawn were altogether partial, missing "the whole truth." In particular, it had generated an "unphilosophical notion": "namely, that FILTH—in some form or other, aerial, fluid, solid, is the sole cause of preventable disease; and that public cleansing and the care of the public health are convertible terms." Echoing wider opposition on the part of doctors to the work of the GBH, Rumsey granted some credence to this; but there were "other less obvious, but no less real, predisposing and excitable causes."[59] Crudely, for Rumsey, the health of the public was governed by *everything.* One instance of this is his vision of the epistemological basis of state medicine, which comprised the generation of statistical information on the following: births, deaths, and marriages; sickness, accidents, and infirmity; occupations and workplaces; dwellings and population density; the production and consumption of different food types; the keeping of animals; changes in topography, climate, and weather; and the planetary movements of the solar system.[60] Nothing was beyond the ken of state medicine as Rumsey conceived it; and as we shall see in the next chapter, he was among a number of critics of the GRO's system of vital statistics, consistently urging more in the way of accuracy and scope.

In administrative terms, Rumsey's argument was that medicine as much as sanitary engineering and civic cleanliness should be the animating force of public health. These elements were aspects of the same project, he argued, developing a position he had originally outlined in 1844 before a select committee and put into print in 1846.[61] At various points in his *Essays*, Rumsey employed the compound term *medico-sanitary* in conjunction with *administration* and *organization*, while arguing for the reform of the medical profession, the medical facets of the poor law, smallpox vaccination, and the legal status of doctors.[62] Crucially, the system he proposed involved the marginalization of political and popular elements in favor of professional and official ones. At the center, he proposed a council of medicine, responsible to a minister of health and composed of nominees of the Crown and those "recommended by learned and professional bodies."[63] At the local level, he proposed a uniform system of enlarged "sanitary districts" containing roughly sixty thousand to eighty thousand inhabitants—roughly double the size of the new poor law unions set up in 1834—governed by sanitary courts composed of elected poor law guardians; representatives of town councils and local boards of health; magistrates and clergymen; and "specially qualified scientific and philanthropic residents" such as "professors of the exact and natural sciences." Furthermore, each sanitary court was to consult with members of a local medical council, as chosen by the registered doctors in each district.[64] Existing local authorities, then, would remain in place, but would be subordinate to supervisory courts, as well as to councils of medical advisors.

As Rumsey stressed on various occasions, this did not amount to a centralized system as such.[65] Rather, it amounted to a localized system subject to central oversight, the day-to-day lynchpin of which was a district MOH. Analogous, he suggested, to the *kreis physicus* of Germany, Rumsey's specialized MOH formed the hub of a localized network of medico-sanitary intelligence comprised of the following agents: registrars of births and deaths, vaccinators, food analysts, poor law medical officers, coroners, sanitary inspectors, engineers and surveyors, hospital surgeons, nurses, midwives, and pharmacists.[66] In terms of the center, each district was subject to assessment via specialized circuit inspectors—medical, engineering, and chemical—while each MOH was required to submit regular reports, so that local knowledge would help to "form the grand national total of information." Still, this was principally a localized system, one attuned to "local conditions and phenomena, which might remain forever unnoticed under mere central action."[67]

Not all professionals in medical and sanitary circles approved of Rumsey's vision of reform. In July 1856, a hostile review appeared in Benjamin Ward Richardson's *Journal of Public Health and Sanitary Review*, established in 1855—one of the first such specific journals— which concluded that it was at once impractical and un-English. "In England we want no State medicine," the anonymous reviewer concluded, for it was much too arbitrary and imperious, and was premised on the creation of a new class of all-powerful "physician-administrators"— a reference to France.[68] In fact, Rumsey's vision was not totally devoid of nonspecialist input. His district sanitary courts, though not directly elected, contained elected officials, as well as gentlemen such as magistrates and clergymen. In an address to the NAPSS in 1857, he lamented that local authorities did not contain more persons "selected on account of position, liberal education, philanthropic pursuits [and] freedom from interest in existing abuses."[69] Like so many among the governing elite, Rumsey evidently believed in the virtues of a generalist education and a degree of financial wealth and independence.

Still, the reviewer had a point, for while Rumsey made frequent reference to the public—he was concerned with its health, after all—this was largely as an object of administration, rather than as a subject. There was no sustained reflection on how to elevate public opinion. For Rumsey, the public was more of a passive than an active entity, devoid of any real, or even potential, authority when it came to matters of health. Moreover, if his system was localized, this was entirely in the service of achieving a full mastery of the facts, close to where they emerged. No mention was made of accountability to local ratepayers, what for others was now a key part of England's constitutional history. If anything, English traditions needed to be abandoned by way of catching up with France and Germany, which for Rumsey were much ahead in terms of their relative progress. Put another way, it was a vision of system and unity which represented the triumph of the professional, expert perspective, making for an almost wholly depoliticized world of technocratic administration. As a letter he published in the *British Medical Journal* (*BMJ*) in 1868 attests, even Rumsey was aware that such a scheme might be regarded as utopian.[70]

Democratic Radicalism

The nonprofessional public was and would remain an active agent, however, not least through the mediation of MPs, pressure groups, the press, and an assortment of elected local authorities. And these multiple agents were not always a force of obstruction.[71] The *Times,* for instance, consistently editorialized in favor of sanitary reform during the late 1840s.[72] But there was also considerable opposition, and it is among ratepayers and radicals that we find some of the staunchest voices opposed to centralization. Certainly some of this opposition was a product of ratepayer parsimony and alarmist rhetoric regarding administrative "tyranny." A common refrain in the local press was that centralization made for "central absolutism," and would promote only a new class of unaccountable officials. In 1848, the *Liverpool Mercury* feared that local authorities would be "degraded into the mere servants of a metropolitan junta."[73] Much of the ire focused on the powers of the GBH to authorize schemes that would lead to increases in local taxation. "With increasing taxation, are we ready to assent to an additional burthen? Shall we surrender the power of electing our assessors, and of taxing ourselves, to a Government too ready to impose vexatious burthens on the people?" asked one self-styled "citizen" in the preface to a collection of newspaper letters and editorials culled from around the country, entitled *Centralization or Local Representation.*[74] There was pronounced skepticism as well toward the "facts" put forward in favor of reform. It was claimed, for instance, that the evidence presented in parliamentary blue books was based on the testimony of "red-hot partisans" and "impracticable theorists." Such evidence could not be trusted, and amounted to a "gross libel" on the competence of existing local authorities.[75]

In part, then, opposition mobilized around the themes of ratepayer autonomy and the efficacy of existing arrangements. But it was also shot through with a sense that institutions such as the MCS and the GBH were an affront to the constitutional traditions of England and the peculiar character of the English. Compared to his European counterparts, "an Englishman feels more deeply the value of, and clings more closely to, the ancient institutions of the land," noted a correspondent of the *Morning Chronicle* in 1848.[76] For the *Daily News,* the attachment to local self-government was one reason why England, unlike the rest of Europe, was not being convulsed by revolutionary unrest.[77] Analogous sentiments were expressed in parliament. In 1847, during the passage of what would become the 1848 Public Health Act, the Tory MP Charles Newdegate argued that centralization was "utterly alien to the constitution of this country."[78] A year later, the radical MP Charles Pearson declared that the bill would deprive local authorities of that "independent action and conduct which was the glory of our Saxon constitution."[79] The most elaborate attack was launched by David Urquhart, a nominal Tory MP but one who shared a number of radical grievances. "Centralisation dissolved the bonds of society," he suggested, pointing to events in France. Furthermore, not only was the bill un-English—an "unconstitutional" attempt "to destroy local self-government"—it was unnecessary, given the powers that already existed under common law: "anyone who would take the time to refer to *Blackstone's Commentaries* would find that the common law provided ample means for putting down all the nuisances to which this Bill referred."[80]

Opposition of this sort was not without consequence. At the center it informed Chadwick's removal from office in 1854, when the *Times*, abandoning its earlier enthusiasm, famously accused Chadwick of "bullying" the nation into health. Locally, questions of ratepayer cost and constitutional precedent informed battles over boards of health. No doubt some of the opposition on constitutional grounds was opportunistic, bolstering arguments that might otherwise have been dismissed as expressions of mean self-interest. It is also the case, however, that for many at the time important principles were at stake. A case in point is the metropolitan barrister Joshua Toulmin Smith.[81] During the late 1840s and early 1850s, Smith emerged as the most outspoken critic of metropolitan Whiggism and "centralization," articulating a localist variant of democratic radicalism. A key figure in the politics of the City of London and the opposition which emerged to the MCS, he was also a supporter of the radical exile Lajos Kossuth, helping to found the London Hungarian Association in 1849.[82] And his views found an audience much beyond the metropolis, including in cities such as Birmingham and Bristol, where he made speeches and wrote articles for the local press. He seems to have been especially popular among radical circles in the West Riding of Yorkshire.[83] In 1852, Smith was nominated to stand for parliamentary election in Sheffield, receiving the backing of the Chartist and Owenite agitator Isaac Ironside. Two years later, alongside Ironside and others, he became a leading voice in the short-lived Anti-Centralization Union (1854–57). As Gregory Claeys has noted, the revival of localist concerns among radicals following the demise of Chartism in 1848 was in part stimulated by the writings of Smith.[84]

As with Rumsey's vision of state medicine, Smith's vision of sanitary governance was about securing unity and system. It is a theme which appears in his two major works on local government—*Local Self-*

Government and Centralization (1851) and *The Parish* (1854)—as well as in the many pamphlets and books he published on nuisance law and the reform of metropolitan government.[85] "Unity is not Centralization," he wrote in *Local Self-Government and Centralization*. National unity was nothing but the aggregate unity of the local units of administration that formed the "real" foundations of the state. Power flowed upward and only upward. Ministers, MPs, and peers might deal with foreign affairs, or act as the final arbiters in legal disputes; otherwise the center had no role in recommending, still less in carrying out, actions at the local level.[86] Nor was Smith averse to writing of efficiency and uniformity. A key part of his argument was that central institutions like the GBH led only to wasteful bureaucracy and the hindrance of "red-tapism." What was required was a "general system" of administration. In one of his early texts, published in 1848, *The Laws of England Relating to Public Health,* he spoke of the need to replace an unruly mass of statute law with "one general and broad system of action": a "machinery" of "universal (not local or partial) application."[87]

What Smith wanted to generalize, however, was a system which turned upon the local and the particular only. Put another way, the administration of "common wants and needs"—public health, but also the poor law, policing, taxation, and highways—was not to be disembedded from where it took place, away from the people it affected. There were no *general,* translocal standards, norms, or models. Drawing on Blackstone, Coke, Glanville, Magna Carta, and rolls of parliament, among other sources, Smith provided a particular reading of the history of the English constitution to make his point: namely, that the essence of England's constitution was common law and, in his reading at least, the small-scale popular assemblies that had sustained it in the past, in particular Saxon shire-motes and folk-motes, and then parish vestries and ward-motes. "Common Law," he declared, "is that Law which springs immediately from the Folk and People themselves, and which is also administered by the Folk and People themselves."[88] Whereas Whiggish histories tended to stress linear development toward the fruition of parliamentary government, Smith, like other radicals, presented something more nonlinear: a zigzagging history comprised of setbacks and deviations, as opposed to cumulative progress.[89] In Smith's case, it was neither the Normans nor the Stuarts that had perverted the constitution. Rather, the rot had set in with the Glorious Revolution of 1688, an event which marked the ascendancy of parliament, executive ministers, and statute law over the popular institutions of common law.[90]

It is not surprising that Smith was sometimes presented in the national press as the antiquarian leader of the "Parish Party."[91] Yet he wrote prodigiously on the subject of public health administration, and he was by no means opposed to all sanitary measures passed by parliament. He granted guarded approval to the 1855 Metropolis Management Act, which set up ratepayer-elected vestry and district boards; and he wrote in glowing terms of the 1855 Nuisances Removal Act, which gave elected local authorities greater powers over matters of sanitation without recourse to central supervision: "What the Nuisances Removal Act does, is, to restore to the Local Authority in every place, that organic life, and some of that action, which, at Common Law, an organized Local Authority in every place has always had; but which has been so much interfered with by multitudinous and empirical legislation as to have become, almost everywhere, paralyzed."[92] And though he made no mention of women, he did advocate the inclusion of *all* resident males in the "practical" administration of a given district.[93] Since each locality was peculiar unto itself, it was only via popular deliberation of each and every problem that the truth would emerge as to the best solution. As he stressed on numerous occasions, truth of this sort was a complex, manifold thing, and was only brought to light when examined from as many angles as possible by those most familiar with the details. By contrast, the "theorists" and "idle schemers" who sat on royal commissions all too readily generalized, looking for bogus analogies between disparate problems while suppressing critical nuances of time and space.[94] In this respect Smith's was a litigious, court-based view of governance.

Perhaps reflecting his own intellectual capacities, which extended to geology, phrenology, history, and the classics, Smith assumed that all residents were, or might become, qualified to discuss matters of administration. Like other political—if not necessarily professional—writers and commentators, he was opposed to the specialization of knowledge and administrative abilities. A "division of labour" might be applied to the organization of economic affairs, he wrote in 1857, but it "has no application to moral, social and political duties." Part of the problem with centralization was that it promoted the idea that "governing must be done by some few who are Brahminically [*sic*] set apart for that purpose."[95] Indeed, if Smith's system presupposed an advanced state of "real public opinion," his system also did much to promote and nurture it. He consistently argued that proper local self-government fostered moral character and collective intelligence and cooperation. The parish, for instance, was as much an educational as an administrative institution. It was "the truest School that can exist: it is the school of men in the active business of life:—it is the school for the highest moral training. . . . [Men] can only become men, and members of a free state, and true 'neighbours' one to another, by the practical school which such Institutions as the Parish keeps continually open."[96]

As Ben Weinstein has argued, Smith shared a number of mid-Victorian preoccupations, not least the development of character and public-spirited citizenship.[97] His critique of centralization was at once political, legal, and moral, and he was by no means the only admirer of Teutonic localism: the prominent historian E. A. Freeman, for example, was another.[98] More importantly, Smith's views informed the metropolitan campaign against the MCS, which was partly about asserting the rights of London's vestries against a Crown-nominated clique of professionals, and his work was widely quoted in the national and provincial press. It was even endorsed in the pages of the professional press. In 1858, the *Lancet* published an editorial entitled "How is the Standard of Public Health to be Raised?" in which it critiqued "the narrow conceits of bureaucracy," while championing "our custom of self-government." It went on to praise the "masterly hand" of Smith in demolishing the "Chadwickian" presumption in favor of central government. "He has exposed with ample sarcasm, but with even more of honest fact and truth, the fallacious quackery of centralism," the editorial declared. "He has shown that if an effective system of sanitary administration is to be carried out, it can only be by calling into free action, the local knowledge, intelligence, and vigour of the small communities."[99]

Smith's vision was also rare and deeply radical. First, it was intensely reverential of the past: a question of modeling the future on the past by way of recovering the liberties of England's historic constitution. For Smith, who was not averse to writing of "progress" and "civilization," one could move forward only by moving backward and reinstating a particular historical legacy, at least as he read it. Second, it was intensely participatory: a form of direct (male) democracy where administrative solutions were not the sole preserve of professionals or officials. In fact, it was a vision where the very distinction between politics and public opinion on the one hand, and specialized administration on the other, had been overcome. In a sense, local self-government *was* bureaucracy. Unity was thus much more than uniformity of administrative means and parts. It was a state of mind: "the consciousness that each man and each Parish is part of a larger whole."[100] Otherwise put, Smith's vision of system represented the triumph of the public, making for a thoroughly politicized—if also unified—world of inclusive, democratic administration.

Whiggish Liberalism

The visions of Rumsey and Smith represent extremes. Somewhere in between we find the Whiggish-liberal vision shared by those among the political and ministerial elite who daily had to negotiate the competing demands of professionals, MPs, pressure groups, and the press. Varied currents of thought fed into the Whig governments of the midcentury, and there was certainly a tension, as Peter Mandler has argued, between those of a more moderate ("Liberal") disposition and those of a more paternalist ("Whig" and "Foxite") sort.[101] Nonetheless, it makes sense to speak of something like a broad consensus regarding the merits of centralization, even if it was by and large promoted by the latter.

The consensus partly was that existing arrangements were woefully inadequate, as demonstrated by the facts and figures that poured forth from the GRO, which were readily quoted; but it also contained a distinctive conception of center-local relations. In brief, the Whiggish-liberal vision was that it was the job of the center to advise local authorities, principally by furnishing knowledge that was "general," while it was the job of the local to adapt this knowledge to "particular" circumstances. Central agencies such as the GBH and the LGAO were not designed to override local initiative, but to augment it and render it more efficient. In this way, unity and system would be forged via the interplay of public accountability and professional expertise, as mediated through the work of central and local levels of governance. It was this vision, then, that best reflected the evolving distribution of governmental parts described in the previous section. Equally, it was this vision that helped to maintain and legitimize this distribution in the face of ongoing resistance and critique.

John Stuart Mill's *Considerations on Representative Government* (1861) is often held to present the most considered formulation of this perspective. This was not the first time Mill had dwelled on center-local relations—it had earlier featured in his *Principles of Political Economy* (1848) and *On Liberty* (1859)—but it represents his most sustained reflections on the matter. Crucially, center-local relations related to a broader conundrum, one which he explored at length in his *Considerations:* how, as Mill put it, "to secure as far as they may be found compatible, the great advantage of the conduct of affairs by skilled persons, bred to it as an intellectual profession, along with that of a general control vested in, and seriously exercised by, bodies of representatives of the entire people."[102] When it came to the administration of the poor law and public health, there was certainly a good case for "management by central government": "local representative bodies and their officers" were "almost certain to be of a much lower grade of intelligence and knowledge than Parliament and the national executive."[103] Yet, it was also the logistical-political case that local authorities and their electors were better placed and naturally more inclined to enact and scrutinize this administration. In Mill's view, local inhabitants possessed a better, more instinctive eye for the all-important details: they lived in the locality after all, and it was their interests that were at stake. Mill's solution is well known: "The authority which is most conversant with principles should be supreme over principles, while that which is most competent in details should have the details left to it. The principal business of the central authority should be to give instruction, of the local authority to apply it. Power may be localised, but knowledge, to be most useful, must be centralised."[104] Like Toulmin Smith, Mill viewed local government as a kind of school for active and informed citizens. Yet for Mill, proper instruction in this respect could only take place on the basis of general knowledge furnished by the center, which would enable local residents "to compare different modes of action, and to learn, by their use of reason, to distinguish the best." Then they could proceed to the more intricate work of adapting this knowledge to invariably peculiar local conditions.[105]

Mill's work was widely read among political and professional elites. Indeed, his views on local government were much cited, and in 1857 Rumsey dedicated a section of an address before the NAPSS to discussing Mill's arguments regarding the "limits to central action" put forward in his *Principles of Political Economy*.[106] Mill's basic premise, however, had first appeared in Chadwick's 1829 article noted above, and it subsequently featured in the arguments of Lord John Russell (as well as Chadwick) in defense of the new poor law in the 1830s.[107] It was deployed again in the 1840s in relation to public health. In 1848, Lord Morpeth, in the course of introducing the Public Health Act of the same year, spoke in favor of a "regulated amount of State control": "The art of central control is to provide indispensable preliminaries, to suggest useful methods, to check manifest abuses, but to leave the execution and detail of the requisite proceeding to local agency and effort."[108] What, on another occasion, he termed an "impartial and scientific superintending authority" was necessary in order to direct and encourage "public opinion" at the local level.[109]

In subsequent years, with the GBH in place, the same argument was made time and again. In 1857, the lawyer Tom Taylor, who in the following year would take charge of the LGAO, delivered a paper to the NAPSS dedicated to attacking Smith's book *The Parish*. Like Smith, Taylor believed that local government should be "animated by a patriotic and unselfish spirit." "Central doctrinarism is absolutely antagonistic to the spirit of England," he suggested, and he heaped scorn on the "ignorance" of existing local authorities.[110] The trouble was that Smith's alternative system was out of date. Even if properly constituted, it would be unable to cope with the conditions created by the advent of "the new industrial economy created by steam power."[111] Amid the chaos of urban growth, what was required was a central department able to shed a "light of wide and general experience." The center was principally a repository of knowledge designed to empower the public: "If, as I contend, [local] powers are a public trust then their exercise ought to be watched and recorded on behalf of the public; the lessons which the experience of each place supplies ought to be deduced and made known for the benefit of all; glaring instances of neglected duty and their consequences should be stigmatised."[112] Similarly, two years later, in 1859, the Whig-Liberal MP and former president of the GBH William Cowper noted before the NAPSS that "the utmost we have in England is a sort of central supervision . . . which is in accordance with our Constitution."[113]

Beyond parliament and the NAPSS, this Whiggish-liberal vision of an interactive relation between center and locality found particular favor among philanthropists, civic leaders, and metropolitan professionals— indeed, among all those who were sympathetic to the Whigs' program of reform of the 1840s and 1850s. Pressure groups such as the Health of Towns Association (formed in 1844) and the Metropolitan Sanitary Association (1847), as well as leading periodicals, helped to counter the assertion that centralization amounted to direct control of local authorities.[114] As one of the leading organs of Whig opinion, the *Edinburgh Review*, argued in 1850: "People say that we are departing from the foundations of the free institutions of our Saxon ancestors—when really we are strengthening them."[115] Particular use was made of organic analogies by way of conveying the kind of unity that was at stake. Central authorities such as the GBH were akin to the head or the brain of the human body, whereas local institutions were akin to the limbs or the hands.[116] Imagery of this sort no doubt resonated with still prevalent ideas of a hierarchical body politic, and Burkean notions of a society composed of intricate relations and dependencies; but it also captured the growing sense that governing must comprise at least some degree of functional specialization and an ability to adapt to ever-evolving new conditions.

The most elaborate presentation of this vision appeared in 1851, in the broadly Tory periodical the *Quarterly Review*. The article was authored by one of Chadwick's close allies, the former surgeon, self-taught engineer, and one-time member of the MCS, F. O. Ward.[117] Entitled "Sanitary Consolidation," the article aimed to dispel "the common but fallacious antithesis between Centralization and Self-government."[118] Far from being opposed, they were the necessary complement of one another. To elucidate this, Ward drew an analogy between society and "the life and organization of Man." As a complex organism, Man was characterized by a twofold "concentration of life": a local and "subordinate" concentration, which determined the adaptation of the body's organs to its environment; and a central and "dominant" concentration, which enforced "the harmonious co-operation of these manifold parts and their subservience to a collective unity." In relation to the latter, Ward referred to the "cerebral" function of the nervous system, which meant that Man manifested "the most strongly pronounced unity" together with "the greatest multiplicity, diversity and individuality of the [body's] constituent organs." Similarly, any developed society—or "social organism"—possessed central and local authorities: the former were "cerebral" or knowledge-based, the latter "ganglionic" or active and practical. "Civilization," he wrote, "is but the name we give to the intense manifestation of this double life, elevating while it complicates the organization of society."[119]

As Ward stressed, this did not make for "Subversive Innovation," but the "CONSERVATIVE DEVELOPMENT OF ORDER," attesting to a progressive development from "primal anarchy to well-knit constitutional government."[120] In particular, the 1848 Public Health Act amounted to an institutional simulation of the natural efficiency of the body. Referring to the right of ratepayers to petition the GBH to begin the process of setting up a local board of health or municipal sanitary department, Ward stated: "Just as a *complaint* of the liver, transmitted in a message of pain along the nerves justifies the ganglionic nervous centre in determining towards it a swifter supply of blood, or of nervous power, for its cure; just so the *complaint* of a parish or town testified in a petition from the suffering inhabitants, justifies the metropolitan sanitary centre in directing thither, by the medium of a commissioner [inspector], the power necessary to abate its disorder."[121] By the same token, there was no place for central dictation, which would override the natural ability of the local to govern itself spontaneously. Central compulsion in fact was akin to the use of artificial drugs, which in time would lead only to "torpor and debility." Popular input at the local level, guided by a central authority, was part of the normal way of things: when "central interference is premature or excessive," Ward wrote, "it acts so as to supersede, instead of regulating or restoring, the normal action of the disordered part."[122]

There was thus little substance to the arguments of the Parish Party, for the principles of the 1848 act were "diametrically opposed" to "the continental system of centralization."[123] Indeed, for Ward, the arguments deployed by the likes of Smith—one of whose works, *The Laws of England Relating to Public Health,* was ostensibly under review in the article—were suspect on empirical grounds as well. As it stood, not only was local government riddled with "jobbing" and "incompetence," it was opposed to the history of the constitution. None other than King Alfred, England's revered monarch of the Dark Ages, had employed central superintendence by way of securing local self-government, in his case by dispatching "Royal *Missi* or Commissioners" to bring "local jobbers" into line: "we must frankly own ourselves indebted to this great king's centralizing vigour for the early development of our popular local freedom," argued Ward.[124] Equally, "natural law" was on the side of sanitary reform, by which Ward meant those "physical laws" of health that had received the "universal recognition of scientific men." He thus drew a distinction between "Political Centralization" based on "controvertible *opinion*" and "public *will*," and "Sanitary consolidation" based on "ascertained *law*." The latter, he argued, "replaces all arbitrary will whatsoever by Natural Law: which substitution, *Lex pro abitrio,* is instinctively felt by the mass of the people to lie at the very root of their progressive enfranchisement."[125]

Though one of the most elaborate defenses of sanitary centralization published at the time, Ward's defense articulated a widely shared sentiment within the Whiggish-liberal elite: namely, that institutions such as the MCS and the GBH were measured innovations, blending the demands of the past and England's peculiar constitutional inheritance with those of the present, most of all the urgent sanitary needs of England's burgeoning towns and cities. And reform was also about securing unity and system; or rather, a kind of organic unity premised on the productive interplay of the popular and professional, representative and ministerial, facets of governance. Put another way, unlike the visions of Rumsey or Smith, the Whiggish-liberal vision sought to affirm, rather than to negate or overcome, the interpenetration of the various parts of England's public health system then in the process of becoming better organized and more distinct. Likewise, the past was to be neither rejected nor idolized, but rather worked with and through by way of affirming the progressive evolution of English institutions. In truth, history was on the side of centralization, which was not intrinsically "un-English"; or at least when it made for more and not less local self-government.

It is somewhat artificial to distinguish between three visions of system. There were variations within each perspective, as well as points of over- lap: Chadwick, for instance, might be placed on the cusp of the techno- cratic and the Whiggish-liberal. Even so, it is evident that the debate was about much more than the relative merits of laissez-faire or intervention- ism, or a bigger or smaller state. Instead, we might point to the interplay of two processes: first, an emerging set of interacting administrative units and agents of governance, including those now thematized as local and central; and second, different and emerging visions of unity, reflecting on and seeking to reform the interrelations of these units and agents.

With this in mind, we can return to the Royal Sanitary Commission, as it became known, formed at the behest of the Joint Committee of the BMA and NAPSS in 1868. On the one hand, the ambitions of state medicine were held in check by the views of the commission, which was dominated by MPs. It recognized a great raft of problems with the system as it stood, even acknowledging that the "governments of France and the United States" furnished "useful hints . . . for systematizing local government in England." Nonetheless, the commission toed a broadly Whiggish-liberal line. "The principle of local self-government has been generally recognized as of the essence of our national vigour," the second report of the commis- sion concluded in 1871. It was a question of working with, rather than against, the grain of England's peculiar institutional history: "Local admin- istration, under central superintendence, is the distinguishing feature of our government." There was no place for an overly meddlesome and ambitious central power, the report noted, "for so completely is self-gov- ernment the habit and quality of Englishmen, that the country would resent any Central Authority undertaking duties of the local executive."[126] With this as its guiding thread, the recommendations offered by the com- mission came as a severe disappointment to sanitary and medical profes- sionals: the Joint Committee immediately raised over thirty objections.[127]

On the other hand, the very genesis and conduct of the commission was complicated by the functioning of a party-political domain of governance. Originally appointed under a Conservative administration, the commission's composition and remit changed following the advent of a Liberal government in December 1868. The number of doctors was reduced from seven to five, while Scotland, Ireland, and London were eliminated from its scope of inquiry, thus moderating what was originally intended as a truly comprehensive inquiry.[128] The commission was not without consequence, it should be emphasized. Most notably, it led to the formation of the LGB in 1871, which did at least bring public health and the poor law under one central office, making for something like a national "medico-sanitary" department, to return to Rumsey. As the commission's report had recommended: "Not only does *economy* forbid any needless duplication of authority, but the greater interests of *efficiency* demand a united superintendence and single responsibility for subjects so closely connected as the Public Health and the Relief of sickness and destitution amongst the Poor."[129] The commission's findings also inspired the 1872 Public Health Act, which paved the way for an expansion in the number of local MOsH and sanitary inspectors. Yet, as processed through the commission, and the agency of ministers and MPs, these measures also amounted to a compromise.[130] They were certainly acknowledged as a step in the right direction, at least given the historical and institutional peculiarities of the English. As Henry Acland argued in 1872, before the NAPSS: "it appears to me that the [Liberal] Government of Mr Gladstone proceed upon the wise principle that instead of waiting until they could construct a perfect theoretical system they should avail themselves of the existing institutions and habits of the country."[131] These same measures, however, also did little to quell calls for reform.

FRAGMENTATION, COORDINATION, AND THE STATE

Simply put, during the late Victorian and Edwardian periods, the struggle for unity and system continued. The dominant perspective remained broadly liberal, to the extent that the Liberal and Conservative parties, for all their differences over particular measures, endorsed a supervisory relation between center and locality. More importantly perhaps, as Christine Bellamy has detailed, the LGB remained committed to a "diplomatic" culture of center-local relations, which was defended in terms that recalled the arguments of Mill.[132] But there also emerged all kinds of new inflections and emphases, including those of a nascent social democratic sort, as in New Liberalism and the varied ideological commitments of an emerging socialist movement.[133] For one thing, centralization was less of a novelty than it had been earlier, and there was a more ready acknowledgment of its longevity and necessity. No longer a foreign peculiarity, it was now recognized as a kind of historical universal, even if in England it had pursued a distinctive trajectory. "The contest is not a new one," declared an article in the *Contemporary Review* in 1879, referring to "the relation of the local to the central government, or in other words, the extent to which self-government is to be allowed," adding: "it has been carried on in most countries from the earliest dawn of history with varying results."[134] At the same time, the search for the historical roots of local self-government continued, probing still deeper into the national past. As J. W. Burrow has shown, it was during these years when a form of historical anthropology developed regarding the origins of the self-governing Teutonic community.[135]

Another development was growing recourse to the notion of the state as an institutional means of either protecting or mediating the freedom of society. The state had figured before, of course; but the earlier preoccupation with England's constitutional inheritance was displaced by a concern with the interrelations of state and society, even if the state—or "State," as it was more often rendered—remained a hugely contested term, susceptible to all kinds of readings. Crudely, on the one hand, as Michael Bentley has argued, the Whiggish organicism of the early and mid-Victorian periods developed into an intensely protean, cross-party form of statist organicism, in which the state secured the conditions in which true self-government—of the self, family, locality, and, ultimately, society—could prosper. According to this line of thought, it was a question of working with and through, rather than against, the state. On the other hand, the state was opposed to society, and posited as an entity that "interfered with" the entrepreneurial and associational instincts of individual citizens.[136] State/society, however, was not the only binary distinction upheld by what was a largely Conservative current of thought: others included collectivism/individualism, and public/private ownership.

To the extent that the public health system remained entangled with the workings of the public and parliamentary spheres, it was not wholly divorced from competing conceptions of the state, which included calls to *bypass* these very same spheres of input. The technocratic impulses of state medicine were given a new lease of life by the emergence of eugenics, coupled with fears regarding national decline and a sense that the health of the poorer sections of society was somehow moving backward and "degenerating." A common refrain among the otherwise diverse advocates of eugenics, which included some socialists, was that parliamentary democracy promoted a slavish attachment to public opinion, which knew nothing of the laws of biological inheritance.[137] Eugenics remained a marginal creed, but more broadly, as Frank Turner has argued, scientists of all stripes grew increasingly critical of the competence of the political classes, while the "cult of national efficiency" that emerged in the wake of the Boer War led some on the radical right to condemn a "nation of amateurs" and campaign for the suspension of normal parliamentary procedures.[138] A strong state needed proper expertise and business-style efficiency, not the bumbling incompetence of generalist administrators and vote-seeking politicians.

Equally, but embodying a decidedly more democratic thrust, public health featured in various visions of "municipalism," based on the civic ownership of public utilities. This was true of Chamberlain's Birmingham-based vision of urban improvement, which was partly premised on the municipal provision of gas and water; and it extended to still more radical variants, such as municipal socialism, which promised democratic control of civic institutions and services.[139] Here public health featured as part of a self-consciously egalitarian vision of political empowerment and material well-being, recalling the democratic aspirations of Toulmin Smith. To give an early example, in 1887 H. M. Hyndman, founder of the Social Democratic Foundation, outlined his vision of a "commune" for London, partly inspired by the Parisian example. Attacking the fragmentary state of metropolitan governance, the inefficiencies of the MBW, and the privileges of the City of London, he called for a unified municipal assembly—a Great Central Council—subject to annual election on a universal suffrage, and the consolidated management of *all* municipal-based services (gas, water, roads, trams, baths, parks, police, poor relief, and education, among others). Hyndman went on: "We may then hope to see a London in which the whole of the people are thoroughly well and wholesomely housed in commodious artistic dwellings ... in which parks and playgrounds and squares, together with good public baths, washhouses and libraries, will be adequately supplied for the whole people; in which the foul smoke that now threatens to poison us outright is kept under rigid enactment in favour of better methods of coal combustion." Such were the many fruits of a "machinery of government" which "would at once uphold a higher ideal of citizenship for the whole population, and would, at the same time, give them a direct interest in the affairs of our great city."[140]

Public health initiatives, such as cleaning streets and the provision of isolation hospitals, were not the principal site of contestation. Debate largely centered on the municipal trading of gas, water, and electricity; and in most cities, municipal ownership was a means of securing greater efficiency, rather than any kind of egalitarian community.[141] Nonetheless, public health was part of a broader fabric of concerns whose management generated heated debate about the "size" of the state and the nature of local government. Pressure groups such as the Liberty and Property Defence Association (LPDA, 1882) and the Industrial Freedom League (1902)—most of whose members were either Tories or moderate Liberals—published a welter of tracts promoting private enterprise and attacking the "socialist danger."[142] "Municipal Socialism is State Socialism writ small," declared one pamphlet published by the LPDA in 1892, speculating that in time, "municipal rule, by reason of its own excesses, will disappear in a State Socialistic rule, more despotic than that of any Monarchy; and the place of local self-government will know it no more."[143] For socialists, municipal control promised quite the opposite. "The main point at issue in London Reform is no mere matter of parks or drains, but whether London shall really become a self-governing community," declared the Fabian socialist, Sidney Webb, in 1894, at that point also a leading member of the Progressive coalition in charge of the LCC. "Government of London by London for London": such was the "watchword" in the ongoing fight "to take its [London's] own collective life into its own hands."[144]

The extent to which these visions informed the everyday workings of the public health system depended, of course, on the actions of various agents, not least members of the public at the ballot box. During the Edwardian period, for instance, ratepayers rebelled against the "collectivist menace" of municipal socialism, nowhere more spectacularly than in London, where the Conservatives (or Moderates) took control of the LCC in 1907 and held on to it for over a quarter of a century. Yet, just as these visions complicated the gestation of England's public health system— among other things, lending it all kinds of contingent local political meanings—so too was the system itself under revision, as professionals, civil servants, and ministers grappled with the question of how to unify its various administrative parts, old and new, local and central. As noted above, the formation of the LGB did little to quell calls for reform, and here the problem of unity developed along two combined fronts: first, there was the question of how the administrative parts of the system should relate to those of a political and representative sort; second, there was the question of consolidating these administrative parts, and placing all of those that had a bearing on the health of the public on a more unified, integrated footing.

One aspect of this was the need for some kind of intermediate tier between central and local authorities, especially outside of boroughs. The problem had first been identified by Rumsey—his sanitary courts fulfilled this function—and it featured again in the criticisms of the Royal Sanitary Commission's report made by the Joint Committee in 1871.[145] Despite lobbying, the LGB proved unreceptive and by the 1880s the leading advocate in professional circles was Ernest Hart, editor of the *BMJ* and chairman of the National Health Society (established in 1871), who delivered numerous addresses on the subject. Like others, Hart's desire was for greater unity and system. "This chaos of areas and chaos of everything else, of which we hear so much, must be turned into cosmos," he declared, in an address to the Sanitary Institute of Great Britain (SIGB) in 1885. "We must have a single area for all local business, administered by one authority, elected on a uniform basis, and exercising identical powers all over the country." "Unification" was all about strengthening local self-government, he stressed, acknowledging that it was something "Englishmen have always vindicated to themselves through every period of their history."[146]

By this point, local government reform was being promised by the Liberal and the Conservative parties, and the result was the Tory-Liberal Unionist 1888 Local Government Act, which created elected and intermediate administrative counties and county boroughs.[147] To be sure, the measure was not without criticism among professionals; but for all the disappointment with the reforms of 1871–72 and 1888, the general consensus was that local government had to be worked with and through, whether in principle, as a good in itself, or as an established administrative fact. As the MOH, Alfred Carpenter, reminded the BMA's public medicine section in 1880, though "the principle of local self-government is so often found to be antagonistic to efficient and really scientific modes of dealing with disease," "the will of the people" could hardly be ignored. For Carpenter, given the brute fact of elected MPs and councillors, popular education rather than legislative coercion was the best way forward, "so that electors may know how to choose the good from among those who ask their suffrage as members of Parliament, as well as local representatives in the assemblies of their particular districts."[148]

In subsequent years, a handful of MOsH called for the appointment of nonelected experts to local health committees and boards of guardians, and there was the occasional flourish of undiluted technocratic hostility toward the populace in general. In 1898, the president of the Midland branch of the Society of MOsH bemoaned the public resistance to smallpox vaccination, confessing that "the phrase 'the government of the people by the people for the people' is a profound mystery to me": "any technical science shows well the folly of trusting a popular vote of the ignorant on a technical truth."[149] But in the main, problems with the system were located less in the constitutional principle or reality of popular representation, and more in the way the system was led at the center and how various public health functions failed to knit together as they might. A crucial focal point in this respect was the idea of a ministry (or state department) of health. The idea had first been mooted by Rumsey in the mid-1850s, and he put it forward again in his evidence to the Royal Sanitary Commission, though in both cases without detailed elaboration.[150] At this stage it was unclear, as Bellamy has noted, exactly what leading public health professionals such as Rumsey and Simon, as well as the Joint Committee, had in mind.[151]

In the event, the 1871 Local Government Board Act, which set up the LGB, did engineer an administrative fusion of the poor law (the Poor Law Board) and public health (the LGAO and the MDPC). But as the LGB began work, the problems immediately highlighted by the Joint Committee were soon joined by others. As political appointees, presidents of the LGB came and went, some staying for a matter of months, others a couple of years, at least until the appointment of Walter Long (1900–1905) and Arthur Burns (1905–14).[152] Meanwhile, the structure of the LGB prevented those with expertise from direct access to ministers (a privilege of the permanent secretaries of Whitehall only); and though some consolidation had been achieved, various health-related functions remained more or less separate. Among other instances, public health and poor law functions were served by separate administrative divisions within the LGB; the factory inspectorate was under the authority of the Home Office; while the GRO, though nominally responsible to the LGB, continued to operate as a distinct office with its own head, the registrar-general. More generally, there was the problem of bureaucratic overload, amid evolving, crisscrossing structures of clerks, assistants, inspectors, and secretaries within the LGB.[153] In 1908, as the new prime minister, Herbert Asquith, set about reshuffling his Cabinet team, Winston Churchill pleaded not to be lumbered with the LGB: "There is no place in the Government more labourious, more anxious, more thankless, more choked with petty and even squalid details, [or] more full of hopeless and insoluble difficulties."[154]

Just these problems featured in the many calls for a ministry of health led by a specialist, *non*political minister. In August 1878, Chadwick addressed the International Congress of Hygiene in Paris on the "Requisite Attributions of a Minister of Health." Drawing on British experiences during the preceding decades, he lamented how central health authorities had been, and continued to be, dependent on "the will of a changing political chief": "for one who was zealous and competent, three were ignorant or apathetic, or positively hostile," he claimed.[155] A similar point was made by Benjamin Ward Richardson, who in October of the same year addressed the SIGB outlining his ideal ministry. Richardson's minister was certainly a man of poise, given the English attachment to local self-government: any minister "who would crave centralising powers" was bound to fail, he suggested. Instead, the minister would be "an authority not a disciplinarian; a judge and director, not a commanding officer; a collator and teacher of all things relating to health, not a dogmatic professor."[156] But he would also "differ from other Ministers of the Crown in almost every particular." As well as boasting a specialist training in health matters, he would "not be a busy party man," despite being of Cabinet rank. In fact, since his role was incompatible "with a mere passing ministerial career and with the worry of parliamentary existence," his appointment would in principle be permanent, something that might be secured via a life peerage in the House of Lords.[157]

Calls for a nonpolitical minister of health continued to appear in subsequent decades, amid widespread misgivings about the impact of "government by party" and the effect of the national electoral cycle on the continuity and cogency of public health administration.[158] Likewise, calls continued to be made for the unification of all public health-related functions. Richardson's ideal ministry had united the LGB, the GRO, the factory and prison inspectorates of the Home Office, the veterinary department of the Privy Council, and the office of Chief Commissioner of Public Works; and although specific institutional remedies differed, the general consensus remained, to quote one MOH, that "the central administration of public health affairs is a thing of shreds and patches."[159] By the turn of the century, the idea of a consolidated ministry had found a promotional home in various bodies, from professional ones, such as the BMA and SIGB, to those of a voluntary and civic sort, such as the Manchester and Salford Sanitary Association, the Childhood Society, and the National Workmen's Housing Association.[160]

Numerous variations on this theme emerged. The 1904 Inter-Departmental Committee on Physical Deterioration, convened to look into the problem of urban degeneration, recommended the setting up of an expert advisory council to the LGB. Modeled on the French Comité consultatif d'hygiène publique, the council would complement the work of the GRO, collecting and digesting anthropometric and sickness statistics, while directing the public health functions of the LGB, giving them "a prominence which the multiplicity of its other functions may have tended to obscure."[161] But it was this latter problem—the general one of how to unify the public health functions of the state, rather than the more particular one of securing a nonpolitical minister—that came to the fore during the Edwardian period, receiving its most thoroughgoing elaboration during the course of the mammoth Poor Law Commission Inquiry of 1905–9.[162] The problem was not only that more needed to be done in terms of resources and manpower. It was also one of coordinating the multiplicity of agents that were now responsible for enhancing the health of the public. MOsH, sanitary inspectors, poor law medical officers, private practitioners, and hospital functionaries (isolation, workhouse, and general); plus more recent additions, such as municipal midwives and nurses, and school medical inspectors: all were playing a role in what was variously styled "public health," "public hygiene," "State medicine," and "the public medical service." The result: "waste," "confusion," "in-coordination," and "want of system."

It was the Fabian double-act, Sidney and Beatrice Webb, and especially Beatrice, one of the commissioners, who took up the question of public health with the most rigor. Notable theorists of a more managerial variant of socialism, the Webbs were also canny networkers. They regularly liaised with government ministers, as well as key public health officials, such as Burns as president of the LGB; George Newman, a leading MOH (and from 1907, chief medical officer to the Board of Education); and Arthur Newsholme, another leading MOH (and from 1908, chief medical officer at the LGB).[163] It was partly owing to these meetings that their vision of reform was crafted outside of the commission. A key facet of what would become the commission's Minority Report, which was principally authored by the Webbs, was presented in late 1906. Speaking before the Society of MOsH, Beatrice ranged over various diseases (such as tuberculosis, measles, and whooping cough) and forms of assistance (isolation hospitals and outdoor poor relief), in all cases lamenting local variations of organization, confused channels of communication, and overlapping responsibilities.[164] At this point her solution was the elevation of MOsH as local supremos of all health-related services, sanitary and poor law.

Almost a year later, a similar argument was presented by Newsholme in an address to the BMA's state medicine section.[165] "At present," he lamented, as part of an argument in favor of greater "coordination," "we have medical officers of health dealing with sanitation and the prevention of infection, Poor-law medical officers dealing with sickness under the most adverse home circumstances, school doctors and nurses knowing nothing or next to nothing of the home conditions which baffle their work, factory surgeons out of touch with local public health administration, and a large body of private practitioners daily in touch with environmental evils that they cannot remove."[166] By 1909, as detailed among the 517 pages of the Minority Report, the Webbs' solution was twofold: first, the replacement of the LGB with a specialized, "self-contained" public health department; and second, nothing less than the abolition of the existing poor law infrastructure, including boards of guardians, and the transfer of all medical and hospital-related functions to local health authorities under the leadership of fulltime MOsH.[167]

In some respects the Minority Report did indeed amount to a "M.O.H.'s Charter," as G.R. Searle has suggested; but such a view requires qualifying.[168] The Minority Report—as with the Majority Report—concerned much more besides the organization of public health services, not least how best to deal with the able-bodied unemployed; and the attitudes of MOsH remained ambivalent, even if their professional journal, *Public Health,* granted the Minority Report editorial approval.[169] More broadly, crucial political principles were at stake. Unlike the more moderate members of the commission, who would eventually support the Majority Report and the setting up of so-called public assistance authorities (essentially revamped boards of guardians), the Webbs wanted to introduce a system based on the type of service required, rather than the type of person in need, poor or otherwise, thus avoiding any kind of "pauperization." To be sure, there were considerable points of agreement between the two reports, including the need to avoid anything that might undermine the moral character of those who required help, and the desire to enhance administrative efficiency and clarity.[170] Yet, the Minority Report also embodied a novel egalitarian premise, which is why some see it as a forerunner of the 1942 Beveridge Report. Put another way, though it empowered nonpolitical, professional agents such as MOsH, the Minority Report remained intensely political.

Neither report was acted upon, however, despite intense lobbying by both sides. As with the findings of the Royal Sanitary Commission almost forty years earlier, the reports had to contend with the workings of the Westminster party system. One problem was finding legislative time in the 1909–10 session in what was an unusually controversial period in parliament.[171] Another was the daunting prospect of having to reform local government finance: in 1911, even Sidney Webb's brilliant bureaucratic brain reeled in amazement at just how complex it had become.[172] In fact, in the short term things only got worse, at least from an organizational point of view. In 1911, inspired by initiatives in Germany, the Liberal ministers Lloyd George and Winston Churchill pressed ahead with their National Insurance scheme, which created another set of central and local authorities—the National Health Insurance Commission, and Insurance Committees and Approved Societies—making for further problems of institutional coordination. Not that these problems escaped notice. Having become dormant following the demise of the poor law inquiry, the idea of a consolidated ministry of state was revived during the war years, and after much struggle the LGB was abolished in 1919. Its successor was called the Ministry of Health.[173]

CONCLUSION

The modern problem of securing administrative unity on a national scale was made of many things. One was the inventiveness of the system. Quite what a "public health system" amounted to as an administrative enterprise was always in flux, evolving as it did in a present packed with initiatives competing for attention. In this respect, the problem was one of catch-up in the context of ongoing innovation: the permanent change that Disraeli spoke of in 1867. Another aspect was the growing organizational complexity of the system; or rather, the accretion of increasingly specialized roles and functions, and a corresponding proliferation of relations that needed coordinating, not least those between center and locality. Yet, as this chapter has sought to demonstrate, these evolving roles and relations were also subject to intense contestation, and from a wide array of perspectives. During both the mid-Victorian period—when the problem of national unity was first posed—and the late Victorian and Edwardian periods—when the distinction between center and local was taken for granted—the system was critiqued from radically different angles. If all were concerned with securing greater efficiency and joined-up, integrated governance, there was little consensus regarding how this might be achieved, and who or what was the most important consideration. Put another way, part of the problem of securing administrative unity was that there was no agreement regarding what, precisely, was at stake. It was always a politicized, multiperspectival conundrum.

It was also a historical problem, and although all protagonists occupied the same open, chronological present, they also had to contend with a past that now stretched over centuries, descending as far back as the Saxons. It is perhaps the Webbs who capture best this peculiar dynamic of modern governance, whereby the openness of the future is affirmed alongside the weight and depth of the past. Immersed in the details of reforming local government—indeed, reforming it radically— the Webbs were also immersed in its history, and it was during their work for the Poor Law Commission when they decided to embark on their mammoth historical study noted above, finally completed in 1929. Their efforts in this respect were especially thorough, but the dynamic had begun much earlier. It was during the 1830s and 1840s when the English tradition of local self-government became an object of politicization, coming into being at the same time that it began to be worked on and reformed; or abandoned, at least according to some Tory and radical interpretations. The English tradition of local self-government, it might be argued, was born only when it started to come apart.

To grasp and dispute the public health system in terms of center-local relations was to operate only at a particular level of abstraction and modern scale and scope. The chapters that follow detail the making and performance of the many other systems that made up the system as a whole. Nonetheless, this particular axis—the intensely politicized, historicized, and contested one of center-local relations—shaped the formation of these smaller, if no less intricate or important, subsystems. As we shall now see, this axis shaped the provision of vital statistics and the measurement of sanitary progress. And yet, conversely, if crucially, these same statistics also shaped how the system was conceived and contested as a modern-historical enterprise comprised of central and local authorities. What had been done, and even what *might* be done, became unthinkable without recourse to numerical facts—if no little amount of opinion as well.

CHAPTER 3

Numbers, Norms, and Opinions

Death and the Measurement of Progress

Public health was not the only system of governance to develop amid an "avalanche of printed numbers." The metaphor is Ian Hacking's, which he uses to capture the unprecedented growth of statistical information in Britain (as well as in France and Prussia) that began in the 1830s.[1] In the case of public health, the principal generator of "official statistics"—the term dates from the 1820s—was the General Register Office (GRO), established in 1837 and located in Somerset House, London. It was this body, much more than any other, that supplied the vital statistics that so engulfed public health. But there were other number-crunching bureaus. In 1881, a Lords committee convened by the Treasury, in order to "simplify and systematize the statistical information supplied [to parliament] from official sources," reported the following: the Home Office (e.g., statistics on court proceedings and prisons); the LGB (poor relief and local government loans); the Post Office (letters and telegraphy); the Committee of Council on Education (elementary schools); and the Treasury itself (public revenue and expenditure).[2] The most prodigious office seems to have been the Board of Trade, which earlier, in 1832, had established a special Statistical Department. By the 1870s, the department was generating numbers on industry and agriculture, and foreign and domestic trade.

Whereas England's tradition of local self-government is seldom seen as modern, this is not true of statistics, which are considered part and parcel of the modern state. It is no coincidence, however, that an avalanche of numbers began falling when it did, just as the English began turning local self-government into a defining feature of their collective, constitutional past. Both were part of a reconfiguration of the spatial and temporal dynamics of governance along modern lines. This is not to suggest a sudden burst of numbers, as if from nowhere. The avalanche that began to fall in the 1830s should certainly be seen as part of a gradual accretion of numerical knowledge dating back to the second half of the seventeenth century with the advent of political arithmetic.[3] In 1801, the longstanding confusion over the precise size of Britain's population was laid to rest with the completion of the first national census. Nonetheless, the accent should fall on novelty. Together with a pronounced increase in the sheer quantity of data, the early Victorian period also witnessed a change in the organization of statistics and their role in the gestation of systems.[4] Put simply, they became fundamental, such that the very being of systems became unthinkable without them. An obvious instance of this is the setting up of specialized, London-based offices—the Board of Trade's Statistical Department and the GRO, for example—to provide numbers on a *permanent* basis. Change in fact would now be assessed through the preprogramed, timetabled production of numbers according to weekly, monthly, quarterly, annual, and decennial rhythms.

What, more precisely, of the spatial and temporal qualities of statistics? In terms of the former, statistics were of general, translocal application, a quality noted and promoted from the start. Particular facts were just that, specific to particular places; but they were also part of a global framework of knowledge, to the extent that these facts could enter into geographical comparisons of any given phenomenon, should it be suitably classified. The initial prospectus of the Statistical Society of London (SSL) founded in 1834—the second of its kind in Britain: a society in Manchester had been established the year before—declared that it sought to collect statistics from "different parts of the empire," and from societies like itself, "foreign and domestic."[5] Later, in 1840, the SSL provided a fivefold arrangement of the different domains of statistical inquiry—geography; industry and agriculture; education; crime; and public health and the poor laws—suggesting that this "system of classification" was "equally available for the most savage or the most civilized community, in any age or country."[6] The statistics that defined the field of public health were of precisely this kind of spatial openness, and they were hardly peculiar in this respect. The same is true, for instance, of the abundance of numbers that surrounded the reform of education, the poor laws, and policing, which also enabled comparisons both within England and with other nations. Indeed, the status of statistical knowledge as a kind of universal language of assessment was quickly confirmed with the staging of the first International Statistical Congress in Brussels in 1853, precursor to the International Statistical Institute of 1885.[7]

Statistical knowledge was also historical, though it has yet to be considered part and parcel of the *temporal* modernity of Victorian governance. The very production of statistics situated society in the same time—the same compressed, clocked present of publication: a given year, quarter, month, or week—as shared by all, regardless of class or location. Equally, statistical knowledge differentiated the present according to a series of variables and their relative degree of attainment, so that some people and places might be judged "ahead," others "behind." In the case of public health, the key variable, of course, was health; or rather, *progress* toward better health. Statisticians, or "statists" as they were initially known, were quite explicit about the role of statistics in this respect. In 1860, Prince Albert addressed a meeting of the International Statistical Congress, the fourth of its kind and the first and last to be held in London. One of the virtues of these gatherings, he told delegates, was that they "pave the way to an agreement among different Governments and Nations to follow up their common [statistical] inquiries, in a common spirit, by a common method, and for a common end." Statistical science, he went on, required the collection of "observations identical in character" and their comparison over "the greatest area," adding:

> And even this comparison of the same facts in different localities does not give us all the necessary material from which to draw our conclusions; for we require, as much as anything else, the collection of observations of the same classes of facts, in the same localities, and under the same conditions, but at different times. It is only the element of time, in the last instance, which enables us to test progress or regress—that is to say, life.[8]

Statistical time, as it might be termed, was thus a particular variant of modern-historical time. If it assumed progress, then progress (or regress) might be a matter of what had occurred in a given space over the course of only a year, quarter, or even week, rather than centuries or ages (though this did not preclude using them in this more expansive fashion). By the same token, it also involved a degree of temporal elaboration that was more than just a bureaucratic statement of clocked particulars (though the generation of statistics depended on a great deal of form filling).

The aim of this chapter is to examine how statistics were used to measure and test the progress of England's public health system. It does so by focusing on the generation and circulation of one fact in particular: death rates. This was certainly not the only fact generated by the GRO. Nor was GRO data the only kind of numerical information mobilized in the governance of public health. Crucially, statistics were generated concerning the *means* of progress. Data circulated on the miles of newly paved streets, for instance, the gallons of water supplied to homes, and annual quotas of smallpox vaccinations. The examples might be multiplied: small or large, micro or macro, every system imaginable was subject to some kind of numerical accounting. The only significant zone of obscurity was a new realm of so-called personal hygiene (see chapter 7). Nonetheless, it was GRO data, and death rates especially, that were preeminent when it came to measuring the success of these means, and where and to what extent they were working. As we shall see, it is here where we might speak of a fully developed process of normalization, in the sense that different localities were now brought together on a common "scale of mortality," and then differentiated accordingly. Otherwise put, death rates articulated the present in the fashion outlined above, differentiating—which is to say, spatializing according to town, city, district or region—national progress toward better health within a standardized, chronological-representational framework.

Two broad points are developed. The first is that the GRO's "facts" were the product of systems and system building. The very generation of death rates turned upon a pronounced self-consciousness regarding the need for system—for uniformity, order, and method—by way of integrating the work of various agents distributed over space. Decisions were made about how to administer and classify death, and which facts to privilege; and these decisions had to be defended and rationalized. As the French historian François Ewald has pithily put it, "normalization begins with vocabulary."[9] The making of these vocabularies, he elaborates, involves agreeing on a common measure, together with a common set of processes that produce this measure. Both types of consideration apply in the case of death rates, and it will be apparent that this chapter shares the view that "facts" are made and put together—which is to say, neither discovered nor invented, but rather composed through multiple practices, and are partly a product of human choices and technologies, and schemas of partial, shifting classification.[10]

The second point concerns agency. In short, the remarkable growth of statistical information was not solely rooted in processes of centralization and bureaucratic empowerment. For one thing, in order to generate its statistical accounts of national health, the GRO depended on the work of localized agents such as registrars and doctors. More importantly, these accounts then informed the actions and arguments of multiple agents, among them MPs, MOsH, ministers, councillors, and local activists. Put another way, the making and circulation of vital statistics empowered all kinds of agents much beyond a central core of officials. It was not simply a matter of "seeing like a state," as James C. Scott has put it in a much-cited formulation.[11] Or if it was, then the statistical eyes were many and multiperspectival, gazing bottom-up as much as top-down. The chapter begins with the administrative labor of making death function as an object of statistical governance.

PROCESSING DEATH

The GRO was established just as a "science" of statistics was emerging as such. During the 1830s, there was much discussion regarding its field of application and its precise ambitions as a science. Among the proponents, all could agree that statistics was beyond "opinion," "rhetoric," and "party politics." As Mary Poovey has shown, partly formed in the eighteenth century, the binary distinction between "fact" and "opinion" was now insisted upon with much more force and regularity, and was crucial to the public authority of this fledgling science.[12] Yet, at this point, quite whether statistics was supposed to speculate about causes and effects was unclear. There was also confusion as to whether it was a science in and of itself, with a particular object of study, or simply a means of furnishing data for all sciences: a kind of semi-science of data collection.[13] In 1840, the SSL attempted to clarify the matter:

> it was not to perfect the mere art of "tabulating" that it [the Society] was embodied;—it was not to make us hewers and drawers to those engaged on any edifice of physical sciences;—but it was that we should ourselves be the architects of a science or of sciences. . . . Statistics, by their very name, are defined to be the observations necessary to the social or moral sciences, to the sciences of the *statist* to whom the statesman and the legislator must resort for the principles on which to govern. These sciences are equally distinct from the purely physical, the purely mathematical, and the purely metaphysical, though the mathematical must lend aid to their pursuit.

In keeping with its founding prospectus of 1834, quoted above, the Society explicitly renounced "opinions," but it encouraged what it called "the proper use of *à priori* reasoning": "The value of hypothesis and conjecture is to point out the direction in which observation will most probably be fertile in discovering truth, demonstrating error, or striking out new paths of investigation."[14]

This meaning persisted throughout the nineteenth century, and it was the one the GRO operated with in furnishing vital statistics. Understood in the singular, statistics was a "social science," self-consciously oriented toward reform, and certainly not averse to speculating about causes and effects, sometimes altogether loosely. At the same time, if it privileged numerical facts, statistics also permitted those of a narrative sort by way of elaboration. Techniques were still rudimentary. Only during the early twentieth century did statistics become associated with the mathematical manipulation of data derived from all kinds of phenomena and that powerful set of tools still in use today, such as correlation and regression analysis, and random sampling.[15] In terms of public health professionals, it was not until the early twentieth century when they were encouraged to familiarize themselves with the work of biometricians such as Francis Galton and Karl Pearson, and the mathematical modeling of statistical variation.[16]

Yet, as Edward Higgs has argued, the emergence of the GRO as a powerhouse of reform-oriented statistics should not be read into its original design.[17] The office was a product of the 1836 Registration and Marriage Acts, both passed in order to overhaul the patchy system of parochial registration that had existed since the sixteenth century. Births, deaths, and marriages were now subject to civil registration, but the overriding impetus was neither the placation of Nonconformist denominations excluded from an Anglican-administered system, nor the collection of statistics in the service of public health. Rather, the impetus was principally legal and actuarial. As Higgs demonstrates, the GRO was conceived as a means of placing the administration of property on a clearer, more comprehensive archival footing. Hence its location in Somerset House, in close proximity to the Inns of Court situated in and around Chancery Lane; the Public Record Office (established in 1838); and later the Principal Probate Registry (1857) and the Land Registry (1862).[18] Furthermore, while the Registration Act provided for the certification of the cause of death—as opposed to just death—this was a product of an amendment lobbied for by Chadwick; and at this point, Chadwick was concerned to enhance the actuarial knowledge of friendly societies and their capacity to act as agents of self-help.

The GRO's actuarial functions would diminish as statistics of this sort were gradually refined by a burgeoning band of corporate actuaries and an increasingly numerate culture of friendly society association. Nonetheless, it was this actuarial rationale that was exploited by the GRO's first compiler of abstracts—later statistical superintendent— William Farr, who transformed its Statistical Department into the nation's principal bureaucratic organ of mortality data.[19] Farr was a doctor and had earlier trained in Paris under the likes of Pierre Louis, a pioneer in the use of statistics to study patient groups. By the time of his appointment in 1839, Farr possessed a growing reputation as a statistician. In 1837, the same year the GRO began work, he published a chapter entitled "Vital Statistics" as part of J. R. McCulloch's *Statistical Account of the British Empire*.[20] Though all of his successors—William Ogle (1880–93); John Tatham (1893–1909); and T. H. C. Stevenson (1909–31)—introduced innovations of their own, it was largely thanks to Farr's efforts that the Statistical Department became a core component of England's public health system. If he could boast a modest degree of expertise to begin with, by the time he retired in 1879 Farr was widely regarded as one of Europe's most able statisticians.

The key function of the GRO remained the bureaucratic management of birth, death, and marriage certificates, and overall responsibility rested with the head of the organization, the registrar-general. Of its four departments, which also included Correspondence (up to 1866) and Accounts, the Records Department commanded the most manpower: in 1895, it comprised forty-five employees to the Statistical Department's nineteen.[21] This compared favorably to an initial four, and under Farr's leadership, with support from the second registrar-general, Major George Graham, the department expanded much beyond its original remit of compiling annual tables of mortality data. The centerpiece of the GRO's output was the *Annual Report of the Registrar-General* (*ARRG*), which presented the registration data abstracted for a twelve-month period. From the beginning, the annual report was supplemented with a "Letter to the Registrar-General," written by the superintendent of statistics. The GRO's statistical functions also grew to include a range of publications, of variable temporal compression, from weekly and quarterly returns to decennial supplements summarizing the experience of England over ten-year periods.

Paginated, tabulated, clocked: so appeared the facts contained in this unprecedented abundance of documents. Their neatness and national scope, however, belies the intricate, localized-centralized work of classification, coordination, and translation that made them possible. When, in 1840, the GRO took over the national census, the then registrar-general,

Thomas Lister, noted the need for "uniformity of system."[22] A similar systematizing impulse presided over death; and as with the census this too proved hard fought and partial—partial to the extent that it involved institutionalizing a particular perspective, and making choices about what to classify and how.[23] Ultimately, from 1911, death in England would be classified according to a schema of French design: Jacques Bertillon's nosology, developed in Paris during the 1880s, endorsed by the International Statistical Institute in 1893, and dubbed the International List of Causes of Death (ICD).[24] Yet this was a schema partly inspired by Farr and his system-building work during the midcentury. It made for a reworked return of something that had begun in England at Somerset House.

In the case of death, there were two key problems: first, making death function as a stable, uniform object of classificatory knowledge across England; second, coordinating the resulting system and its multiple procedures and agents. Each of these can be taken in turn.

Naming, Simplifying, and Classifying Death

One of the first tasks carried out by Farr was just this: the establishment of a uniform system of names for causes of death (nomenclature), coupled with a uniform system of classification (nosology) by which to group these causes in order to facilitate statistical analysis. The two went together, as Farr pointed out in his letter of 1839, where he presented his first "statistical nosology." "The advantages of a uniform statistical nomenclature, however imperfect," wrote Farr, after having set out his classificatory schema, "are so obvious that it is surprising no attention has been paid to its enforcement in Bills of Mortality": "Each disease has in many instances been denoted by three or four terms, and each term has been applied to as many different diseases; vague, inconvenient names have been employed, or complication registered instead of primary diseases. The nomenclature is of as much importance in this department of inquiry, as weights and measures in the physical sciences, and should be settled without delay."[25]

The same point was made by other statisticians. Their empirical raw material had to be uniform and comparable if, like other scientists, they were to make general statements about phenomena, and the regularities and causal relations that governed their existence. Crucially, this meant demanding only a single piece of uniform data; or in the case of the GRO, a single cause of death, as described according to the prescribed nomenclature. From the start, the GRO encouraged the registration of "primary" and "secondary" causes; but only the primary—where primary was understood as the most important—cause was processed by the GRO. This is not to diminish the significance of the statistical inquiries this made possible; simply to suggest that these inquiries were premised on the exclusion, at the point of registration, of the particularity of a given death, and the complex, multicausal ingredients and unique morbid events that had preceded it.[26]

This is one reason why statistical reasoning was regarded with suspicion throughout the century (and beyond). Suspicion of this sort was especially acute during the early Victorian period, when the likes of Charles Dickens and Thomas Carlyle criticized the way statistics quantified and classified the complex, thereby reducing by abstraction objects of study that were composite, situated, and particular—and not least the "Condition-of-England-Question," as Carlyle famously dubbed it in 1839.[27] Unsurprisingly, Toulmin Smith chose not to do battle in statistical terms during the midcentury, making much the same point. Statistics were manifestations of "theory," he argued, entirely subordinate to the political desire to uproot the governance of collective affairs from its "practical" embedding in the local.[28]

Equally, statistical enthusiasts made similar criticisms and directed them quite specifically at the GRO's registration system. It is significant that Rumsey was among the earliest and most prescient critics of the GRO, and this was partly on account of its limited informational reach and ambition. In 1860, he spoke before a meeting of the NAPSS in Bradford, where he critiqued "the assumption that the last phenomena of mortal disease may be correctly reported as the 'cause' of death." "They are, in general, but the penultimate effects of the real cause, or at most the last link of a chain of secondary causes."[29] As noted in chapter 2, in his *Essays on State Medicine* Rumsey called for panoptic-like powers of statistical scrutiny, including statistics of sickness and not just cause of death. The absence of knowledge regarding preceding bouts of sickness was thus one defect, and so too was the absence of information regarding congenital factors, the quality or not of any medical treatment, as well as socioeconomic variables, such as poverty and overcrowding. And yet it was altogether reasonable to suppose that they too might have played a causal role. (These criticisms were not without consequence, for, as we shall see in chapter 6, what became known as the "notification of infectious diseases" has its roots in calls for the registration of sickness.)

Farr himself was aware of this. He was not surprised, for instance, that in some cases no cause could be provided by a medical attendant, given the complexity of a single death. As he noted in the *30th ARRG* (1869): "Now, when it is considered how multitudinous and complex the causes are, not of the one phenomenon, but of the many phenomena of death, for death has its many phases as well as life, it can scarcely be surprising to find that out of nearly half a million deaths no causes were assigned in eight thousand or more instances." "In many cases," he added, "the primary cause can, but in many cases it cannot, be discovered"; and this was partly because it was not always clear how far the causal chain of a particular death might be traced back.[30] Nonetheless, Farr also reminded his readers that the science of vital statistics was impossible without this kind of reduction: indeed, it was constitutive of what it was as a science. He opened the second decennial supplement, published in 1875, by stating that his domain of inquiry was "the gloomy kingdom of the dead, whither have gone in twenty years [nine hundred thousand] English children, fathers, mothers, sisters, brothers, daughters, sons . . . each having left memories not easily forgotten; and many having biographies full of complicated incidents." To which Farr added: "Here, fortunately for this inquiry, they appear divested of all colour, form, character, passions and the infinite individualities of life: by abstraction they are reduced to mere units undergoing changes as purely physical as the setting stars of astronomy or the decomposing atoms of chemistry."[31] It was about collecting the "elementary facts" and working from there. How else could one get at the multiplicity of causal relations that obtained at the *collective* level, as evident in general patterns and regularities? There followed almost six hundred pages of commentary and tabulated information.

It was not, then, a simple process of simplification. Rather, the registration system reduced complexity at one level—the unique death of an individual—while enabling it at the abstract level of the population, and its statistically rendered variables, which could then be combined and computed for epidemiological purposes. It was a necessary trade-off: one kind of complexity for another; particular complexity for general complexity. But there was still the question of how death should be classified if the GRO was to function as an engine of this kind of abstract statistical inquiry. As Simon Szreter has argued, Farr's pioneering work in nosology—the classification of diseases—was driven by a commitment to its utility in terms of preventing disease.[32] This reflected two things. The first has been detailed at length: namely Farr's broadly environmentalist—if ultimately idiosyncratic—understanding of disease causation, based on the role of processes analogous to fermentation (or "zymosis").[33] The second is perhaps still more important: the practical orientation of statistics as a social-administrative science. And Farr certainly considered himself first and foremost a statist.

Farr devised his first system in 1839, revised it in 1842, and introduced a third in 1856; and he was always intensely self-conscious regarding the partial nature of the task and of the existence of other nosological perspectives. In his 1839 letter, he was entirely forthcoming on this score. After considering various nosologies then in use—including William Cullen's still popular system, which originated in 1775, as well as more recent ones, such as John Mason Good's *A Physiological System of Nosology* (1817)—he explained the rationale of his own "statistical nosology." Of particular importance was the decision to present a separate class of "epidemic, endemic, and contagious diseases"; or what, after 1842, became known as the "zymotics," which included cholera, smallpox, measles, scarlet fever, influenza, and typhus. In Farr's view, "this great class of maladies is the index of salubrity . . . they can be controlled and almost always admit of prevention or mitigation. Of the utility of keeping this class of diseases distinct in a practical sanatory [*sic*] report there can be no question."[34]

Farr made the same argument in 1856, when he first presented the nosology that would structure the GRO's abstracts from 1860. It developed out of an ultimately abortive scheme commissioned by the first International Statistical Congress to develop a standardized system for use around the world; and unlike his nosology of 1839, which contained three classes, Farr's new one of 1856 contained five: zymotic diseases (class 1), constitutional diseases (2), local diseases (3), developmental diseases (4), and violent deaths (5), plus further subdivisions, or "orders," within each.[35] "Classification is a method of generalization," he stated: "Several classifications may, therefore, be used with advantage. . . . The medical practitioner may found his main division of diseases on their treatment as medical or surgical; the pathologist, on the nature of the morbid action or product; the anatomist, or the physiologist, on the tissues and organs involved; the medical jurist, on the *suddenness* or the *slowness* of death; and all these points well deserve attention in a statistical classification." However, his own "eyes" were those of a "national statist," fixed on "the improvement of the race of men." And it was the zymotic class of diseases that had "a special claim to the attention of statists, inasmuch as by prophylactic measures, of which vaccination is an example, and by hygienic arrangements, the ravages of epidemics may be greatly diminished. They are more than other diseases under public control."[36]

Farr maintained this self-consciously practical-statistical orientation throughout his tenure as superintendent, as did his successors. It could hardly have been otherwise. That causes of death might be named and classified differently was a matter of ongoing discussion, as agents beyond the GRO offered alternatives. In 1869, the Royal College of Physicians published its first "approved" *Nomenclature of Diseases,* based around a broadly anatomical nosology; revised editions followed in 1885, 1896, and 1906.[37] In 1875, Rumsey summarized the criticisms that had arisen since the 1840s, which included those of James Stark, Farr's counterpart at the Scottish GRO established in 1854, who objected to the internal differentiation (the "orders") of the zymotic class in particular.[38]

New names and distinctions were thus introduced—from 1869, for instance, "typhus" was divided into "typhus," "enteric," and "simple continued" fevers—as were new orders and classes.[39] In 1883 (for the year 1881), Ogle modified some of the names used for designating death in line with the College's nomenclature and introduced a new eightfold system of classification, which included new orders, as well as the addition of separate classes for dietetic and parasitic diseases. Later, in 1903 (for 1901), Tatham replaced Ogle's system with a fourfold classification, again updating names and orders. Like Ogle had before him, Tatham stressed that it should be regarded as only a "provisional" system of classification and that it was intended for public health purposes. It was on this basis that the crux of Tatham's system was the broad distinction between "general" and "local diseases." Although it did away with Farr's zymotic class, general diseases were nonetheless considered more preventable than local diseases, and indeed now included variants of tuberculosis, which had previously been placed under the "constitutional" class. Provisional as well as practical: for Tatham, his own system followed in the statistical tradition established by Farr, whom he dubbed a "genius."

Working the System

It was these shifting classificatory systems that governed the production and presentation of the GRO's mortality data—systems indeed that determined the official-statistical form of the deaths of millions. Making these designs work was another matter. Although the new system was more comprehensive, ambitious, and better resourced than the old, it was also more organizationally complex and demanding. Spatially, the system was composed of registration districts that mapped onto the administrative landscape of the reformed poor law, which comprised over six hundred unions. Each district was further divided into subdistricts, manned by a local registrar. A superintendent registrar was responsible for a district as a whole, and it was his job to collate the certificates collected locally and forward them to the GRO. Throughout the century, there were roughly 620 superintendents and 2,000 local registrars at work, most appointed by boards of poor law guardians. The paperwork was immense. Between June 1837 and June 1838, clerks in the GRO processed 399,712 birth certificates; 111,481 marriage certificates; and 355,956 death certificates. By 1888, these same figures had risen to 879,868; 203,821; and 510,951, respectively.[40]

Various initiatives emerged by way of managing the novel complexity of the system. At Somerset House, the growing volume of information that required handling spurred technological experimentation. In 1857, the GRO purchased a Scheutz's calculating machine, similar in design and conception to Charles Babbage's difference engine. Scheutz's machine proved only of modest use in the calculation of life tables, and in 1870 the GRO purchased an arithmometer, a much smaller desktop device and precursor to the handheld calculator. The first of several acquisitions, Farr wrote to the Treasury in 1872 praising the arithmometer, claiming that it "enabled a clerk to perform probably twice as many calculations as he can perform without it."[41] By contrast, data processing—the sorting of data, as opposed to its mathematical computation—remained manual throughout the Victorian and Edwardian periods. The so-called ticking system involved the use of large sheets of paper, one for each subdistrict, and the placing of an individual tick in a column according to the variable in question (a particular disease, for instance); the ticks were then added up and the data transferred to a sheet for the district as a whole. It was a time-consuming process. In 1856, the GRO reported that it had taken one clerk four days to abstract the mortality data of Lancastrian females for the year 1854—a labor which involved dealing with 310 sheets of paper and a total of 29,063 ticks.[42] Only in 1911 was data processing mechanized, with the introduction of a punch-card system imported from the United States to help manage the census of that year.

Similarly, initiatives were introduced by way of managing the proliferation of points of potential resistance and confusion. In 1845, Farr

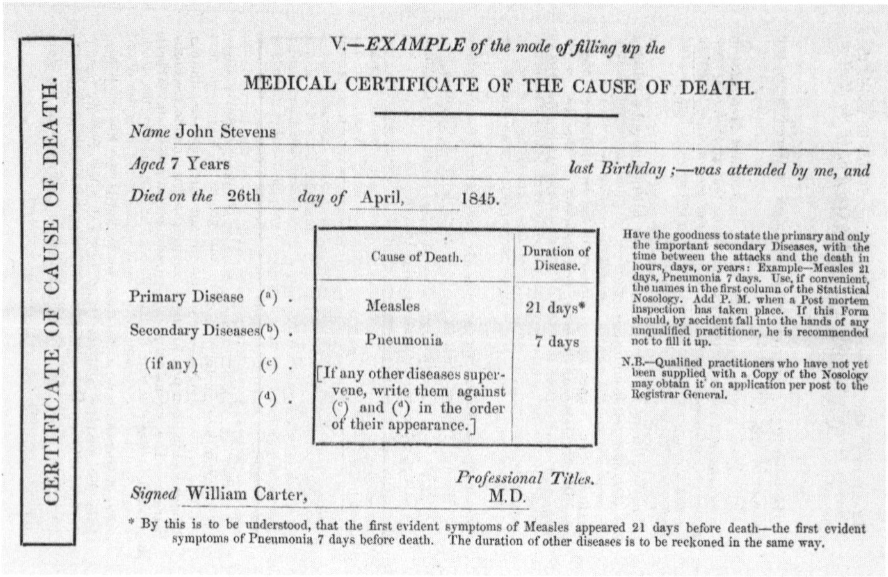

CERTIFICATE OF CAUSE OF DEATH.

V.—*EXAMPLE of the mode of filling up the*

MEDICAL CERTIFICATE OF THE CAUSE OF DEATH.

Name John Stevens

Aged 7 Years *last Birthday ;—was attended by me, and*

Died on the 26th *day of* April, 1845.

	Cause of Death.	Duration of Disease.
Primary Disease (a) .	Measles	21 days*
Secondary Diseases(b) .	Pneumonia	7 days
(if any) (c) .	[If any other diseases supervene, write them against (c) and (d) in the order of their appearance.]	
(d) .		

Have the goodness to state the primary and only the important secondary Diseases, with the time between the attacks and the death in hours, days, or years: Example—Measles 21 days, Pneumonia 7 days. Use, if convenient, the names in the first column of the Statistical Nosology. Add P. M. when a Post mortem inspection has taken place. If this Form should, by accident fall into the hands of any unqualified practitioner, he is recommended not to fill it up.

N.B.—Qualified practitioners who have not yet been supplied with a Copy of the Nosology may obtain it on application per post to the Registrar General.

Signed William Carter, *Professional Titles.* M.D.

* By this is to be understood, that the first evident symptoms of Measles appeared 21 days before death—the first evident symptoms of Pneumonia 7 days before death. The duration of other diseases is to be reckoned in the same way.

FIGURE 2. A model death certificate circulated by the GRO in 1864 and based on the initial circular of 1845. Source: *Registration of the Causes of Death: Circulars to Medical Practitioners, and to Registrars* (London: George E. Eyre and William Spottiswoode, 1864), 8. © The Bodleian Libraries, The University of Oxford.

issued a curricular to all local registrars and qualified physicians, surgeons, and apothecaries detailing his nosology and nomenclature, the correct way of filling out certificates, and the meaning of "primary" and "secondary" causes (see figure 2). Hereafter, the GRO distributed register books to local registrars, supplemented with up-to-date instructions and preprinted certificates. Regulatory initiatives also extended to the public. The 1874 Registration Act, for instance, tightened up procedures relating to the communication of information. In particular, the act stipulated that nearest relatives had to notify the local registrar of a death within five days of its occurrence, accompanied by a medical certificate, which doctors were now obliged to supply should they have attended the body at some point before or after it had expired.

Problems remained, however, and were especially acute at the local level, where they turned on the use and abuse of certification forms. The high point of critique came in 1893, when, after years of lobbying, MPs agreed to form a select committee on death certification. The flaws of the system were laid bare in particular detail, with the committee collecting almost 240 pages of testimony.[43] The fact that burials could take place without the provision of a death certificate meant that bodies might be disposed of without any kind of registration, which for some was an invitation to infanticide (and it seems the system did indeed allow for this).[44] It was also noted that doctors filled out false certificates at the behest of a relative worried about loss of public face. This was especially so when it came to suicide, alcoholism, and syphilis. Given that it was relatives of the deceased, rather than the doctor, who forwarded the certificate to the local registrar, the system encouraged what one MOH called "errors of commission," a "form of evasion" which "statesmen call diplomacy."[45] Solutions from abroad were duly considered: first promoted by Rumsey and Farr in the midcentury, the French municipal office of *médecin vérificateur,* responsible for confirming, certifying, and communicating all deaths without exception, was a particular favorite and featured in the testimony of several witnesses before the select committee.[46]

The 1893 committee was only a momentary, if concentrated, manifestation of a rolling culture of critique that had been present from the start. As elsewhere, systemic problems were not only noted; they were systematized, becoming internalized, critical elements of classification and counting. In 1845, for instance, local registrars were instructed to distinguish deaths reported without certification by a registered doctor as "not certified."[47] In 1860, the figure stood at roughly 20 percent of the total number of certificates; by the end of the century it had been reduced to below 2 percent.[48] Considerable progress was made on this front, but even certified deaths could prove problematic. Still at the end of the century doctors were using obsolete terms; providing a medley of causes (occasionally as many as ten); detailing symptoms rather than causes; and mistaking "primary" for "secondary" causes.[49] The term in use from 1839 was "not specified," and from the 1860s "not specified or ill-defined." In 1881, Ogle instituted a system of investigating certificates of this sort, and in 1883 he elevated the "ill-defined and not specified" into one of the eight classes of his new nosology; Tatham too maintained it as a separate class in his design of 1903.[50] During this period the number declined from roughly 6 to 4 percent of the total number of certificates received by the GRO.[51]

Another troublesome point in the system arose when uncertified deaths were referred to coroners' courts, the same courts charged with investigating deaths by violence and those judged suspicious. The number of deaths subject to a coroner's inquest was never especially significant, flitting between 5 and 7 percent during the Victorian and Edwardian periods.[52] Nonetheless, in deaths not attributable to violence

or accident, the verdict was often of no use in terms of the GRO's statistical requirements, even if it might have settled legal questions and
quelled local intrigue. It was common for juries to return a verdict of
"sudden death" or "death by the visitation of God." In Norwich, during 1882, of the fifty-five nonviolent deaths subject to a coroner's
inquest, some forty-two were then certified as "died of natural causes."[53]
Complaints of this kind were first voiced during the 1840s—Farr called
for reform as early as his third letter in 1841—and were still being made
in the Edwardian period. The fundamental problem was that the inquest
remained an institution whose priorities were legal rather than statistical; and while critics were certainly conscious of the inquest's conflicted
sense of purpose, few could resist noting how coroners seemed to disre-
gard their "scientific" responsibilities. More often than not, noted the
MOH for West Riding in 1901, the coroner "is satisfied if the evidence
appears to show that death has not resulted from criminal violence,
forgetting the other purposes, medical and scientific, to which inquests
are intended to be subservient."[54]

Given the elaborate labor of translating a singular dead body into an
abstract, tabulated fact, these criticisms might be regarded as unduly
harsh. If anything, the system worked remarkably well. Yet, it was just
these modern, systematizing impulses that helped to build and improve
a system composed of multiple parts, all of which required standardiz-
ing and integrating on a national scale before death could assume an
official-statistical form: nosologies, names, paper forms, and acts of
writing and computing. The most contestable element was the nosological one; but as was affirmed at the time, the GRO's perspective was a
statistical one, and as such concerned with governing. When, in 1911,
the then statistical superintendent, T. H. C. Stevenson, introduced the
ICD, he took care to note, as all of his predecessors had before him, that
there was "much room for difference of opinion according to the point
of view from which it [the classification of disease] is approached." In
this case, "considerations of general utility and convenience" were in
play. Apart from furthering the cause of national uniformity—the LGB
was using it for collating the reports of MOsH—it made for a more
integrated system of global statistics, facilitating "the comparison of
English mortality with that of other countries."[55] By this point, the ICD
was in use in France, the United States, and Canada, and was already in
its second incarnation. In 1899, the International Statistical Institute
had agreed on a revision cycle of ten years so as to keep up with the

latest diagnostic and etiological innovations.[56] What had been taking place on an ad hoc basis in countries such as England was thus systematized, becoming a preprogramed act of revision.

THE "NATIONAL SYSTEM OF COMPUTATION"

The great profusion of documents that emerged from these intricate, systemic processes opened up what might be characterized, after John Pickstone, as an analytical mode of interrogating national health. For Pickstone, the essence of analytical sciences—of which Antoine Lavoisier's chemistry and Xavier Bichat's pathological anatomy are exemplary instances—is a concern to deconstruct complex objects into their constituent elements.[57] The task then is to group and classify these elements, compare their relative frequency, and examine them in terms of their different qualities and structural relations. The GRO's publications might be seen in this light, as might nineteenth-century statistics more generally (by contrast, twentieth-century mathematical statistics conforms more to Pickstone's experimental way of knowing, premised on controlling carefully defined variables, and focusing attention on a single causal link and hypothesis). Statisticians often described their science in these terms. In 1847, Joseph Fletcher of the SSL, a pioneer of criminal statistics, acknowledged that the "man who studies society" could hardly manipulate his object of interest in the manner of a laboratory-based chemist. Society was "in a state of unceasing change," "wholly beyond his control": "Analysis, therefore, in the sense of the chemist, is absolutely impossible." Even so, statistics made possible an analogous mode of investigation: "by the exhaustive enumeration of facts we get a means of detecting the excess or deficiency of certain social elements in definite classes or localities, and by multiplying these lines of observation, and the combinations in which they are arranged for purposes of comparison, we gradually arrive at higher and safer inductions."[58]

With respect to death, the analytical operations undertaken by the GRO routinely generated the following: gross averages of total deaths; the relative frequency of fatal diseases, both individually and in their nosological classes; rates of mortality for different age groups (birth to age four, five to nine, etc.); average life spans; the relative mortality of males and females; and the ratio of births to deaths. All were computed for periods of variable chronology (one, five, or ten years, etc.) over areas of variable geographical scope, including regional divisions, and registration counties and districts. The GRO's statistical work was thus characterized by a kind of analytical suppleness, capable of zooming in or out over different admixtures of time and space, and with respect to particular elements, singly or in combination with others. It opened up a new and incredibly rich domain of governmental critique, in which progress could be assessed via a medley of numerical measures, and in degrees of movement away or toward national averages and standards—a truly modern world of intricate statistical density only glimpsed prior to the 1830s, but which was now subject to continuous, timetabled bureaucratic reproduction.

In broad terms the role of the GRO's Statistical Department was to keep the nation up-to-date and fully furnished with precisely this kind of analytical information. The most accurate and comprehensive documents were the *ARRGs* and decennial supplements, although these could take years to prepare. More regular documents were supplied in the interim. In 1840, the GRO began publishing weekly returns of mortality data for metropolitan districts, a service that gradually expanded from the mid-1860s onward: by 1873 it had extended to twenty towns and cities; by 1895, to thirty-three; and by 1914, to ninety-seven. Beginning in 1842, quarterly returns were also provided, appearing within a month of each quarter's end. Initially covering the 114 most populous districts, by the early 1850s they were of national scope. Finally, from the mid-1860s, annual summaries of London and "other large cities" were provided, which normally appeared the following March or April. At the end of the century they included over one hundred towns and cities.

Amid this mass of published data, the GRO chose to publicize one fact above others as a means of measuring public health in any given area: the "rate of mortality" or "death rate," summarizing the cumulative total of deaths as expressed per thousand of the population (or as per hundred in the early *ARRGs*). Crucially, its promotion turned on a causal claim as well: simply that death rates bore some relation to the efficacy of sanitary actions undertaken locally. It was also, then, a means of probing the efforts of local authorities as much as normalizing collective health according to a common scale of measurement. The rate of mortality was not the only available indicator. In the early 1840s, Chadwick made a bid for the average age of death, and others included the ratio of deaths to births and births to population.[59] Nor was it the most precise measure of health. The most accurate data was contained in actuarial life tables, which presented the probability of dying for each year of life within a given population. Under Farr, however, the death rate was promoted as the principal "numerical test" of public health, assuming a prominent place in all the office's publications, weekly, quarterly, and annual. In 1863, in a formulation that would persist, the GRO's use of death rates was dubbed the "national system of computation" by two members of the Manchester and Salford Sanitary Association (MSSA). "By means of these figures," they suggested, referring to an earlier *ARRG*, "we could at once see the amount of mortality occurring in any particular place, and compare it in this respect with other places; or mark how far it departs from any ideal standard of health which we might have fixed upon."[60]

Why foreground just one particular figure? Statistics was a self-consciously reformist enterprise, and for the Victorian GRO this meant serving the mixed constituency of agents empowered within the broadly liberal system of modern center-local relations detailed in the last chapter. The promotion of death rates should be understood in just this context, and it was partly about serving professionals and advancing the aims of sanitary science. "As political economy rests upon the idea of value, so our science [sanitary science] rests upon the idea of health, and it is as important to us to find a measure of health as it is to the economist to find a measure of value," Farr explained in 1866 before the NAPSS: "That measure must be simple and applicable to all countries. Now, the measure that is in universal use is the rate of mortality."[61] Put another way, it was about constituting a common field of comparative analysis that all spaces might inhabit, whether small (towns) or large (nations), foreign or domestic. Death rates functioned in precisely this fashion and were quoted at length at national and international sanitary gatherings throughout the second half of the century. Meanwhile, the GRO worked hard to expand (spatially) and intensify (temporally) their collection and circulation in England. In 1865, just as the GRO started to publish the weekly death totals of ten British cities beyond London, it began to include those of Vienna, thanks to the cooperation of the city's chief statistician, Dr. Glatter.[62] Later, during the 1870s, it started publishing quarterly and weekly death rates for twenty-four cities in Europe, the United States, Africa, and Asia—among them New York and Bombay—in what it dubbed a "great International Statistical Return."[63] By 1914, its reach extended to thirty-two cities across the world, which now included Moscow and Rio de Janeiro.

At the same time, the GRO also sought to serve and stimulate the more popular and political parts of the system; or in terms of agents, so-called nonprofessionals, such as MPs, councillors, civic activists, and ratepayers. This was apparent from the start in both the form of its tabulated information and in the explanatory passages of its multiple reports. Informing meant prodding and probing, and the GRO did not refrain from pointing to all manner of problems relating to overcrowding, air pollution, water and food supplies, and emerging sewerage systems. Death rates were by no means the only figures quoted or discussed: even weekly returns contained much more besides, including disease-specific rates and the price of coal and food. But they formed the key figure when it came to making introductory comparisons. Here the virtue of "general death rates," as they were also known, was less their ability to unify different spaces and times on a common scale of measurement and more their ease of computation and comprehension.

This included presenting what today (in the United Kingdom at least) we would call "league tables," which rank the performance or success of particular units of administration. The first of these tables appeared in the 7th ARRG (1846), where county-by-county mortality rates were presented in descending order—from worst to best, rather than vice versa—and they featured in subsequent ARRGs (see figure 3). It was the more accessible annual summaries that emerged as the principal place where this sort of tabulated ranking occurred; and if not in tabulated form, then with narrative descriptions to that effect. In the summary for the year 1872, for instance, two tables appeared, one ranking twenty cities "in their order of mortality," the other fifty large towns. The GRO was keenly aware of the legislative context, noting the requirement (following the 1872 Public Health Act) to appoint MOsH and sanitary inspectors: "mayors and town councillors should give themselves no rest until they have done their utmost by sanitary precautions to save life," it stated after the first table. "They are now on their trial. They will be questioned at the bar of public opinion." Following the second table of large towns, it noted that "Preston, Walsall, Northampton, Bolton and Dudley enjoy here a painful preeminence, which cannot fail to awaken the attention of their respective authorities" (see figure 4).[64]

As we shall see in the next section, death rates were readily mobilized in the public sphere, informing debates in parliament and at the local level. Posing problems in this fashion, however, was not unproblematic, and the GRO's national system also had its critics, in particular among doctors and MOsH. They were especially vocal during the 1860s and 1870s, when lobbying for state medicine was at its height, as detailed in the last chapter. At root, the problem was one of inference, and what, if anything, might be deduced from a single fact in the absence of further

Average Annual Marriages, Births, and Deaths to 100 Persons living, in the Divisions and Counties of England; arranged in the order of the mortality—beginning with Counties in which the mortality is highest.

(Facts from Table A.)

No.	DIVISIONS.	COUNTIES.	To 100 Persons Living (50 Males and 50 Females).			One Marriage	One Birth	One Death
			Marriages.	Births.	Deaths.	To Persons living.		
8	North Western	Cheshire; Lancashire	·859	3·612	2·616	116	28	38
1	Metropolis	Middlesex (part of); Surrey (part of); Kent (part of)	·968	3·084	2·547	103	32	39
	ENGLAND		·773	3·215	2·189	129	31	46
6	Western	Gloucestershire; Herefordshire; Shropshire; Worcestershire; Staffordshire; Warwickshire	·771	3·228	2·188	130	31	46
9	York	North Riding; East Riding; West Riding	·802	3·438	2·186	125	29	46
10	Northern	Durham; Northumberland; Cumberland; Westmoreland	·710	3·353	2·107	141	30	47
3	South Midland	Middlesex (part of); Hertfordshire; Buckinghamshire; Oxfordshire; Northamptonshire; Huntingdonshire; Bedfordshire; Cambridgeshire	·697	3·260	2·091	143	31	48
7	North Midland	Leicestershire; Rutlandshire; Lincolnshire; Nottinghamshire; Derbyshire	·734	3·259	2·072	136	31	48
4	Eastern	Essex; Suffolk; Norfolk	·696	3·083	2·021	144	32	49
5	South Western	Wiltshire; Dorsetshire; Devonshire; Cornwall; Somersetshire	·706	3·014	1·957	142	33	51
11	Welsh	Monmouthshire and Wales	·700	3·002	1·948	143	33	51
2	South Eastern	Surrey (part of); Kent (except Greenwich); Sussex; Hampshire; Berkshire	·684	2·933	1·918	146	34	52

No.	COUNTIES.	To 100 Persons Living (50 Males and 50 Females.)			One Marriage	One Birth	One Death
		Marriages.	Births.	Deaths.	To Persons Living.		
34	Lancashire	·903	3·707	2·680	111	27	37
33	Cheshire	·649	3·167	2·322	154	32	43
27	Warwickshire	·734	3·331	2·288	136	30	44
38	Durham	·800	3·651	2·252	125	27	44
26	Staffordshire	·795	3·526	2·250	126	28	44
35	West Riding	·797	3·606	2·232	125	28	45
42	Monmouthshire	·762	3·245	2·224	131	31	45
13	Cambridgeshire	·784	3·429	2·210	128	29	45
22	Gloucestershire	·847	3·003	2·192	118	33	46
36	East Riding (with York)	·903	2·978	2·189	111	34	46
28	Leicestershire	·751	3·292	2·185	133	30	46
11	Huntingdonshire	·794	3·636	2·141	126	28	47
8	Buckinghamshire	·671	3·302	2·132	149	30	47
25	Worcestershire	·817	3·533	2·129	122	28	47
10	Northamptonshire	·790	3·457	2·129	127	29	47
31	Nottinghamshire	·738	3·290	2·126	136	30	47
32	Derbyshire	·714	3·204	2·125	140	31	47
12	Bedfordshire	·803	3·586	2·122	125	28	47
9	Oxfordshire	·721	3·163	2·094	139	32	48
23	Herefordshire	·633	2·685	2·071	158	37	48
16	Norfolk	·710	3·029	2·065	141	33	48
39	Northumberland	·714	3·256	2·051	140	31	49
21	Somersetshire	·688	3·014	2·040	145	33	49
24	Shropshire	·655	2·697	2·040	153	37	49
17	Wiltshire	·643	2·959	2·029	156	34	49
14	Essex	·648	3·070	2·020	154	33	50
5	Berkshire	·664	2·967	1·985	151	34	50
40	Cumberland	·567	3·095	1·976	176	32	51
7	Hertfordshire	·596	3·224	1·974	168	31	51
2	Kent (except Greenwich)	·710	3·019	1·974	141	33	51
15	Suffolk	·727	3·170	1·968	138	32	51
43	South Wales	·721	3·173	1·958	139	32	51
41	Westmoreland	·621	2·885	1·950	161	35	51
6	Middlesex (part of)	·465	2·534	1·945	215	39	51
20	Cornwall	·688	3·305	1·940	145	30	52
30	Lincolnshire	·740	3·266	1·937	135	31	52
4	Hampshire	·770	2·881	1·934	130	35	52
18	Dorsetshire	·680	3·018	1·917	147	33	52
37	North Riding	·705	3·015	1·908	142	33	52
29	Rutlandshire	·646	3·095	1·879	155	32	53
19	Devonshire	·771	2·854	1·878	130	35	53
3	Sussex	·673	2·967	1·839	149	34	54
44	North Wales	·648	2·676	1·830	154	37	55
1	Surrey (part of)	·499	2·697	1·809	200	37	55

FIGURE 3. The order of mortality of English and Welsh registration divisions and counties during the year 1845. Source: *7th Annual Report of the Registrar General of Births, Deaths and Marriages, in England*, No. 727 (1846), xxvi. © The Bodleian Libraries, The University of Oxford.

THE 50 LARGE TOWN DISTRICTS.

The mortality of these town districts, 24·8 in the year 1871, was at the rate of 23·8 in 1872; higher, in the aggregate, than the mortality of London, but somewhat lower than the mortality of the great cities. They follow arranged in groups according to the order of mortality:—

ANNUAL RATE of MORTALITY per 1,000 Persons estimated to be LIVING during 1872 in 50 LARGE ENGLISH TOWNS; ranged in the order of the rates from the lowest to the highest.

Cheltenham	17·6	Birkenhead	20·5	Plymouth	22·3	Carlisle	24·6	Wigan	26·6
Hastings	17·8	Derby	20·5	Lincoln	22·4	Stoke-upon-Trent	24·8	Macclesfield	26·6
Maidstone	18·0	Shrewsbury	20·6	Cardiff	22·5	Dover	25·2	Ashton-und'-Lyne	26·6
Chatham	18·8	Brighton	20·9	Bath	22·7	Blackburn	25·5	Merthyr Tydfil	26·7
Reading	19·2	Chester	21·0	Yarmouth	22·7	Stockport	25·8	Exeter	26·8
Oxford	19·3	Swansea	21·3	Halifax	22·9	Gateshead	25·9	Preston	27·9
Colchester	19·3	Worcester	21·4	Newport (Mon.)	23·0	Bury	26·3	Walsall	28·9
Southampton	20·3	Coventry	21·8	Rochdale	23·4	East Stonehouse	26·3	Northampton	29·7
Devonport	20·4	Gosport	21·8	Ipswich	24·0	South Shields	26·4	Bolton	30·0
Cambridge	20·4	Huddersfield	22·2	York	24·2	Tynemouth	26·4	Dudley	32·3

FIGURE 4. The order of mortality of fifty large town districts during the year 1872. Source: *Annual Summary of Births, Deaths and Causes of Death in London, and other Large Cities, 1872* (London: HMSO, 1873), x. © The Bodleian Libraries, The University of Oxford.

information; and this was especially crucial given the assumption of the efficacy of local authority agency. The GRO acknowledged the limitations of death rates in this respect, and it supplied a wealth of other facts; but for some the office's foregrounding of general death rates was an invitation to fallacious reasoning. Once more, Rumsey led the way, first noting the problem in his *Essays* and expanding on it thereafter. His broad point would have been evident to any competent MOH, or indeed any studious consumer of GRO literature: simply that the death rate of a given area depended on a host of other variables beyond the sanitary efforts of a local authority. These included the relative proportion of males to females; the number of those living at each age; the habits, migrations, and occupations of a given population; differences of climate and season; and the distribution of institutions where people might die, such as hospitals. Furthermore, in urban areas especially, the boundaries of registration districts failed to correspond to those of sanitary authorities.[65] Such was the "preposterous abuse of published death rates that often characterizes popular statements and pleas for 'sanitary' reform," stated Rumsey in 1860, that it "almost justifies the opponents of the science [of statistics] that 'you may prove anything by figures'"—a reference to Carlyle's essay on Chartism (1839).[66]

The problem, then, was partly about what might be tolerated at the level of popular engagement and interest, and not all professionals agreed with this hard line. Notably, given his prominent status, John

Simon defended the use of death rates. If not entirely accurate, he suggested in his *Ninth Report* to the Privy Council (1867), they still made for "a rough and ready, but fairly trustworthy, comparison of degrees of health" and the efficacy of sanitary reforms.[67] Criticism continued, however, peaking in 1874, when the president of the Society of MOsH, Henry Letheby, launched an especially aggressive assault, summarizing the problems that had been highlighted in the preceding decade or so, and adding some of his own.[68] Editorials in the *BMJ* and the *Sanitary Record* condemned Letheby's intervention, partly on the grounds that the problems were already well known.[69] It was also sufficiently stinging to prompt a riposte from the GRO, which had hitherto refrained from engaging directly with these arguments. In a paper to the SSL, Farr's deputy, Noel Humphreys, made explicit the office's pragmatic rationale, as shaped by the need to serve a varied constituency of agents: "The population standard [death rate], by its very simplicity, offers many inducements for its acceptance, and is not only thoroughly comprehended by the public, but has been so far endorsed by the Government and Houses of Parliament as to have been recognized as a safe basis for legislative enactments in health matters."[70] Taking aim at "authorities upon State Medicine," who, he claimed, "lacked the special training necessary to the statist," he went on to demonstrate how those factors that undermined the utility of general death rates operated within tolerable limits for the purposes of comparison.[71] For Humphreys, in short, the death rate was an accessible and reasonably, if not perfectly, accurate measure; and it would be difficult to find a better test of the health of towns, given the need to work with the public and its representatives. To be sure, as Humphreys later acknowledged in 1884, before the NAPSS, "false and misleading deductions might be based upon them [death rates]; but it would be difficult to prove that any real or lasting mischief has therefrom resulted which could for a moment be held to counter balance the good that has arisen from their general use," not least their role in stimulating "public interest in health matters."[72]

These exchanges were not without consequence, even if the GRO's national system remained in place. Crucially, it meant that within professional circles, more so than elsewhere, death rates were used in a critical fashion, often with caveats and alongside other measures. These measures included the zymotic rate, disease-specific rates, and age-specific rates, especially rates of infant mortality. This more considered use of mortality rates intensified from the 1870s, when the term *crude death rate* was first used, and when the number of MOsH underwent a marked expansion. "Death-rates are the only test at present available of the efficacy of sanitary action, and probably our readers will need no caution that right conclusions cannot probably be drawn from death-rates," noted an editorial in the *Sanitary Record* in 1884.[73] Professional textbooks further heightened awareness: the first extensive primer on the subject, Arthur Newsholme's *Elements of Vital Statistics,* published in 1889, dwelled at length on the matter.[74] The GRO also introduced some crucial innovations. In 1883, under Ogle's leadership of the Statistical Department, the GRO began to "correct" and "standardize" the death rates that appeared in its annual summaries by way of incorporating age and gender differentials.

Corrected or otherwise, death rates served a normalizing function, just as the GRO intended, inscribing the local within the national and the international. Professionals certainly took an interest in death rates from abroad, but it was England that provided the principal framework of scrutiny. Again, all of the GRO's returns, weekly, quarterly, and annual, provided much more besides: by the 1880s, for instance, the quarterly returns contained subsections regarding "Urban and Rural Mortality," "Mortality at Different Ages," and "Zymotic Diseases." Yet, it was death rates that occupied the foreground, almost always opening up dense pages of analysis that helped to popularize a particular kind of descriptive language that talked in numerical aggregates and statistical averages. The national aggregate was usually referred to first, as in the following from a quarterly return for 1856: "The deaths in the three spring months were 100,310; and the annual mortality was at nearly 21 in 1,000; the average annual rate of the season being nearly 23 in 1,000. The mortality has been, during the whole of the half year past, much below the average."[75] But as the GRO would elaborate, the national average was the product of multiple averages that might be grasped at various levels, including at the level of registration districts and cities. To give but one example, from the third quarterly return for 1907: "In 76 great towns, the death rate was 12.2 per 1,000 living, or 0.1 above the death rate of the country as a whole. The rate in the several towns ranged from 6.5 in Hornsey, 7.5 in Kings Norton, 8.0 in Willesden . . . to 15.0 in Hanley and in Stockton on Tees, 15.6 in Great Yarmouth and in St. Helens, 15.9 in Sunderland, and 16.4 in Liverpool."[76] Synchronically, then, one might compare the death rate of a given space with that of others, or in relation to a national average; alternatively, one might compare the death rate of the same space over time. Such was the official statistical point of departure for analyzing the progress of England's public health system.

Death rates inhabited various official publications that circulated within the public health system. Besides featuring in the reports of other central offices, such as the GBH, MDPC, and LGB, they also prospered at the local level, most of all in the annual reports of MOsH, where they served as the prelude to incredibly detailed analysis. National and local figures were routinely brought together amid textual reference to statistical "rises" and "falls," and "higher" and "lower" positions. The report for Liverpool in 1861 began by invoking the national picture, as described by the GRO's returns, before noting how the city's mortality rate was up on the previous year, adding: "although it did not rise above the average of the previous five years, and was considerably lower than the average of the years preceding 1856."[77] Although much less elaborate than reports for cities, those for towns and rural districts contained similar passages. "The total death rate in 1896 was 17.1; in 1895, 17.8; in 1894, 16; in 1893, 17; so the past year [15 per 1,000] will compare very favourably with its immediate predecessor, and the averages for twenty years," stated the 1897 report for the Devonshire coastal town of Torquay. It then quoted the national average of 17.4 per 1,000.[78]

The passages quoted above hardly make for stirring stuff. It is worth recalling a few instances, however, simply because this history-by-numbers, as it might be called—a mode of narration, that is, whereby progress and regress, and relative continuity and change are matters of statistical degrees—was absolutely crucial in terms of how different localities obtained their temporal and spatial bearings. For officials and professionals, at least, it was an unavoidable part of their routine informational diet. Indeed, time series of death rates also featured in the pages of the professional press, including in the *Lancet*, the *BMJ*, the *Sanitary Record*, and *Public Health*, all of which mediated between various sources of official information, local and central. In 1873, two years after the establishment of the LGB, the *BMJ* began publishing a section entitled "Public Health and Poor Law Medical Services," which provided a space for commentary on MOH reports, as well as (from 1884) digests of GRO returns; from 1905, the quarterly returns of the GRO were summarized in a section entitled "Vital Statistics."

Just as crucially this history-by-numbers enabled criticism. Readers of these reports were free to draw their own conclusions; yet, as in GRO literature, there was no shortage of critical embellishment, not least in the pages of the professional press. In 1878, for instance, in an editorial entitled "Sanitary Inaction in Bristol," the *Sanitary Record* began by referring its readers to an earlier report which had "contrasted the stationary death rate of Bristol with the decline shown in the death rate of most of the other large English towns during the same period [1865 to 1876]." It went on: "Compared with London, Bristol has lost much ground as regards their relative sanitary condition, estimated by their mortality statistics. It is difficult to urge any reason why this state of things should be accepted as satisfactory by the ratepayers, the Town Council, or the medical officer of health of Bristol."[79] Similarly, in the following year, the *Sanitary Record* reprimanded Preston's town council, which it claimed had "conceived the notion that there is nothing of concern in the fact that the death-rate of their town for the last quarter was nearly 42 per 1,000." The complacency of the town council was such that it had caused Preston "to vie with Dublin in possessing the unenviable distinction of having the highest death-rate of any place in the kingdom."[80]

In this way, the timetabled circulation of death rates fostered a normalized consciousness of comparative health and the position of a given town or city in the flow of time toward better things. On the one hand, death rates provided a common scale of comparison, rooted in a common time of chronological periodization and publication. On the other hand, rooted in a sense of historical progress, the multiple differences of degree they revealed also pointed to those spaces that were ahead and those that were behind; or as it was sometimes expressed, those that were winning and those that were losing. Ultimately, civic pride was at stake, just as the GRO intended. In 1888, in a paper read before the Manchester Statistical Society, the doctor and leading member of the MSSA, Arthur Ransome, commented on a table in the GRO's 1883 annual summary that ranked England's twenty-eight major cities according to their death rates. Ransome was principally concerned to highlight the importance of using corrected death rates, but the lowly position of his own locality was painfully obvious: "I fear, however, that the patriotic, or perhaps more correctly the civic, feelings of many of us will be shocked at seeing the place of Manchester and Salford in this table." For all the efforts of the two councils, he went on, "these twin towns are sadly lagging behind in the race after health. Manchester is still the worst town in the kingdom and nearly 60 percent of her inhabitants die over and above the average lost in 28 towns."[81] Ransome was a professional and was relatively numerate; his audience was much the same. But what of the other agents targeted by the GRO?

DEATH RATES IN THE PUBLIC SPHERE

The Foucauldian wisdom is that statistics provide a form of authority by which to objectify and normalize populations.[82] This is true, but it captures only one aspect of their modernity. In the case of death rates, although they served to objectify geographical units of variable scope (divisions, cities, districts, etc.) on a common scale of measurement, they also circulated throughout the various parts of the public health system, empowering MPs, councillors, activists, and ratepayers, just as much as professionals and bureaucrats. As we have seen, the very promotion of death rates was an acknowledgment of this unruly mix of agents. Otherwise put, a statistical means of turning communities into *objects* of governance doubled as a means of empowering them as *subjects* of governance. Equally, statistics were far from universally trusted. It was not only professionals who were critical. Politicians, pressure groups, and members of the public might be suspicious of the very use of statistics as a means of argumentation. In 1857, Benjamin Disraeli captured existing misgivings, declaring that it was an "age of statistical imposture." By the early 1890s the phrase "there are lies, outrageous lies and statistics"—a modification of "there are liars, outrageous liars and scientific experts"—was common enough for statisticians to take note.[83] The result was that there was little the state could do to determine the precise appropriation or reception of statistics.

Death rates certainly enjoyed a popular profile. National newspapers such as the *Times* and the *Daily News,* as well as local ones such as the *Manchester Guardian,* the *Birmingham Daily Post,* and the *Leeds Mercury,* featured digests of the GRO's quarterly and weekly returns. They were much less elaborate than those that featured in the professional press. By the Edwardian period, the *Manchester Guardian*'s weekly digest, which had begun in 1865, amounted to only a brief statement of the national average coupled with an alphabetized list of towns and cities and their respective death rates. It was little more than a couple of column inches in length. Even so, for interested parties, digests of this sort made for a regular and relatively cheap means of keeping abreast of variations in national health, offering a window on the working of the system in much the same way as other columns of figures. By midcentury, it was common for various series to be integrated within the same clocked pages of a single newspaper, including share prices, crime rates, poor law returns, and the financial flow of goods into and out of the country. Public health was by no means the only system whose fluctuating fortunes—peaks and troughs of performance, and degrees of continuity and change—could be tracked in dense, corseted rows of printed statistics.

In the pages of newspapers, death rates were also situated amid editorials, readers' letters, and reports of parliamentary speeches. To borrow from the Victorians, these might be regarded as embodying "opinion" as opposed to "fact." As noted above, from the inception of statistics as a science during the 1830s it was common to distinguish numerical facts from the abstractions of theory, the rhetoric of party politics, and the whims of popular opinion. The binary distinction fact/opinion was often mobilized, as authors reminded their readers that they were dealing with something epistemologically harder than mere words: "figures of arithmetic," not soft, slippery "figures of speech." It is no coincidence that tedious fact-grubbing became an object of popular derision in the Victorian period, most famously perhaps as Thomas Gradgrind of Dickens's *Hard Times* (1854). In practice, however, death rates were open to appropriation by agents armed with just this: opinions, theories, rhetoric. To be sure, the GRO might exercise some interpretive control, besides its classificatory foregrounding of the zymotic class. As noted in the previous section, its weekly, quarterly, and annual reports were not averse to highlighting problems that needed attention. Furthermore, as Higgs and Szreter have described, Farr's letters sometimes indulged in emotive evocations of the plight of the poor, and his successors toed a broadly environmentalist line amid rising currents of eugenic thinking.[84] Beyond this, there was little the GRO could do, not least when it came to user-friendly death rates. This was not necessarily antithetical to the cause of public health; but it did mean that death rates were used to support all manner of arguments, of varying degrees of popular purchase and credibility.

The range of these arguments increased the more death rates mixed with other statistical measures, and so were part of more general diagnoses of the state of society. This included damning, even shrill, evangelical Christian assessments. In the general election year of 1874, death rates were part of a battery of statistics—vital, educational, judicial, commercial, and poor law—invoked by William Hoyle, a leading member of the temperance organization, the United Kingdom Alliance. Subtitled *Facts and Figures for Electors and Politicians*, Hoyle argued that the rising tides of pauperism, crime, ignorance, and ill health were the product of one particular cause: the "powerfully bewitching . . . seductive and dangerous" availability of alcohol.[85] Universal prohibition was

Hoyle's solution. Arguments in favor of no significant reform, of course, were just as political as quite the opposite, and other general assessments that mobilized death rates were of a more mainstream, liberal sort. In 1883, the economist, free trade advocate, and pioneering statist (he had earlier founded the journal, the *Statist,* in 1878) Robert Giffen presented an address before the SSL to mark his inauguration as its president. The title of his address said it all: "The Progress of the Working Classes in the Last Half Century." Average wages, food prices, the monetary value of savings deposits, as well as general death rates (drawn from a paper by Noel Humphreys): all of these facts demonstrated that, contrary to the assertions of socialists and "land nationalizers," the working classes were in much better shape than they had been, and that the accumulation of capital "in a few hands" was a force for good. This, he contended, was the only reasonable conclusion that might be made once the statistics had been studied properly, and not used as "instruments of political warfare."[86]

Giffen's paper was much cited, and he went on to publish further papers that upheld his initial reading; but clearly everything depended on how particular statistics were used, combined with others, and then interpreted. Death rates, for instance, also featured in Seebohm Rowntree's study of York (1901), where he attempted to redefine the problem of poverty and demonstrate that it was far more prevalent than most imagined.[87] An especially notable instance is Robert Blatchford's *Merrie England,* and not simply on account of its popularity. First published in 1893, this unrelenting attack on urban-industrial capitalism sold more than one million copies during the 1890s and helped to consolidate his journal, the *Clarion,* as the leading organ of late Victorian socialism. It is also notable for the way it mobilized death rates as part of a peculiar mode of delivery that was at once aggressively didactic and painstakingly descriptive. The polemical force of *Merrie England* resides just here, and the text was addressed not to an anonymous public but to a particular—and partial, fictionalized—embodiment of it: "Mr. Smith," a committed Liberal and an opponent of socialism, but also a "hard, shrewd man" with a taste for facts. Accordingly, in "these letters," wrote Blatchford, "I shall stick to the hardest of hard facts; and the coldest of cold reason."[88]

Death rates were among the various facts pitched at Mr. Smith, coming into play in the section where he attacked "the evil effects of the factory system on public health."[89] "Look through any great industrial town ... and you will find hard work, unhealthy work, vile air,

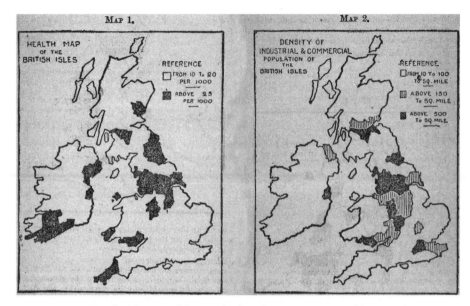

FIGURE 5. Two health maps of the British Isles. These maps were crudely "copied," according to Blatchford, from Bartholomew's *Gazetteer of the British Isles,* published in 1887, which featured a more elaborate scale of shading. Source: Robert Blatchford, *Merrie England* (London: Clarion Office, 1895), 24–25. © The Bodleian Libraries, The University of Oxford.

overcrowding, disease, ugliness, drunkenness, and a high death rate. These are *facts,*" he emphasized, before displaying two maps of the British Isles that demonstrated a correlation between high death rates and "the distribution of manufactures" (see figure 5). Further death rates generated by the GRO were then quoted and commented upon, among them the average death rates of eight agricultural counties compared with the death rate of industrial Lancashire.[90] And yet, while the text drew on the authority of statistics, it also critiqued their abstraction. Later on, Mr. Smith is encouraged to use his imagination by way of visualizing the peculiar lives which official death rates reduced to a single figure: "Cast your eyes, then, my practical friend, over the Registrar-General's returns, and imagine if you can how many gentle nurses, good mothers, sweet singers, brave soldiers, and clever artists, inventors, and thinkers are swallowed up every year in that ocean of crime and sorrow, which is known to the official mind as 'The high death-rate of the wage-earning classes.'"[91] The passage was sandwiched between others urging sympathy, compassion, and solidarity. "Hard" facts, evidently, could only do so much.

Another possibility was for death rates to pass unread. In some cases this was a product of what might be called considered indifference. Death rates played a crucial part in the debates over compulsory small-pox vaccination and the Contagious Diseases Acts, but some opponents argued they were an irrelevance, given the moral and political principles at stake. Whether or not these measures worked was beside the point.[92] More straightforward kinds of indifference doubtless greeted a large proportion of the death rates that appeared in the busy pages of newspapers. Not even local representatives could be relied upon to play the part of the informed citizen. As MOsH complained, there was no guarantee that their reports would be studied properly by councillors. Speaking at a conference in 1890, one metropolitan officer urged his colleagues to restrain their literary instincts and write strictly factual reports, for "their [annual reports'] general destination is the waste paper basket."[93] Eastbourne's MOH later suggested that "not one of us, I think, can be without the experience of being asked questions about matters as if they were new when they have been dealt with in report after report." Other councillors, he suggested, seized on only one or two paragraphs that affected their property or business interests.[94]

Nonetheless, for all these variations of use and reception, death rates *did* function as the GRO's national system intended, helping to fashion and promote public health matters both within and beyond parliament. During the midcentury exchanges on sanitary centralization, Whigs in particular invoked death rates by way of urging the need to adapt to new urban conditions. In March 1847, when Lord Morpeth introduced what would become the 1848 Public Health Act, he began by "placing before the House" the "main facts which have developed in the progress of those [sanitary] inquiries, official, parliamentary and statistical."[95] His principal source of facts was the GRO, whose quarterly returns constituted the "documents of most authority on these subjects," drawing further on death rates that had been commented upon in two lectures delivered under the auspices of the Health of Towns Association in 1845. This in fact would become common parliamentary practice. Certainly GRO literature might be drawn on directly by MPs and ministers when introducing or discussing a bill; but this did not preclude drawing on GRO statistics that had passed through the analytical hands of others. In 1883, at a conference on the dwellings of the poor held at London's Mansion House, Ernest Hart presented a table he had constructed based on GRO data, which ranked the corrected death rates of forty metropolitan districts. A year later, in the *Sanitary Record*, Hart boasted that his figures "have since been much inquired for, and have fallen into the hands of sanitarians and statesmen," including William Gladstone and William Harcourt, both of whom had quoted them in parliament.[96]

Death rates also featured in the evidence gathered by select committees and royal commissions. It was at the local level, however, where death rates really prospered as a tool of critical interrogation, doing so on a more consistent basis. In Liverpool, the impact of GRO statistics was felt with some force during the early 1840s, largely owing to the energies of a local doctor, W. H. Duncan. In 1843, a year after some evidence of his had featured in Chadwick's *Sanitary Report,* he delivered two lectures to the city's Literary and Philosophical Society, which sought to correct a "prevalent impression among not only the professional, but the non-professional part of our own community, that, as compared with other large towns, Liverpool occupie[s] a favourable place in the scale of mortality." The truth was otherwise: "Now, the fact is, judging from the annual proportion of deaths to the population [as supplied by the GRO], Liverpool is the unhealthiest town in England."[97] There followed much recrimination in the pages of the local press and among the city's elites as to why this was the case. Duncan offered a broadly environmentalist explanation; others blamed the city's large Irish population. In 1847, the Tory-Anglican *Liverpool Mail,* following the publication of another damming return from the GRO, suggested that the city's high death rate reflected the ongoing influx of "the scum of Ireland," attracted by "the prodigality of our benevolence."[98]

The issue of public health was much less contentious than the question of education, which had long aroused sectarian conflict, and Liverpool's Tory-led council proved more than receptive amid a barrage of statistics and criticism. In 1845, with the blessing of the mayor, the national Health of Towns Association established a local branch, and in the same year started to publish the *Liverpool Health of Towns' Advocate,* a monthly digest of sanitary information.[99] In 1846, parliament passed a private public health bill for Liverpool, providing much the same powers as the general statute of 1848; and in the following year, one of the country's first MOsH—none other than Duncan—began work. Indeed, Liverpool was soon receiving plaudits as a pioneer sanitary city, but as elsewhere the council was kept on its toes. The proceedings of its health committee were published in the local press, and it was not uncommon for councillors to seize on bad statistics. In April 1867, the recently elected Liberal councillor for the ward of St. Anne's, William

Dawbarn, published an open letter to the Conservative mayor, John Grant Morris, complaining of the "abnormally" high death rate for the previous two years.[100] He conceded he was not a member of the council's health committee and so was hardly "acquainted with all the various reasons that direct the counsels of this body." Even so, equipped with the data contained in the annual MOH reports and the measure of authority this provided, he launched a full-scale attack on the record of the council:

> I observe that in the year 1860, when the late Dr Duncan was our medical officer of health, that under his oversight we had a report published showing the death rate of 1860 to be 24.3 per 1,000. I have now in my hands a report for 1866, of the present medical officer of health, Dr Trench, giving us the awful death rate of 41.7 to a 1,000. What a contrast! . . . Now, Mr Mayor, what I want to draw your attention to is the fact that, in 1860, we had arrived at a good normal point for Liverpool, when we had arrived at a death rate of say, in round numbers, 25 per 1,000. . . . Now, Mr Mayor, why has this not been our average death rate? Have we not spent enough on officers, and all kinds of imaginary useful appliances to obtain a better state of things?[101]

Various "deductions" followed, the principal one being that the "old midden [cesspool] system, when properly worked," was much more effective than the "new water-closet system." He advised the council to concentrate on the task of regulating overcrowding, rather than lavishing money on new sewers.[102]

It was not all about numbers. In the early 1860s, the journalist Hugh Shimmin made a name for himself and his paper, the *Liverpool Porcupine,* by highlighting the insanitary conditions of the city's slums using detailed descriptions of the poorest districts.[103] Slum literature of this sort featured prominently in the provincial press, just as it did in its metropolitan counterpart, thanks to the likes of Henry Mayhew and George Sims.[104] But if, as was noted at the time, numbers lacked the emotional punch of narrative accounts, they remained a touchstone, swirling in and around general assessments of a given council's performance, as much as specific projects. Joseph Chamberlain's three-year period as Liberal mayor of Birmingham during the mid-1870s, for instance, was steeped in statistics, principally those regarding municipal expenditure and rental values, but including death rates. His flagship Improvement Scheme was born and nurtured amid death rates. The scheme entailed the demolition of some inner-city slum areas, such as Rope Walk and Lower Priory, and their replacement with a boulevard, modeled on those of Haussmann's Paris, and later christened Corporation Street. In March 1876, Chamberlain acted as counsel for the corporation at the initial LGB public inquiry, where he made great use of death rates. On the opening day, he presented a list of the streets earmarked for demolition, "in which the death rate varied from 28 to 97 in the 1,000, the normal death rate for Birmingham in healthy times being about 22 in the 1,000." The city's MOH then gave evidence, contending that "the death rate in Birmingham might be as low as in Portsmouth or Norwich, where it was 17 or 18," should sanitary work of this sort be carried out, adding that there "was a striking difference in the death rate in the area under discussion and other parts of the town. The death-rate in Edgbaston was only 13 per thousand."[105]

By the time the scheme was finished during the mid-1880s, Chamberlain was almost a decade into his parliamentary career. In the meantime, it was left to his Liberal successors on the city's improvement committee and those in the local party to fight for a scheme which Conservatives, shopkeepers, and landlords opposed at every turn—much in fact as they opposed the work of the city's health committee more generally. Amid the exchange of claim and counter-claim, it must have been hard to tell who was right and wrong, statistically speaking. In October 1877, shortly before a new round of municipal elections, Liberal councillor Edwards addressed the voters of Duddeston ward, which he had represented for the past three years. The council had done good sanitary work, he claimed, during his tenure: "While the birth rate had gone up at a rapid rate, the death rate had gone down, so that it might be said that the town was growing at both ends. (Laughter.)"[106] A month later, a meeting of the St. Martin's Ward Conservative Association was presented with an altogether different picture by its chairman, who claimed that, "from the returns of the [local] registrar, the death rate had gradually increased" over "the past few years": "The work of the Health Committee had been a complete failure."[107]

Despite their conflicting invocation, death rates remained the measure of choice when it came to assessing the sanitary effects of the Liberals' Improvement Scheme. In 1882, the improvement committee, in a report which was circulated in the local press, laid out figures relating to the scheme's cost, impact on rateable values and rents, and "sanitary results." With respect to the latter, the report presented a table detailing the average death rates, street by street, for the years 1873–76 compared to those for 1879–81: in Rope Walk, there had been a shift from 42 per 1,000 to 24.9; in Potter Street a shift from 44 to 28.8. Some credit, it went on, should be accorded the work of the health committee; but the improvement committee was also deserving of praise, having constructed "a wide and open street," and "let in light and air in the neighbourhood affected by the scheme."[108]

Although statistics were promoted as a means of quelling party conflict, even of bypassing it completely, it was impossible to disentangle facts such as the death rate from increasingly organized party-political struggles to reform the present. This was partly by design: death rates were meant to be accessible, thereby enabling public debate and scrutiny. Yet Rumsey's midcentury misgivings were valid, for rarely were the kinds of caveats supplied by professionals noted by nonprofessionals. There was in fact little progress on this front, and by the end of the century death rates were a routine feature of municipal electioneering, where they mixed freely with its overblown rhetoric. During the 1898 LCC elections, a Progressive leaflet illustrated the "Misery of Slumdom" with reference to London's differential death rates, while claiming that the Moderates (Conservatives) "would leave the housing of the labouring classes entirely to Private Enterprise," "wrecking the Housing Policy [of the Progressives]" and leading to "the permanent continuance of overcrowding and slums."[109] In party-political terms, however, statistics cut both ways. In the 1910 LCC elections, the London Municipal Society, an aggressive home of Tory-inspired antisocialist sentiment, published a mighty seven-hundred-page compendium of statistical information called *Facts and Arguments for Municipal Reform Speakers and Candidates*. Among the barrage of facts relating to every aspect of the council's affairs, it noted "the remarkable reduction" in the death rate since the assumption of power by the Moderates in 1907, detailing a drop from 15.9 in 1905 to 14.5 in 1908. Quoting the 1908 MOH report for the County of London, it was also pleased to announce that in only two other major cities, Bristol and Leicester, was the death rate lower than in the metropolis.[110] "No better testimony," it declared, "can be secured than this decrease in the death rate, for bad administration is quickly followed by a rise in the death rate."

Death rates also empowered the voluntary parts of the public health system, which might have no particular party axe to grind, nor even a denominational one. In December 1889, the sanitary committee of Newcastle's council was presented with a "Memorial Relative to the Death Rate," signed by fifty-four of the city's clergymen. They represented "every body of Christians in the city" and the sentiments of all those engaged in pastoral work.[111] Quoting various kinds of death rate—general, infant, and zymotic—the basic charge of the memorial was that not enough was being done to safeguard the health of the city's poor. Stung by the claims, the sanitary committee commissioned reports by the MOH and the borough engineer, and in the following February published a point-by-point statistical refutation. It was altogether erroneous, it suggested—and quite rightly—deducing either an annual general or an annual infant death rate from the figures for the seven weeks up to November 23, 1889. In any case, there was good reason to suppose that Newcastle's population had grown more than the estimates of the GRO, meaning that the death rates were in fact less than stated; and so it went on.[112]

The controversy lasted only a few months and the clergymen failed to respond with any further statistics. But it was not an exceptional instance, for public health was made of statistical skirmishes of this kind, which might be remarkably dense, even at the local level. According to Newcastle council's twelve-page rebuttal, some of the "facts" contained in the memorial were simply incorrect; some were correct but had been interpreted wrongly; others interpretations were generally correct, but required nuancing; some statements were "unsupported by evidence"; other facts awaited confirmation, as in the question of Newcastle's death rates, which would only be "definitely settled next year when the census is taken." For all that, the committee conceded "that there is room for improvement in many matters affecting the health of the city," and it looked forward to receiving the "cordial support of the memorialists" in future years.[113] This is one example among many of the local conflicts and coalitions opened up by the circulation of the GRO's official statistics.

THE "NORMAL"/"NATURAL" DEATH RATE

A final function of death rates that might be discussed resides just here, in helping to pose the question of what might be achieved; or, to quote Newcastle's sanitary committee again, the question of "room for improvement." Death rates were used in this fashion from the start. As early as the 1840s, Farr spoke of "excessive" rates of mortality, as did those beyond the GRO who drew on its statistics. In 1845, professor of forensic medicine and member of the SSL, William Guy, gave a lecture on behalf of the Health of Towns Association in which he spoke of the "unnecessary" and "fearful sacrifice of human life continually taking place." Drawing on statistics for the year 1841, he put a figure on the amount of life that might be saved with better sanitary arrangements:

"If the sanitary state of the entire country could be raised to the condition of the healthiest counties, so that instead of one death in 46 inhabitants there should be only one death in 54, we should have an annual saving of no less than 49,349 lives, or about one-seventh of the whole number of deaths!" Given that such a claim might appear "extravagant," he reminded his audience that there were a number of districts, principally small agricultural ones, where the rate of mortality was not just below the national average for 1841 (one in forty-six), but below even the desirable rate of one in fifty-four. It was a "reasonable assumption" in fact that with "proper sanitary measures" in place the national average might be one in fifty.[114]

The broad assumption that underpinned assessments of this sort, of course, was that the public's health might be enhanced as part of the broader movement of historical progress and human civilization. The altogether modern problem was specifying a *reasonable* standard of attainment, given that so much might be achieved, ultimately, in the future. Farr was no philosopher, but as a statist he was certainly a dedicated theorist of the preventable and the practical. His zymotic class is one instance of this. Another is the way he grappled with precisely this modern standard-setting conundrum. The conundrum is partly captured in the modern notion of the normal, which, as Hacking suggests, slips between two meanings. Whereas it can be used to refer to what *is* the average, it can also be used to refer to what *ought* to be the average, were things as they should be; or, as it was often put at the time, as things were "naturally."[115] The former, of course, is intrinsically reasonable and was deployed at the time. As described in the previous sections, excess mortality was commonly measured in terms of deviations above an achieved average death rate—the current national average, for example, or a past average specific to a particular town—as things stood at a given point in time. The latter, the normal as "ought" or "natural," is more open, simply because it is subject to competing conceptions of what *might* be achieved. Ultimately, one might opt for something "extravagant," to quote Guy again, which did in fact happen in the form of the utopian visions of Richardson noted in chapter 1. His city of Hygeia would lead eventually, he suggested, to a "natural" death rate of only five per thousand; and by this measure, which "approached" perfection, everywhere in England was excessive, and by some margin.[116]

Quite self-consciously, Farr opted for a reasonable standard that had been achieved in a minority of districts. In a quarterly return for 1843, he set the standard against which excesses might be measured at

2 percent (or twenty per thousand); in a subsequent quarterly return for 1847, he revised this to eighteen per thousand.[117] In the end, during the mid-1850s, he opted for seventeen per thousand, which became known as the "healthy district standard." As he explained in a supplement to the *16th ARRG* (for the year 1855), in some sixty-four districts, almost all rural, the death rate ranged between fifteen and seventeen: "Upon going over these districts it will be found that the health and circumstances of the population by no means approach any ideal standard of perfection. Nature, however, does much for the inhabitants. The fresh air dilutes the emanations from their nuisances, and infectious diseases are not easily transmitted from their person to person in detached houses." He then stated that "it may be assumed with certainty, that the mortality of the English people, in very variable but generally favourable conditions, does not exceed 17 in 1,000 deaths." It followed that the "deaths of 17 persons in 1,000 may therefore be considered, in our present imperfect state, natural deaths; and all deaths above that number may be referred to artificial causes." The rate of seventeen per thousand was thus established as the benchmark, or point zero, of a new means of making normalizing judgments, in which one could group districts according to their "degrees" of divergence above or below a healthy standard.[118]

Szreter writes that Farr's healthy district standard was an "ingenious rhetorical invention" whose "ultimate ploy" was to intensify rivalries between local authorities.[119] No doubt Farr was concerned to do precisely this, in keeping with the GRO's broader strategy of probing and prodding the newly differentiated level of the local. The problem with this reading is that it obscures the way Farr wrestled with the modern conundrum outlined above. Indeed, Farr's healthy district standard can also be understood in terms of the "self-referential"—and, ultimately, arbitrary—epistemology of setting normative technical standards that Ewald has argued characterizes modern governance more generally. As Ewald elaborates, standards of this kind are not defined in an a priori fashion. Rather, they are empirical, "immanent" valuations and represent the "one best," or relative best, as revealed by experience at a given point in historical time. They do not involve any ideal of perfection, transcendental or utopian, mobilizing instead a more pragmatic, situated sense of the possible and the good.[120] It follows that although these standards may hold for a while, their historically situated character means that they are "destined to disappear" in the wake of further progress.[121] Put another way, Farr's healthy district standard can also be understood as an attempt to establish some sort of statistical benchmark for a system of governance without any ultimate measure of success.

Farr formulated his healthy district standard in precisely this manner, as is clear from a passage in a quarterly return from 1857, which detailed, once again, how he had arrived at the figure. It merits quoting extensively:

> The mortality of England and Wales in 1857 has been compared with the mortality of England and Wales in the ten previous years and it may be compared with the mortality (22.36 per 1,000) of the 19 years 1838–56. It is below that average. But is that average itself, it may be asked, the true standard? What is the natural rate of mortality among Englishmen under favourable sanitary conditions? . . . No direct answer can be given to these questions. No large body of Englishmen is breathing pure air, living on a perfectly sound diet, free from all defilement, and free from vice, expressing duly the mind and body generation after generation. We can point to no model city—to no model caste; we can discover no model parish in the country. . . . What course then remains open to the inquirer? Only one. The mortality of the districts of England, in which the sanitary conditions are the least unfavourable, can be employed as the standard measure until happier times supply the real standard of vitality. Sixty-four districts in various parts of the country are found where the mortality of the people ranged on an average extending over ten years from fifteen to seventeen deaths in 1,000 living. This is not an accidental event; the mortality only fluctuates in such places slightly from year to year, and the death rate under the same circumstances will not be exceeded.

After suggesting the figure of seventeen per thousand, Farr posed the question of whether it would be right, on the basis that it was possible to *imagine* people living in more favorable circumstances, to posit a lower rate. But this would be contrary to his empirical reasoning: "17 in 1,000 is supplied as a standard by experience. Here we stand upon the actual."[122] The standard of seventeen, then, was neither an average nor a perfect rate of mortality. It was the (relatively) best rate that could be generated on the basis of the available evidence. It was, as Farr later put it in the *20th ARRG* (1859), referring to a life table he had constructed from the same set of districts, "the nearest approximation we can obtain . . . of the human race in the normal state."[123]

Farr's healthy district standard remained at seventeen throughout the rest of his tenure, and indeed throughout the 1880s, thereby stabilizing a particular point of reference that had begun to be formulated in the 1840s: namely, a reasonable sense of what might be considered excessive, and by extension achievable, above and beyond the multiple and shifting average death rates of England. The measure featured in the full range of the GRO's publication, from its decennial supplements to its weekly returns, where it mingled with characteristically critical commentary. "The Authorities of the 20 great cities deserve applause for what they have done," declared the annual summary for 1872, "but they are far from having attained the stage of the traveller who can rest and be thankful," it went on, for almost fifty-four thousand people had perished unnecessarily according to the standard.[124] It made for a simple message: "Wherever the mortality exceeds 17 in 1,000 there is much sanitary work to be done," as a weekly return put it in 1874.[125]

Beyond the GRO's publications, Farr's standard enjoyed much less currency compared to death rates per se, and indeed some questioned whether any kind of measure of excess mortality should be framed in such a crude way—including Rumsey.[126] But in much the same fashion as death rates, the standard slipped and spilled into various arenas. It seems John Simon during his brief period as medical officer to the GBH was alone in using the standard as a prelude to an extended discussion regarding the precise boundaries of what constituted natural deaths on the one hand, and artificial and preventable deaths on the other.[127] The dominant practice was to accept the standard as it was, and to use it by way of assessing performance and outlining something to aim for. It was, after all, a kind of performance target. In November 1866, for instance, Nottingham town council was presented with the annual report of its sanitary committee, which included the good news that "whilst in other towns the mortality was *considerably* in excess of the normal rate, Nottingham was *very little* above it." Addressing his fellow councillors in the town's guildhall, the alderman presenting the report added: "It was no doubt impossible to define exactly what was the normal death-rate; but scientific men laid it down that all deaths above 17 per 1,000 were preventable; if that were so, then Edinburgh had got to reduce the death rate by 20 per cent, whilst Nottingham, according to the returns, had got to reduce it only three per cent (Hear, hear)."[128] MOsH also mobilized the standard. Bradford's MOH, Thomas Whiteside Hime, even featured a bar chart in his annual report for 1884, where each bar for a series of subsequent years was differently shaded above and below the normal point of 17. It was sufficiently striking for the town's surveyor to share it with fellow professionals at a district meeting of the Association of Municipal and Sanitary Engineers and Surveyors in 1886, having added a bar for 1885 (see figure 6).

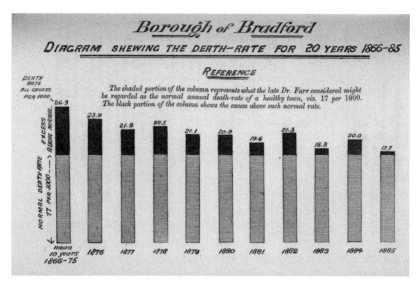

FIGURE 6. Bar chart of the death rate in the Borough of Bradford, 1866–85. Source: J. H. Cox, "Municipal Work in Bradford," *Proceedings of the Association of Municipal and Sanitary Engineers and Surveyors*, vol. 12, 1885–86 (London: E. and F. N. Spon, 1885), 107. © The Bodleian Libraries, The University of Oxford.

Neither Ogle nor Tatham shared Farr's enthusiasm for the standard, and its use petered out in the 1880s. It did, however, feature briefly in the bulky pages of decennial supplements. As noted above, the standard was always a *relative* measure, and this did not escape notice; and in fact it could hardly have done so, given the progress taking place. In the decennial supplement of 1885, covering the period 1871–80, Ogle noted how 101 districts now met Farr's healthy standard; but it was Tatham, in the supplements of 1897 and 1907, that actually revised the standard, first to fifteen and then to fourteen.[129] As Farr had before him, he drew up a healthy district life table for each new standard. In 1907, he noted how the lower rates of mortality for the period 1891–1900 meant he could either expand the number of districts included in the life table or, more exclusively, "fix a more rigid standard of mortality as a test of healthiness." In the end, he "decided to further raise the standard of healthiness," drawing up a table with three fewer districts than the one of 1897, which had contained 263 districts, and at the lower rate of fourteen per thousand.[130] Why had he chosen this latter option, and indeed the standard of fourteen? Earlier, in the supplement of 1897, which covered the period 1881–90, he had made clear that ultimately such decisions were "arbitrary." He detailed the general spread of death rates, which ranged from twelve to thirty-six per thousand, and the number of districts where these applied, adding:

> Speaking generally, districts with low rates of mortality may be called "healthy," while those with high rates must be considered "unhealthy." For the present it will be advisable to designate as healthy only those districts with the lowest death rates, and to regard all other districts as more or less unhealthy, the excess in the death-rates over those of healthy districts constituting the measure of unhealthiness. But in any case only *comparative* healthiness can be dealt with and the line dividing districts which are to be taken as healthy from those which are to be taken as unhealthy must always be an arbitrary one.

He plumped for the standard of fifteen per thousand, though even at this point, as Tatham noted, he could have opted for fourteen per thousand, the rate he would adopt ten years later.[131]

CONCLUSION

Evidently, measuring the success of the public health system depended on a hugely elaborate administrative system in its own right. This was not the only function of the GRO, and it supplied much beyond mortality data. But this was certainly among the GRO's core functions, and it was no less complex than any other. In particular, it combined systems of registration, classification, and selective factual promotion and publicity. And none of these systems escaped criticism: all were revised and updated. Measuring progress was always a work in progress.

Chapter 2 examined the emergence of a broadly liberal culture of modern center-local relations, and this clearly impacted on how the GRO—and Farr especially—developed its statistical brief during the Victorian period. The promotion of death rates is a clear instance of this. But it also worked the other way, in the sense that the GRO's statistics came to inhabit and define the functioning of this all-important administrative axis. Most of all, the GRO enabled the public health system to reflect on itself in terms of a statisticalized variant of modern-historical time. At the risk of repetition, the dynamic was as follows: while the GRO's publications *unified* different cities, towns, and districts according to the same compressed temporal clock and statistical means of measurement, they also *differentiated* these spaces in terms of their variable rates of progress and advance. It is no coincidence that a new language of "centralization" and "local self-government" flourished at the same time as a new culture of statisticalized administration. Both were crucial to contesting and historicizing the administration of public health.

The dynamics of this are not best captured by thinking in terms of a modern state. Besides obscuring the novel spatial and temporal dimensions of what developed, it also obscures the way death rates redefined how multiple agents—central and local, professional and nonprofessional—reflected on their own and others' agency. To be sure, we might speak of a process of normalization. One effect of the GRO's national system of computation, for instance, was to inscribe the local within the national, meaning that local *self*-government was routinely mediated via statistical reference to *other* localities, or in relation to a national average or standard. Nonetheless, this new language of normalizing, numerical critique was also a popular language, one that was pitched at the many and not the few. As we have seen, the result was less the triumph of fact over opinion, and more the emergence of dense admixtures of the two. There was no necessary advance toward factual clarity. And yet, we might argue, it could hardly have been otherwise, for the rise of official, objectifying statistics was also accompanied by the development of more organized and inclusive forms of political association. In a way, the disputed and overburdened Victorian sanitary "fact" marks the modern spot where these two processes met.

Certainly the term *bureaucratic* captures something of the way the GRO functioned, not least its reliance on millions of standardized registration forms. But what is bureaucracy, precisely? The next chapter explores one instance of this: the lowly officialdom of the local sanitary inspector.

CHAPTER 4

Officialism

The Art and Practice of Sanitary Inspection

Much like statistics, bureaucracy is commonly regarded as a defining feature of the modern state. Certainly the public health system relied on what the Victorians began calling just this: "bureaucracy," or, alternatively, "red tapism" and "officialism," all terms that emerged during the 1830s and 1840s. It meant that the public health system was forged not only amid invocations of historical progress and a barrage of statistics, but also amid the routine production of official reports and returns, and millions of letters and standardized forms. This is not to suggest a sudden eruption of practices of writing and recording. Marriage, baptism, and burial registers; land and hearth tax records; or the printed proceedings of assize courts and quarter sessions, among other examples: all were generated during the early modern period.[1] Likewise, various agents had long been charged with inquiring and documenting, from parish beadles to portside customs officers. "Clerks" were already at work, such as those employed to document the deliberations of the general courts of London's seven sewer commissions, which date from the 1530s. Self-styled "inspectors" were not unknown by the eighteenth century, such as inspector-generals of imports and exports, and inspectors of corn returns.

Nonetheless, the logistical scale and material density of bureaucratic practices intensified considerably from the 1830s, just as they were designated as such—as "bureaucracy": see below—and just as governing more generally was assuming a modern spatial-temporal form and dynamism.

Indeed, bureaucracy flourished at both central and local levels of governance, and was partly about managing the relations *between* these two newly articulated elements. The best-known example of this is growing resort to central inspectorates. The first central public health inspectorate was established in 1848 under the auspices of the GBH, and at this point it was principally concerned to promote Chadwick's vision of sanitary reform. Others included inspectorates for the poor law (1834), prisons (1836), and police forces (1856), as well as for commercial practices, such as the management of fisheries (1861) and the manufacture of explosives (1875). By the 1870s, there were roughly five hundred inspectors working for "the Government." The creation of new areas was also accompanied by reform of the old. Created in 1833, the factory inspectorate based at the Home Office comprised a team of nineteen inspectors, four chief and fifteen regional. By 1900, the system had grown to include one chief inspector, five regional superintendents, forty-seven district inspectors, thirty-seven junior inspectors, and thirty-one assistants.[2] Further support was provided by a medical inspector and a principal lady inspector, herself in charge of six female subordinates.

Another example is the LGB based in London's Whitehall district, where a different kind of bureaucratic diversification developed. In particular, the LGB inherited from the Poor Law Board the distinction made in the Northcote-Trevelyan report (1854) between "intellectual" and "mechanical" grades of what was now being called the "civil service." It made for two broad fields of administrator: generalist, Oxbridge-educated permanent and assistant secretaries, and a cadre of lower grade clerks charged with office management (indexing, filing, and copying), compiling statistics and accounts, and typing letters.[3] By the end of the century, members of this lower tier numbered over 130, between them serving five principal subdivisions: a Poor Law Division; a Legal and Order Division; an Audit and Statistical Division; a Public Health, Local Finance and Local Acts Division; and a Sanitary Administration and Local Areas Division.[4] A third and more technical field comprised central inspectors, including a chief engineer and a chief medical officer, each in charge of their own specialist departments.

This chapter examines a further twist in this increasingly dense field of public health bureaucracy: the practice of sanitary inspection. It was a peculiar bureaucratic art, as we shall see: among other things, it involved weighing up considerations of health and amenity, and the use of a medley of microtechnologies. Yet, if one variant among many, sanitary inspection exemplifies some of modern bureaucracy's defining features.

Two might be highlighted. One of these has been mentioned already: practices of writing. Like other bureaucrats, sanitary inspectors were concerned with communicating standards, and regulating their adherence over time and space. Crucially, in so doing, they also served an archival function, and it is here where—to recall the variants discussed in the previous two chapters—modern-historical time reached its greatest degree of *compression*. To be sure, inspectors might read an article in the sanitary press invoking England's long history of local self-government; and their annual reports, or those of their superiors, MOsH, might rely on statisticalized narratives spanning a few years or so. Otherwise sanitary inspectors were required to generate something more basic, factual, and chronological: that is, records detailing dates, times, and places, with little or nothing in the way of embellishment, or else similarly chronicled notices, letters, and memoranda. Like other bureaucrats, especially of the clerical sort, much of their time was spent clocking and recording the minutiae of governance. They did much more besides, but inspection systems would have been impossible without this kind of temporally compressed paperwork.

The genesis of the term *bureaucracy* is instructive in this regard. Another French innovation, it emerged in Britain during the 1830s to describe a centralized form of government.[5] Derived from the French for office or writing desk (*bureau*), it also carried an association with technologies of inscription and correspondence (pens and paper especially), as well as the red tape that for centuries had been used to bind administrative dossiers. "N. where the power is in the hands of centralizing red tapists or government clerks, as in Prussia" was one definition given in 1855. A "bureaucrat," it followed, was "a member or an advocate of such administration."[6] Chadwick was deemed exemplary. "Was there ever a better bureaucrat than Mr Chadwick?" declared an editorial in the *Morning Chronicle* in 1848, this man who wants "to regulate the world from his writing-desk."[7]

A second feature is the differentiation of bureaucracy from a public domain of opinions and commercial interests, and a party-political domain of ministers, MPs, and councillors. Perhaps the best instance of this is the reformed civil service that emerged over the second half of the century. For the permanent and assistant secretaries in the upper tier at least, the new code of "anonymity" was about negotiating, even transcending, the worlds of parliamentary struggle and journalistic intrigue.[8] But even lowly bureaucrats like sanitary inspectors presented themselves as independent servants of the public good, much above the fray of political bickering, squalid financial interests, and electioneering. Beginning with John Stuart Mill's reflections in his *Considerations on Representative Government* (1861), "bureaucracy" came to mean just this, shedding its initial association with continental-style centralization: a paid, professionalized, and nonpartisan domain of administration.[9] In 1910, Ramsay Muir, a professor of modern history, published an essay called "Bureaucracy in England." "Bureaucracy means the exercise of power by professional administrators, by trained and salaried experts," he wrote. "It has never existed, and will probably never exist, by itself; but it can thrive equally well under any form of government, monarchic, aristocratic or democratic."[10]

Both of these qualities capture the modernity of what developed during the Victorian period, not least the institutionalization of bureaucratic practices on a *permanent* basis and the advent of routine systems of official reporting and archiving. As with statistics, change was now captured and administered according to more intense, pre-programed rhythms, which here extended to daily note keeping and filing practices. Yet, as will be argued here, the modernity of practices like sanitary inspection also resides in the way they remained entangled in those public and political domains from which they were otherwise distinguished. This affected all facets of England's burgeoning public health bureaucracy, and it was not only a source of frustration. After all, the very formalization of these offices was partly a product of parliamentary statutes and the cooperation of ministers and MPs; but it also worked the other way. A case in point is the LGB, where a commitment to ensuring a degree of parliamentary control and accountability made for struggle. In 1876, Simon resigned as medical officer to the LGB, complaining of a lack of resources and an aversion toward appointing properly trained inspectors. "Mr Stansfeld's system," he later wrote, invoking the resistance of his former political boss and president of the LGB, the liberal-radical MP James Stansfeld, was composed of only ill-qualified, "walking gentlemen."[11] It is one instance among many of frustration on the part of the LGB's more specialist teams of medical and engineering officers.[12] Likewise, even the lofty, liberally educated permanent and assistant secretaries were brought down to earth on a regular basis, mediating as they did between the demands of their changing political masters on the one hand, and those of professional associations, pressure groups, and local authorities on the other.

The world of the sanitary inspector made for a stark contrast to that of metropolitan Whitehall, which was then in the process of becoming the administrative and ceremonial hub of Britain's far-flung empire. It was local, public-facing, and altogether grubby by comparison. Yet, as we shall see, its demands were just as intense and born of the same modern dynamics and systemic relations. Indeed, the complexities of inspection—the nuances of conduct, professional association, and the application of technical knowledge—were a product of their multiple relations with elected representatives, members of the public, and fellow officials. This was not necessarily a bad thing, for support was forthcoming from all of these agents; but it could also make for conflict. One day, inspectors might be reading about their professional autonomy in the sanitary press; the next, filling out forms and contending with obstructive councillors and landlords. It was a varied job, despite its routine nature. The chapter begins with the expansion of sanitary inspection and its formalization as a technical task.

EXPANSION AND SPECIALIZATION

The office of inspector of nuisances—or sanitary inspector: inspectors came to prefer the latter—first appeared in the 1847 Towns Improvement Clauses Act, and developed as part of the emerging system of modern center-local relations detailed in chapter 2. Ultimately, compulsory appointments were the product of the frustrated campaign for a systematic system of state medicine, and in particular the 1872 Public Health Act, which also made compulsory the appointment of MOsH. In the meantime, major cities had begun appointing inspectors, besides those employed on a temporary basis during epidemic crises, such as when cholera struck. The first official appointments were made in Liverpool and London in the late 1840s, and by the 1860s both cities could boast extensive teams of inspectors working under the superintendence of MOsH. In Liverpool, there were no fewer than forty-two at work by 1866. Small towns had also begun to appoint inspectors, although rarely in conjunction with a MOH.[13] The 1872 act also formalized earlier arrangements: simply that inspectors were responsible to the local authority that appointed them, whether a corporate sanitary committee, a board of health, a metropolitan vestry, or a board of guardians. These bodies—and in urban areas especially, their MOsH as well— were empowered to "direct" the work of inspectors and "require" their attendance at meetings, where their actions would be discussed. In general, inspectors in urban areas reported to a MOH, while in rural districts they reported direct to the sanitary authority, usually a board of guardians.

One novelty after 1872 was thus the employment of inspectors in rural districts, commonly one but occasionally two: by 1880, for instance, the rural sanitary district of Stroud, Gloucestershire, was home to a duo of inspectors, which between them patrolled a population of roughly twenty-nine thousand.[14] Another novelty was the involvement of the LGB in appointment processes. In 1872, the board began subsidizing salaries—normally half, out of an annual grant voted by parliament—and as part of the bargain vetting appointments. There was some resistance to begin with. In 1873, of the 1,104 authorities that had appointed MOsH and inspectors, just over 50 percent were receiving half-pay from the center. The LGB could also prove difficult. In 1889, one inspector complained of "the flagrant exhibition of red tapism indulged in" by the LGB, which had insisted on a one-year contract for an inspector in the Shipton and Silsden areas of Yorkshire, even though the local authority was willing to appoint for three.[15] Still, if not without vexation on all sides, numbers expanded and by 1895 roughly 90 percent of authorities were receiving financial subventions.[16] The bureaucracy was as follows. Using a standardized LGB form, the town or district clerk would forward details of the size of the population and administrative area in question, along with proposed salary and tenure. Once agreed, confirmation came in the form of a typed letter, dated and numbered, and signed by an assistant secretary from "Whitehall, S. W." Supplementing statute law, LGB orders issued in 1872, 1880, 1891, and 1910 provided the principal frame of reference in terms of job specifications.

At the local level, the pioneers remained cities, where it became common to employ chief inspectors along with subordinates with their own sanitary specialisms. Something of this had been apparent before, even outside of large urban centers: by the mid-1860s, Brighton was home to a chief inspector, an inspector of slaughterhouses, and an inspector of common lodging houses (CLHs), essentially cheap hotels catering for the very poor.[17] Yet, in cities at least, this proliferation of inspectorial roles intensified considerably during the latter decades of the century. By the mid-1890s, for instance, Manchester council was employing twenty-eight residential inspectors; four smoke inspectors; two food and meat inspectors; and six factory and workshop inspectors. Figures for 1896 give an indication of their industry. In total, some 46,270 dwelling houses, 2,480 workshops, 451 slaughter-houses, and 29,984 "miscellaneous" sites were inspected.[18] The biggest employer was the LCC. In 1900, there were some 260 sanitary inspectors, of all descriptions, working in the metropolis.[19]

A key driver was thus the demographic growth processed by the GRO, which among other things enabled scrutiny at the local and central (LGB) levels regarding the ratio of inspectors to population. Expansion and specialization were also propelled by the emergence of a thicket of crisscrossing sanitary initiatives, coupled with a more precise—if ultimately eclectic—appreciation of the variables that affected the public's health. The crucial development was the reformulation of nuisance law. The term *nuisance* had originated in the medieval period, and as developed under common law referred to a variety of offences that infringed upon civic amenity and decency; and while these offences might be environmental—and as such a possible threat to health—they might also be social and civil. As codified by William Blackstone in the eighteenth century, disorderly inns and eavesdropping neighbors were as much nuisances as unwholesome waterways and ill-managed pigsties.[20] The statute law that developed in the wake of a series of cholera epidemics (in 1831–32, 1848–49, and 1853–54) was focused on sanitary offences, finding its principal expression in a series of Nuisances Removal and Diseases Prevention Acts between 1846 and 1855.[21] By the late 1860s, following the 1866 Sanitary Act, there were seven types of nuisance altogether, including insanitary dwellings and business premises, and noxious chimneys and furnaces.[22]

These nuisance laws at once reflected and anticipated various currents of regulatory activity. The power to inspect premises connected with the production of "meat, poultry, game . . . fruit, vegetables, corn, bread, or flour," to quote the 1855 Nuisances Act, was further developed with legislation that targeted the adulteration of food, notably the 1875 Sale of Food and Drugs Act. One consequence was the appointment of public analysts to undertake laboratory investigations of suspect items.[23] Similarly, powers to enforce "sufficient privy accommodation, drainage and ventilation" dovetailed with an emerging mass of centrally vetted bylaw regulations regarding the built environment, including minimum volumes of domestic air space and the correct positioning of soil pipes. By the 1860s, local authorities were authorized to condemn dwellings judged "unfit for human habitation," thus enabling slum clearance, at least in theory. Finally, the power to "cleanse, whitewash, purify, and disinfect" business premises and homes was amplified by the onset of germ theories and texts dealing with the science of disinfection from the 1870s. Environmental sanitation was lent a new chemical and microbiological precision, while the notification and isolation of infected persons was gradually placed on a more rigorous footing.

The sprawling nature of these powers did not escape notice at the time and eventually led to the passing of the mammoth 1875 Public Health Act, designed to "systematize" the legislation which had accrued over the previous three decades; and it was this act which provided inspectors with their main source of statutory guidance through to the interwar period. The same period also witnessed the first attempts to formalize sanitary inspection as a technical task, complete with institutional certification. The first inspectors were an eclectic bunch, drawn from a variety of backgrounds, including tradesmen, post office clerks, constables, carpenters, and soldiers. In places such as York, Hereford, and Carlisle police officers simply added nuisance inspection to their list of duties; and when it came to making appointments, local authorities prioritized good character and common sense over any kind of formal expertise.[24] These qualities continued to be important and were prized by inspectors themselves, as we shall see; but by the 1860s the general consensus among leading public health advocates was that inspectors required some kind of specialized instruction and examination.

The first exams were carried out in 1877, under the auspices of the SIGB, later the Royal Sanitary Institute (RSI).[25] The exams covered four topics: elementary physics and chemistry in relation to air, water, and soil; rudimentary statistical methods; practices of municipal hygiene, such as refuse removal and disinfection; and statutes and bylaws relevant to inspection. Aside from a profusion of professional handbooks, candidates could also benefit from texts such as *The Student's Guide to Success in Sanitary Inspectors' Exams,* published in 1901 by Grimsby's chief inspector.[26] The success rate, it seems, was a little over 55 percent: by 1898, of the forty-nine hundred or so candidates examined, some twenty-eight hundred had passed.[27] One breakthrough came in 1891, when the LGB ordered that all inspectors appointed in London after 1894 would require valid certification. This prompted the formation of another exam board in 1899, the Sanitary Inspectors' Examination Board, which comprised representatives from the LGB, the Society of MOsH, the Royal Institute of Public Health, and the Worshipful Company of Plumbers.[28] In 1910, after much lobbying, the LGB made the possession of a certificate of competency a compulsory component of all appointments across England.

INSPECTION SYSTEMS AND THE IDENTIFICATION
OF PROBLEMS

In some crucial respects, then, the evolution of the office beat a typically modern pathway of growing technical formalization. It is no surprise that by the turn of the century MOsH and inspectors were noting how much an earlier common law culture of regulation had been displaced by one which was more specialized and sanitary. "The legal definition of a nuisance defined by Blackstone is a very much larger one than the practical nuisances with which a Sanitary Inspector has to deal," wrote one provincial MOH in 1901, adding that "the suppression of disorderly inns, the prevention of eavesdropping, and the punishment of common scolds, do not come within the province of the Nuisance Inspector." "He is really a health officer; he is one of the skirmishers of the great 'preventive medicine army' engaged in pushing forward the attack upon disease into the enemy's country."[29] The technical status of inspection was affirmed elsewhere, not least in the periodic pages of the professional press, which formed such a key component of their culture of association. Numerous journals—the *Sanitary Record* (established in 1878); *Public Health* (1889); the *Journal of State Medicine* (1892); the *Sanitary Inspectors Journal* (1895)—ensured that inspectors could keep informed of the latest innovations in the theory and practice of disease prevention. By the Edwardian period, germs were widely recognized in inspection circles as pathogenic agents, while inspectors would attend or read lectures on other sciences of professional interest, such as chemistry, anatomy, and statistics.

It also involved considerable bureaucratic empowerment. In contrast to common law procedures, which normally involved recourse to court-based deliberations of one sort or another, sanitary inspectors were equipped with summary powers of abatement. As Simon noted in 1869, "the system of summary procedure is the essence of our modern nuisance law."[30] In the case of most inspections, full proceedings involved two stages: first, the issuing of a preliminary notice following an inspection; then, in the event of noncompliance, the issuing of a legally binding formal or statutory notice. In the second stage, initiating action simply required that an inspector and his employer, the local authority, were "satisfied of the existence of a nuisance."[31] To be sure, the use of two kinds of notice, coupled with noncompliance, could make for a sluggish system. In 1895, an inspector for the London borough of Lambeth lamented that he and his colleagues were "fettered with the red tape of procedure and harassed by the law's delay." Depending on how regularly the local sanitary committee met—which might adjourn for six weeks in the summer—it could take up to forty-nine days to issue a formal notice; and if this was not complied with, up to seventy days to proceed by court summons; and then a further four weeks for the police to enforce the order, should a magistrate have decided that this was appropriate. "In other words, it takes, in the case of a neglectful or obstinate person, any time between 6 and 14 weeks before we can legally get a nuisance abated, although the Act says they are to be abated 'summarily.'"[32] Yet, recourse to court proceedings was only occasional and the overwhelming majority of nuisances were resolved using either preliminary or statutory notices.[33] The *threat* of legal action was evidently more important than its actual use. Both preliminary and statutory notices made clear the consequences of noncompliance (see figure 7).

This explains why inspectors were able to accomplish so much. Even outside of cities the figures are impressive. In the rural district of Bromley, the town's inspector identified over 750 nuisances in 1881 alone, most of which (some 599) arose from defective drainage and overflowing cesspools. In addition, he ordered the disinfection of seventy-eight houses, thirteen slaughterhouses, and two CLHs.[34] One might regard inspectors, then, as roaming, normalizing officials, as they were to some degree. They were equipped with summary powers and a great battery of standards; some may even have received certified training. Yet, as we shall see in the sections that follow, just as modern were the frustrations they endured owing to the empowerment of MPs, councillors, and members of the public. Furthermore, it was never a matter of applying some pure form of technical-inspectorial knowledge. Rather, in practice, something more bureaucratic, discretionary, and sensory was at stake, as inspectors grappled with multiple demands, while moving back and forth between their offices and a variety of spaces. We turn now to each of these aspects of the role—the bureaucratic, discretionary, and sensory—all of which served not so much to dilute their expertise—which, in any case, was quite lowly—as enable it to function as part of necessarily mobile, site-specific inspection systems.

Logistics and Bureaucracy

As with other systems of inspection, central or local, sanitary inspection was premised on the assumption that things were not as they should be. The problem was finding out where and to what degree. On the one

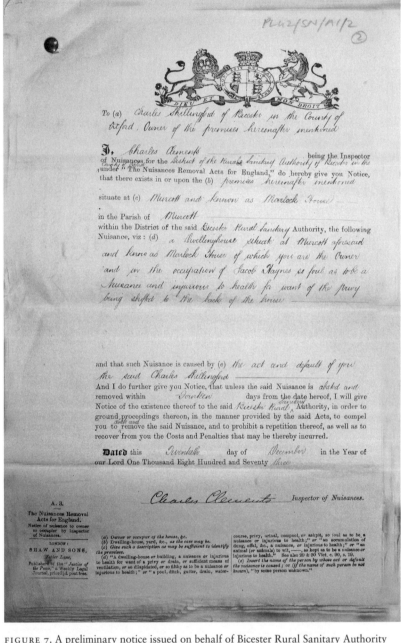

FIGURE 7. A preliminary notice issued on behalf of Bicester Rural Sanitary Authority on December 20, 1873, ordering the owner to relocate a privy midden. The consequences of noncompliance are detailed in the final paragraph. The standardized form was printed by the legal stationers, Shaw and Sons, based in London. Source: Oxfordshire History Centre, PLU2/SN/A1/A2.

hand, this demanded spatial coverage and temporal regularity; or as statute had it, the inspection of a district "systematically at certain periods, and at intervals as occasion may require." Professionals were more specific. An inspector "ought to have a personal knowledge of every house in his district," urged one MOH before the BMA's public medicine section in 1880, "and to make an inspection at least twice a year."[35] Others recommended a more class-specific disposition. Earlier, in 1873, one of the first inspection manuals had suggested that it was "probable that it [the regularity of inspection] should vary with the known requirements of a locality; for it would be a waste of time to inspect a neighbourhood of genteel residences . . . as frequently as streets or localities inhabited by the poor, and abounding in unsanitary conditions."[36] Certainly some of their work might be regular: CLHs had to be limewashed every April and October, and this normally required enforcement. Yet inspectors consistently complained of unwieldy workloads (see below), and it seems unlikely that twice-yearly visits were always made in relation to every domestic dwelling in a given area. In rural districts especially, inspectors had to contend with scattered properties, meaning that horses and pushbikes were required. Even so, as a matter of routine, inspection involved traversing space and visiting and revisiting premises of one sort or another.

On the other hand, some archival record had to be kept of where had been inspected and when, and any notices issued and letters received. Given the growing volume of work, inspection systems could hardly have functioned as systems without relying on clocked paperwork: work might be duplicated; initial notices might go unchecked; and problems identified by either the public or MOsH left unattended. This, too, was a statutory obligation, with statute law specifying record keeping on a "systematic," "day-to-day" basis. The same paper-related diligence was required of MOsH. "All orders given should be in writing, and all letters, reports and other written documents should be copied and properly classified and preserved," urged one manual for MOsH published in 1873: "Nothing should be left to memory."[37] A daily journal formed the principal record of an inspector's work, but an inspector also had to fill out notices of abatement, as well as those regarding the occurrence of any infectious diseases he came across. Further duties included keeping track of letters from members of the public and councillors. And paperwork bred paperwork: notices might be logged in a special register of notices; letters in a special letter book. There was some relief. By the 1870s, standardized forms and journals, requiring

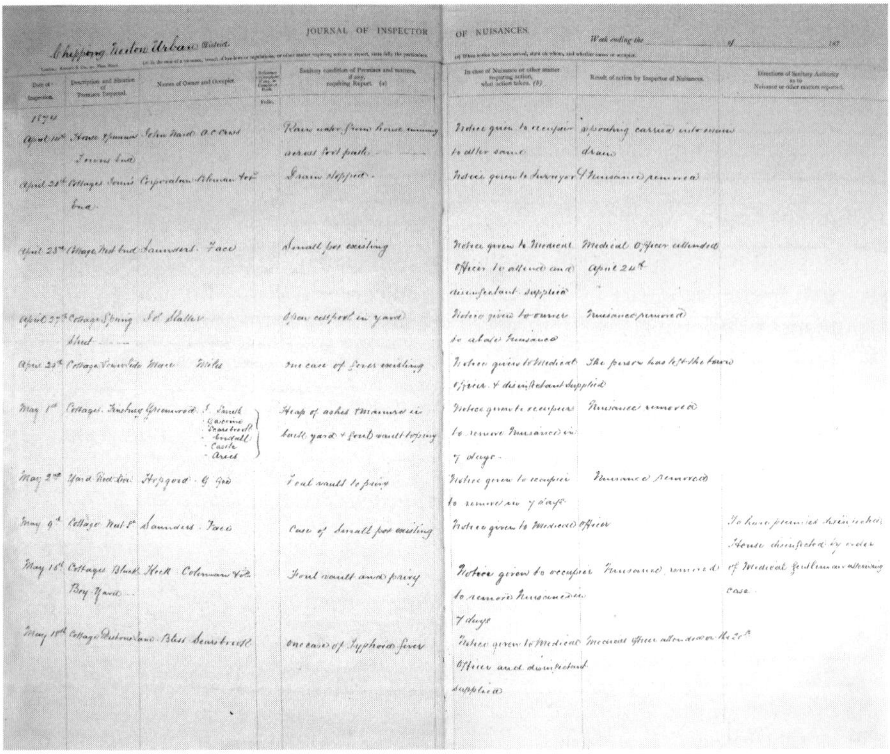

FIGURE 8. Two pages from the journal maintained by the inspector of nuisances for Chipping Norton urban district covering the years 1873–76, on pre-prepared stationery supplied by Knight and Co. It is one of three volumes for the years 1873–83 detailing the notices that were issued and corresponding dates, properties, owners, problems, and remedial actions. Source: Oxfordshire History Centre, BOR1/20/A2/4.

only the details to be filled in by hand, were being mass-produced by LGB-approved publishers such as Knight and Co., based in Fleet Street, London (see figure 8).

Some of this paperwork was completed on-site, where inspectors would fill out pocket-sized notebooks and standardized observation forms, detailing the date, address, and details of any infringement or problem. The job of updating records and reading and writing letters was necessarily office-based, or at least off-site, in a room of a town hall or vestry and in the company of other records. These were the local centers of England's public health system; and as with the central centers, as it were, one of their key functions was to provide a space where paperwork could be assembled and ordered. Specialized sanitary offices—or what might be dubbed the Inspector's Office—first emerged in cities such as Liverpool and Leeds during the 1850s, and seem to have become common in large urban areas by the 1870s, when they could be found in places such as Newcastle, Blackburn, Sheffield, Bristol, Leicester, and Huddersfield. Most were located in town halls, where they nestled alongside the office of the chief municipal bureaucrat, the town clerk. Alternatively, in rural districts, offices might be situated in the headquarters of boards of guardians: in 1880, Stockton-on-Tees opened a new poor law office, comprising a meeting room and administrative facilities for the local GRO registrar, MOH, and sanitary inspector.[38] By the Edwardian period, an inspector's office might be one of many contained in a municipal health department. In 1909, the department at St. Helens opened a new suite of offices in the town hall. Located next to the offices for the health visitors and school nurses, the office comprised four rooms in all: two offices for the inspectors—one for the chief inspector; another for his subordinates—plus further offices for the MOH and borough engineer.[39] Elsewhere, as in Blackpool, where a new set of offices was opened in 1911, laboratories for chemical and bacteriological analysis featured among the facilities.[40]

Note taking, letter writing, form filling, and record keeping: all inspectors required these basic skills by way of managing the logistical dimensions of their role and generating a bureaucratic memory of what had been done. Doubtless some inspectors were more diligent than others; but however diligent, the employment of clerks helped to lighten the load. Clerks were commonplace in urban areas by the end of the century. In 1898, the City of London's sanitary department was home to one clerk; by 1908, the number had increased to four, serving a team of twenty-two inspectors.[41] Equally, practices varied, and in some places elaborate systems of archival management developed. In 1899, F. J. Allan, MOH for London's Strand district, boasted of the card-index system he had devised. Numbered envelopes containing records of correspondence and notices were kept for all dwellings in the district, and stored in sequence in a cabinet. A corresponding card index presented brief abstracts of what Allan termed the "sanitary history of each house," including dates of notices, cases of infectious disease, and the number of occupants at times of inspection. A similar system, he was pleased to announce, had been adopted in 1894 by the municipal council of Paris, and its principal benefit was that it allowed for ease of reference and the quick assembly of evidence in relation to court cases and slum clearance projects.[42]

Record keeping and issuing notices formed one means of coordinating action; another was conversing in person. This too might take place on-site. In cases of infectious disease it was common practice for inspectors and MOsH to visit dwellings together. Otherwise the office seems to have provided the principal location. In 1891, the Finnish doctor Albert Palmberg in his Europe-wide survey of public health systems (translated into English in 1893), detailed what he termed the "daily programme in an urban sanitary office." It began at 9:00 A.M. with the arrival of the MOH, inspectors and the clerk: "He [the MOH] reads his correspondence, gives orders arising out of it, hears the verbal reports of the Sanitary Inspectors . . . and arranges for meeting them later in the day at any spot where his presence may be required." The inspectors then filled out any reports and notices, before leaving at 10:00 A.M., at which point the clerk began updating their journals.[43] Once again, there were variations and not all departments required daily attendance at the office. G. Petgrave Johnson, MOH for Stoke-on-Trent, bemoaned the fact that some authorities had embraced a "measure of decentralization," whereby inspectors were required to attend only once a week, supplemented with the use of divisional inspectors to check the work of subordinate district inspectors. The problem was that it was overly bureaucratic: "All day books are duplicated and messengers are employed to collect and distribute these books." The dominant system, however, seems to have been the "centralized" one Palmberg had earlier described, and which was much preferred by Johnson in the interests of efficiency.[44]

Health, Injury, and Comfort

On-site, away from the office, inspectors dealt with a variety of scenarios, including houses where people were sick or dying (see chapter 6). In the main, however, the role was a proactive one: a question, that is, of searching out and dealing with problems before they caused sickness and injury. The idea that bylaw infringements and sloppy hygiene might lead to ill health was an intrinsic part of their calling. As one inspector noted in 1895, in terms of the temporal-causal chain of infection, inspectors came "even before the doctors, because if we were called in before the doctors there would be no need for them to come and cure that which they [inspectors] can and do prevent."[45] This basic assumption was manifest both in the structure of local sanitary administration, which accorded MOsH main responsibility for dealing with outbreaks of infectious disease, and in the summary nature of an inspector's powers.[46] More broadly, the evolution of these powers via the nuisance statutes of the 1840s and 1850s was underpinned by the authority of epidemiological investigations regarding the links between dirt, overcrowding, and disease, and especially the zymotic class. Subsequent developments in food hygiene and the chemical analysis of water and air further enhanced this preventive rationale, providing inspectors with a modicum of scientific authority.

In practice, the rationale of inspection was decidedly more mixed and mutable; and though sanitary science—itself a composite of various disciplines—may have underpinned its general ethos of prevention, much depended on the nature of the problems encountered. For one thing, sanitary standards doubled as moral ones, making inspectors agents of decency as much as health. This was especially so in cases of overcrowding, which was associated with all kinds of moral ills, including drunkenness, pauperism, and even incest. Equally, though the standards they were charged with enforcing might be based on sanitary science, their formulation in statutory and bylaw terms invariably left much to the discretion of inspectors. One instance is the condition of toiletry accommodation, a routine concern of all authorities. Statutes such as the 1875 Public Health Act simply prescribed "sufficient" accommodation; and though bylaws might be considerably more specific—such as insisting on ventilating windows—the meaning of "sufficient" remained open to interpretation. As one inspectors' exam primer noted, "all hinges on the word *sufficient*."[47] Certainly some inspectors seem to have exploited this room for maneuver. In 1893, it was reported that the inspector of Folkstone, which contained roughly five thousand houses, had ordered the replacement of over two thousand water closets, prompting complaints from residents.[48]

Whether bylaws were imprecise or not, the professional press played a crucial role in translating broad statutory standards into technical norms and model arrangements. Handbooks and periodical articles dwelled at length on the minutiae of best practice and the latest innovations in the design of technologies such as chimneys and water traps. Technical guidance of this sort no doubt sharpened an inspector's sense of the pathogenic possibilities contained in defective sanitary arrangements, but it by no means extinguished older common law considerations regarding civility, safety, and property. In fact, it could be argued that they became *more* and not less important. It is not so much that considerations of this kind provided more impetus than considerations of health, as that they could not be easily distinguished. Statutory nuisance law recognized something of this ambiguity, providing a twofold definition of a nuisance. By the mid-1860s, of the seven statutory nuisances, five were defined as either a "nuisance or injurious to health," with a further one—overcrowding—described as either "dangerous or injurious to the health of the inmates." Quite where health ended and comfort and safety began was by no means clear, despite the disjunctive *or*. As one High Court judge affirmed in 1881, the law meant to strike at "anything which would diminish the comfort of life though not injurious to health, and anything which would in fact injure health."[49] Inspectors were accordingly urged to take into account what was termed, altogether loosely, the "degree of annoyance" of a putative nuisance.

This was a widely acknowledged feature of nuisance administration. On the one hand, nuisances could be just that: irksome annoyances which impinged upon civility and the enjoyment of property. On the other, they might be health-related or only half so, or even just possibly. Discomfort *might* lead to injury and ill health, and it was entirely in keeping with the preventive ethos of public health to err on the side of caution. Testifying in 1877 before the Royal Commission on Noxious Vapours, Simon, by then a recognized authority on all matters sanitary, medical and administrative, made the following observation in relation to nuisances:

> I think the expression "injurious to health" in many of these discussions has been used in a sense to impose upon the person who is charged with the duty of protecting health, an obligation to prove that some named and catalogued disease, such as typhoid fever, or small-pox, or dysentery, or epilepsy, or something, is produced by these vapours. I do not think we are bound, when it is a question of sanitary injury, to show injury of that circumscribed kind. To be free from bodily discomfort is a condition of health. If a man gets up with a headache, *pro tanto* he is not in good health; if a man gets up unable to eat his breakfast, *pro tanto* he is not in good health.[50]

The pliant nature of nuisance law was affirmed elsewhere as a matter of ongoing comment. Professional handbooks dwelled on the subject, while sanitary journals reported court proceedings that weighed up the claims and interrelations of health and comfort.[51] Similarly, the idea that identifying a nuisance might require the application of only crude probabilistic reasoning—the assertion, that is, that a given condition or bylaw transgression would probably, at some point, somehow, injure the health of those exposed to it—was acknowledged, even finding its way into legislation in the shape of the 1891 Public Health (London) Act. Previously, only overcrowding had been distinguished as "dangerous"; but the term now featured in six of the seven offenses, empowering inspectors to act when a given scenario was either a "nuisance or injurious or dangerous to health"—or some combination of all three.[52] As one lecturer in sanitary law noted in 1893, the act had at last made it clear "that future as well as present health is to be taken into account."[53]

Inspection, then, was not entirely driven by the imperative of health, and even when it was, considerations of health might combine, in varying degrees, with those of danger and comfort. Quite what considerations were in play in the case of particular nuisances is difficult to reconstruct. Inspectors were under no obligation to provide a detailed record of their reasoning, only a brief bureaucratic trace of the nuisance they had encountered. The weekly reports of the inspector for the rural district of Bicester during 1873—who seems to have visited anything between one and five properties a day—contain the following, for instance: "very offensive privy"; "one small bedroom, badly ventilated"; "cottage sewer blocked with mud and weeds."[54] Similarly brief descriptions can be found in the records of the inspector for the urban district of Chipping Norton during the early 1880s.[55] Anything up to thirty notices a month were issued regarding offenses such as "sloppage in drain," "privy vault very full," "bedroom very foul," and "occurrence of dung."

What is clear is that considerations of comfort and amenity played a key part in the determination of at least some nuisances. In 1878, an inspector for the district of Epping in Essex explained that he dealt "not only with nuisances against health, but also against convenience, street nuisances and obstruction of the footpaths, persons loitering and goods placed on footpaths, carts standing in or driven on the wrong side of the road, or with sleepy drivers and chimneys on fire."[56] Action was also taken against businesses which caused "distressing noises." Cases were brought against stables, builders' yards, boilermakers and piano teachers on account of the noise they created.[57] Offensive smells were another target. During the 1890s, Bermondsey vestry launched a successful crusade against the unsavory arts of fur pulling, leather making, and bone boiling. "Bermondsey has had an evil reputation for bad smells, which was probably deserved about fifty years ago," declared the local MOH in 1899, "but such is not the case now, and has not been for many years." Gone were the "animal dusts" and "peculiar smells" of drying hides and rotting fish offal that had earlier offended residents.[58]

The majority of nuisances were no doubt compound problems in which it was difficult to disaggregate health from comfort and safety.

Indeed, given the volume and variety of work, it seems likely that each problem embodied its own particular amalgam of concerns; and certainly in some instances the relative weight of these concerns was the subject of deliberation. In 1896, W. Dyson Wood, the county MOH for Oxfordshire, dealt with two cases he had been asked to advise upon by Mr. Pratt, the nuisance inspector for Henley. One was a piece of land containing five pigsties, which in the end he deemed a nuisance. "It seemed to me," Wood reported the following year, "that the smells complained of were liable occasionally to be actually injurious to the health of delicate persons living in the neighbourhood and that in other cases there was a nuisance at any rate preventing various occupiers from having the free enjoyment of pure air in their house and in their gardens." The other was a set of stables which had given rise to a complaint from a nearby cottage; but in this case Wood "was not able to satisfy [himself] that, from a sanitary point of view, there was any nuisance."[59] In general, however, given that most notices were complied with without too much trouble, it was not necessary to provide a detailed rationale; and in any case, definite epidemiological danger was difficult to prove. Discretion and a kind of safety-first, speculative reasoning were crucial.

Looking, Touching, and Testing

Finally, what did inspectors do when they visited a site and how did they go about determining a problem? Different kinds of inspection demanded different kinds of engagement. In the case of food inspection, it was a question, not of finding a problem as such, but of *suspecting* one, in this case an instance of adulterated food or drink. It then entailed purchasing the suspected item so it could be sent to a public analyst for laboratory-based investigation. Following the statutory legislation of the 1870s, the number of samples obtained increased dramatically. According to the LGB, which required analysts to submit quarterly reports to its offices in Whitehall, during the five years 1878 to 1882 over 88,000 samples were subject to scrutiny. Of these, the majority were of milk (31,605), spirits (9,058), coffee (6,226), and butter (5,956).[60] By the mid-1890s, over 40,000 samples were being analyzed every year.[61] After 1875, the procedure was as follows: an item was purchased by an inspector and divided into three parts (one each for the vendor, inspector, and analyst); the part for the analyst was placed in a suitable container (normally a glass jar or tin) and dispatched by person or post; the analyst then carried out his work, and returned a certificate to the inspector detailing the composition of the item and whether or not it contained an abnormal amount of "foreign ingredients"; and if so, a prosecution was launched.[62]

In these instances, inspectors were but a single point in a complex system composed of hearsay and suspicion; the science of chemistry and a medley of laboratory instruments (test tubes, pipettes, drying ovens, and centrifuges); bureaucratic regulations governing the production of paperwork; and, in cases of prosecution, court proceedings and the authority of a judge.[63] With other forms of inspection, it was the inspector who determined whether or not a problem existed; and here it was a matter of marrying the kinds of consideration outlined above—health, comfort, and safety—with the performance of the body's senses. Inspectors were sometimes characterized as the "eyes, ears and nose" of a local sanitary authority, and all three would be mobilized, quite literally, on-site, making for a form of bureaucratized, embodied empiricism. They were routinely encouraged to develop a "habit of close observation," as Francis Vacher, MOH for Birkenhead, put it in 1894.[64] Pipes, floors, and chimneys had to be carefully scrutinized in the case of houses, each of which demanded different sensory combinations. "In descending the cellar steps notice would, of course, be taken of the amount of air and light in the passage, and of any smell of coal gas," stated one MOH in 1901. "The flooring of the basement should be carefully examined for signs of damp, [and] should be tapped for hollowness."[65]

Meat inspection is another instance.[66] Inspectors normally confronted slaughtered animals which had been skinned and dressed, and where the carcasses were either hanging from hooks or laid out on large tables. It was a delicate art, despite the enormous volume of flesh some of them had to contend with: in 1882, Liverpool's inspectors condemned roughly sixty-four tons of meat; in 1908, some forty tons were seized in Leicester.[67] Color, texture, and smell were all crucial variables. "Good meat," noted one handbook, was "florid in hue in the case of young adult animals, brighter before eighteen months, and darker after six years, but it is never dark red or patchy."[68] Another noted the following: "Healthy meat should possess a sweetish odour. The muscle substance should be firm, florid, and elastic. It should also be mottled or marbled by an intimate mixture with fat."[69] Particular organs could also require particular forms of palpation. In the case of tongues, which might display symptoms of "lumpy jaw" (actinomycosis) and foot-and-mouth disease in the form of nodules, it was best, so the MOH of Cumberland wrote, "to seize the tongue with the left hand near its root, then grasp the organ firmly with the right, and while continuing to grasp it firmly, run the hand over it from root to tip."[70] Here especially touch was critical. If all five senses had to be "trained," as Vacher encouraged in his *Food Inspector's Handbook,* it was sensitivity of touch that most distinguished the able meat inspector: "Touch will accomplish so much that a really skilful inspector might almost be entrusted to examine a roomful of carcasses blindfolded, and pick out the diseased ones."[71]

The embodied nature of inspection meant that it was at the mercy of a number of variables, not least the sensory competence of a given inspector. The weather might also play a part: observing the extent of smoke pollution was made much more difficult by strong winds and heavy rain. But where some control over the environment might be exercised, attempts were made to facilitate inspection. As Chris Otter has described, built spaces were increasingly designed in the interests of "inspectability."[72] Some of this emerged as part of efforts to enhance the legibility of towns and cities. Street names and door numbers, for instance, meant that inspectors could negotiate their districts with greater fluency. Other interventions were more calculated. The municipal abattoirs which began to emerge during the late nineteenth century were lit by gas or electric light, allowing for the clustering of carcasses next to one another in a line or semicircle. From the 1870s, domestic sanitary inspection was facilitated by the introduction of "inspection chambers" or "manholes" situated to the side of houses or on footpaths, which enabled access to junction points receiving the drains of premises before they entered the main sewer.[73]

An inspector's senses would also combine with the agency of various instruments. Key devices included those used to prise and penetrate. A meat inspection might involve the use of a scalpel, bowel scissors, and a pocket lens.[74] Incisions might be made into organs in order to reveal lesions; skewers might be inserted into carcasses by way of probing for putrefaction. Also important were gauging tools such as tape measures, rulers, and portable scales. By the 1890s cameras were being used to capture smoke pollution. Testing drains and domestic plumbing networks was a further facet mediated via miniature mobile devices. A basic test consisted of placing a strong-smelling liquid or gas into a water closet or sink, followed by a pail of hot water; should the smell become apparent it was sure evidence of a defective drain or fractured soil pipe. The "scent test" might be performed using peppermint or even a Banner drain grenade, a phial containing pungent gas, which

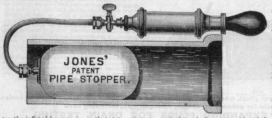
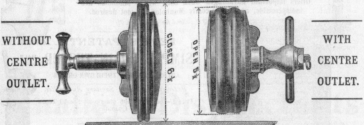
FIGURE 9. "Jones' Patent Drain & Pipe Stoppers." This was a regular advert that featured in the *Sanitary Inspectors Journal,* often alongside adverts for disinfectants, disinfecting machines, and sanitary ware. Source: *Sanitary Inspectors Journal* 4, no. 2 (1898): v. © The Bodleian Libraries, The University of Oxford.

entered the market in 1887.[75] Other tests included the use of smoke; but the most reliable, so it was claimed, was the hydraulic test, which involved stopping up a pipe—perhaps using a Jones's expanding screw stopper—and then monitoring the level of water. If the level dropped, it meant joints were sweating or a pipe had cracked (see figure 9).[76]

Paper forms; the body's senses; a jumble of technologies; and a medley of standards: inspection systems combined all of these elements by way of regulating—and archiving—particular localities and trades. Equally, inspectors combined and mixed various considerations. Indeed, even when acting in the name of health, an inspector might double as an agent of civility and amenity, articulating a confluence of concerns to do with comfort, morality, and property. This was especially so when it came to nuisances, and there was the occasional plea for the abolition of the term on account of its wide remit, including one made in 1910 that complained of the administrative overload it entailed.[77] Yet, the capacious nature of the term was also bureaucratically *useful*, enabling the law to be applied in a flexible fashion, open to the interests of property holders, as well as to problems that might ensue even when there was no immediate danger.

It is no surprise that some inspectors struck a decidedly skeptical note when it came to the microbiological intricacies of germ theories. In 1908, in an address to a conference of inspectors organized by the RSI, the chief inspector of Middlesbrough urged colleagues not to pay any heed to the existence of germs. His worry was that inspectors were becoming unduly distracted by "invisible" agents at the expense of established sanitary concerns: "We must not be led away by the fascination of the unknown and attempt to obtain useless credit for dabbling in the mysteries of, say, tuberculous germs in milk." Partly this was because it was the role of MOsH to keep abreast of scientific innovations; mostly it was because cleanliness was at the root of so much that was essential to a healthy and respectable lifestyle. He reminded his listeners that "Cleanliness is next to Godliness," and ended on a note of reassurance: "Our work will still be required when all germs have been localized and duly allotted to their special function, and their life history defined and understood."[78]

Explicit calls such as this to overlook germ theories were rare, but they reflect the persistence of a capacious, wide-ranging environmentalism which we might otherwise associate with the common law tradition and Chadwick's *Sanitary Report*. Above all, they reflect the demands of sanitary inspection as a complex system of administration that was both on-site and proactively preventive. It was thus, for the most part, a task which combined speculation, discretion, and the application of embodied thinking; and although animated by a regulatory, normalizing ethos, it would be wrong to speak of anything like a science of inspection. Furthermore, as we shall now see, its status as a professional task was compromised, as inspectors struggled through a modern field of multiple agents, competing interests, and informational inputs.

THE STRUGGLE FOR PROFESSIONAL INDEPENDENCE

The first national gathering of sanitary inspectors was held in 1876 as part of the inaugural congress of the SIGB. It henceforth became an annual conference, attracting inspectors from around the country and extensive coverage in sanitary journals. The other key development was the establishment in 1883 of the London-based Association of Sanitary Inspectors.[79] Over the next decade a nationwide confederation of regional branches was established, and in 1907 the association was affiliated with NALGO. By 1887, the London branch could boast 240 members; by 1909, the association as a whole just over 1,500.[80] Each branch held monthly meetings, while each year the association staged a national conference. By the late Victorian period, sanitary inspection was a career open to considerable progression, at least for the ambitious and mobile. In 1897, Albert Taylor—also author of the popular *Sanitary Inspector's Handbook*—was acting as chief sanitary inspector to the vestry of St. George's in London; and he had earlier served as chief inspector of nuisances in Wigan, and before that as sanitary inspector of Wallasey, near Liverpool. In the same year, J. J. Bryan, a Mancunian inspector, took up a three-year post as a sanitary surveyor in Hong Kong.[81]

Sanitary inspectors lacked the social distinction of the central inspectors acting for the LGB. Much like their Oxbridge-educated superiors, the assistant and permanent secretaries, central inspectors laid claim to a certain gentlemanly detachment. In 1888, the German judge P. F. Aschrott published his *English Poor Law System, Past and Present*, which queried the grounds on which LGB inspectors were appointed. He was told by one LGB insider that "they must, above all, be gentlemen, who, on account of their previous occupation and their position in life, enjoy consideration and are accustomed to exercise authority."[82] Sanitary inspectors, by contrast, were part of an expanding corps of officers employed within an increasingly formalized and complex sphere of local governance, and whose authority lay in their technical-bureaucratic aptitude and membership of an institute or association. Associations of this sort flourished during the mid- to late Victorian period, and included the Metropolitan Rate Collectors Association (established in 1882) and the Corporate Treasurers' and Accountants' Institute (1885). In the case of public health, the first associations were established in the 1850s and 1860s, most notably the Metropolitan Association of MOsH (1856; from 1873, the Society of MOsH) and the Poor Law Medical Officers' Association (1868). Later ones included the Association of Municipal and Sanitary Engineers and Surveyors (1873) and the Institute of Public Cleansing (1898).

Central to the self-organization of these professions was ongoing reflection on their status as such, and sanitary inspection was no exception. Its culture of association comprised a number of strands that served to *differentiate* sanitary inspection from other spheres of governance and modern forms of authority. Besides routine review of their professional practice, inspectors affirmed their status as specialized, nonpartisan agents of administration. In common with other professionals, inspectors conceived of themselves as "public servants" acting in the "public interest."[83] They too, according to one inspector in 1883, aspired to act "fearlessly, disinterestedly and independently for the public good."[84] Rhetorically at least, inspectors regularly laid claim to that sense of ethical superiority that distinguished the public servant from the vote-seeking politician and the self-interested businessman. Another facet was the translocal nature of their association, and not least the way the pages of the professional press—much as with the press more broadly, of course—assembled and served up all manner of details and developments disembedded from their local point of origin. Over the course of a few pages in the *Sanitary Record* or the *Sanitary Inspectors Journal* one might read articles entitled "Sanitary Inspection in Paris," "Alcohol and the Health of the Army in India," and "Cremation in Leeds." Perhaps it was taken for granted; but this kind of routine reporting and information gathering was crucial to the elaboration of a specialist pool of knowledge and the affirmation of a common set of experiences.

Meat inspection was one area where all kinds of intricacies were gathered together in this fashion. In 1894, T. M. Legge published some "notes" on continental abattoirs in the pages of *Public Health*—research in fact that would later feature in his *Public Health in European Capitals* (1896)—praising the rigor of meat inspection abroad and especially the pronounced involvement of veterinary professionals.[85] Likewise, in

1899, a piece appeared in the *BMJ* on meat inspection authored by the assistant MOH for Liverpool. "Both in arrangements for slaughtering and meat inspection, England is very far behind when compared with Continental countries," began one section called "Regulations in Foreign Countries," before detailing the construction of German abattoirs and methods of stamping meat.[86] Ten years later, the MOH Hugh Macewen published a handbook on meat inspection which drew on his experience of methods employed in Berlin and the packing houses of the United States. References were made to the work of Professor Robert von Ostertag, head of the veterinary department in the Reich Health Office, Berlin, whom Macewen described as "the Father of Modern Meat Inspection."[87]

Inspiration was also sought closer to home, and the association routinely organized periodic fact-finding missions to local sites of interest. In 1899, for instance, visits were paid to Enfield's new isolation hospital and Lincoln's sewage works.[88] The latter was part of that year's annual conference, which also included a health exhibition patronized by the then president of the LGB, the Tory MP Henry Chaplin (see figure 10). Less regularly, the association also tapped into global networks of knowledge. In 1895, the association attended the International Sanitary Congress in Paris, which included a reception at the French Interior Ministry.[89] Two years later, over one hundred inspectors traveled to Belgium for the next conference. Hosted by King Léopold II (then the cruel custodian of the African Congo), the six-day event included discussions and papers—three were presented by English inspectors—and visits to Antwerp, Bruges, and Brussels.[90] Inspectors were quite explicit about the utility of such gatherings in terms of comparing different systems. In 1900, a delegation from the RSI attended an international meeting hosted by the Société française d'hygiène, which included an address by W.H. Grigg, inspector of Fulham. "We are citizens of the world," he declared, before noting that the "great object of these Conferences is, of course, the enabling of every attentive participator to improve his knowledge of the subjects discussed, and to compare experiences in order that the best system or systems of work might be arrived at."[91]

Meanwhile, all could agree they were participating in a common administrative endeavor that was progressing through time, historically. Annual presidential speeches in particular, which were then published in the press, nurtured a shared sense of historical purpose. Reference might be made to falling GRO death rates, Richardson's utopian city of Hygeia, or other fields of governance where the progress of

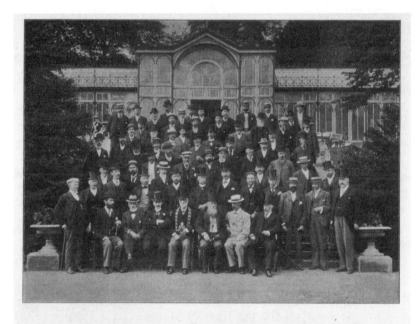

THE SANITARY INSPECTORS ASSOCIATION,

LINCOLN, 1899.

FIGURE 10. A selection of the hundred and more delegates that attended the annual conference of the Sanitary Inspectors Association, in Lincoln in August 1899. The front row includes the city's mayor, MOH and chairman of the sanitary committee. Source: *Sanitary Inspectors Journal* 5, no. 3 (1899): 41–42. © The Bodleian Libraries, The University of Oxford.

public health could be discerned. "We may strengthen our principles, by considering and revising our results," declared Chadwick in 1886, a president of the association in its early years: "Take, for example, our prisons, once the chief seat of pestilence, now by sanitation with the means of water carriage and cleanliness in every cell the seat of the highest health."[92] On another occasion Chadwick concluded by stating that "greater triumphs have been achieved for the enhancement of the health, the strength, the prosperity, the happiness of nations, than in any previous age in the history of the family of man. (General cheering.)"[93]

The labor of inspection, then, was the very stuff of history and not just in terms of its archival-bureaucratic qualities: it was also part of a grand narrative of progress at once local, national, and global. Grandiose visions of the forward march of time mixed with the generation of petty paper traces. And yet, this progress was hard fought and another function of the professional press and association meetings was to reflect on the multiple ways the independence of inspectors was being frustrated, thereby preventing anything like the "systematic" action prescribed by statute. It was a product of the same modern, dialectical dynamic described in the previous chapters. As inspectors, they were public servants, charged with promoting public health and public well-being. Equally, as part of this very same status, they were also answerable to the public and its representatives, whether local or national. This latter aspect underpinned all they did. Parliamentary statutes defined their role; their employers were elected local authorities. The result was a modern system of inspection where professional-bureaucratic empowerment mingled with quite the opposite: public accountability and political interference.

Their ambiguous status in this respect—as with other modern professionals, at once independent of, and dependent on, political connections and relations—made for a peculiar relation to elected institutions; or rather, an *ambivalent* relation of alternating praise and criticism. Much of their professional disinterest derived from what was sometimes called the "non-political character of sanitary reform," by which was meant its basis in sanitary science.[94] Yet inspectors could hardly remain aloof from an institution—parliament—which passed the laws that defined their office and its powers. On some occasions, parliament was the subject of reverence and respect. The annual dinners of the association began with a series of toasts to national institutions, including parliament, the monarchy, and the British Empire; and a handful of MPs always featured among the association's honorary members. Association discussions often praised the wisdom of parliament in passing landmark measures such as the 1848 and 1875 public health acts. Inspectors were fiercely protective of this patriotic image: suggestions that the association aspired to act like a trade union were vehemently rejected.[95]

Equally, a "keen eye," as one association meeting put it, was kept on parliamentary matters likely to affect inspectors, such as bills under scrutiny.[96] Criticism was accordingly measured. As inspectors, they could hardly denounce an institution upon which their own office depended; at the same time, as independent professionals, they had to abstain from pointed partisan criticism. Thus, when they broached the subject of party politics, they preferred to distinguish between the progressive and the regressive elements of parliament, rather than particular parties. In

1886, at the association's third annual dinner, one speaker speculated that forthcoming sanitary legislation would receive mixed support from across the political spectrum—"Conservative, Liberals and Home Rulers"—but added: "There was a party of progress and cleanliness, and there was a party who loved to stew in their own juices."[97] Similarly, when urged to lobby parliamentary candidates during general elections no reference was made to advocating particular parties, only "public men," and the "political platform" as a whole.[98]

The same tension governed the inclusion of MPs within the association along with revered sanitary figures—besides Chadwick, Richardson also served as president during the 1880s—by way of providing a point of contact with the world of politics and parliamentary influence. Greater access to ministers does seem to have been achieved via the patronage of eminent gentlemen: in 1886, Chadwick headed up one of many deputations to the LGB, where he presented a detailed list of grievances to the then minister in charge, James Stansfeld, who had recently returned to the post for a second time.[99] Bills were also sponsored in parliament by honorary members. During the session of 1899–1900, the Liberal MP for West Aberdeenshire, Robert Farquharson, put forward a bill—to no avail, as it happened—which provided for security of tenure for all inspectors and MOsH.[100] Yet this was also a world that inspectors were supposed to be detached from. The dual status of the association in this respect would often emerge in the course of acknowledging the support it received from MPs and mayors. At the same annual dinner of 1886 quoted above, another speaker, referring to the association's honorary members, noted: "They had in their ranks gentleman of every shade of politics, yet as a body they were free from all political bias or prejudice."[101]

A similar ambivalence is apparent in their relation to political institutions at the local level. It was not uncommon for inspectors to praise councillors for the support they offered. Taylor's *Handbook* commended Manchester council for issuing a circular stating that the city's sanitary committee "desire it to be distinctly understood that every inspector will be expected to do his duty towards the public with absolute impartiality."[102] Support of this kind was certainly forthcoming in places. During the 1890s, the Progressive (Liberal-radical) coalition in charge of the LCC championed the cause of inspection and the number of inspectors increased accordingly, from 188 in 1893 to 301 in 1903.[103] In the 1900 metropolitan borough elections, the Fabian Society issued a set of "questions for candidates," the first of which read: "Will you insist on: 1. An immediate increase in the number of Sanitary Inspectors, at least up to a minimum of one for every 2,500 houses?"[104] In any case, whatever their political complexion, local authorities were responsible for all kinds of sanitary improvements, as was duly appreciated. In 1908, at the twenty-fifth annual dinner of the association, the Liberal MP Llewellyn Atherley-Jones proposed a toast to local government, noting that "for the healthier state of the population . . . we are in the main indebted to the local government system of this country."[105]

Yet, just as much opprobrium as praise was heaped on local government, principally on account of the hostility inspectors might face at this level. As inspectors pointed out, many of those elected to the committees or boards that authorized their work also owned property in the same areas under scrutiny. The pecuniary interests of elected councillors and guardians were often at odds with those of public health. "Earnest men, anxious to do good work," noted one inspector in 1883, "become *marked* men, and are looked upon as meddling and officious persons." Such was the anxiety resulting from this "antagonism" that he feared many inspectors hesitated to report nuisances occurring on the property of their de facto employers.[106] Intimidation of this sort certainly took place. In Brighton, a civic crisis erupted in 1894 when members of the town's sanitary committee, all with links to the local butchers' association, disputed the status of a carcass deemed diseased by an inspector. Resignations ensued and the committee had to be hastily reconstituted, though not before an outpouring of criticism in the local press.[107]

Dramatic incidents like this were rare, and the well-documented parsimony of local sanitary committees was of more significance.[108] This hardly resulted in total obstructionism, but in some towns and cities it did make for a culture of administration which was more reactive than proactive. Either way, one source of contingency was the local electoral cycle and the annual turnover of councillors and guardians. "One year there may be one or two gentlemen who take great interest in all sanitary matters," noted one inspector in 1883:

> From these gentlemen one meets with considerate treatment, and encouragement to be energetic and alive to one's duty; and to an officer they are in every sense a very help in times of trouble and difficulty. But then the next year, the committee may be formed of very different metal [*sic*]. . . . These men take a seat in the committee room, and come there with personal motives, pledged to oppose the officers in every way they can, ever ready to protect their own immediate friends, owners of property, or their brother tradesmen from the lawful sanitary requirements that may be needful.[109]

The entanglement of inspection in the vagaries of local political systems thus introduced an unwelcome element of uncertainty; and though it hardly made for chaos it certainly prevented the systematic continuity of leadership and direction craved by inspectors.

Further complications were opened up by the ambiguity of statute law, which failed to specify precise terms of employment. Beyond the need, "from time to time," to appoint "fit and proper persons," parliamentary statute specified little else.[110] National variations of status accordingly formed another point of professional reflection; and although LGB orders introduced a greater degree of specification, there was still much that central officials were unwilling to impose on local authorities. Few inspectors were given permanent contracts, for instance. As the chief inspector of Torquay asked in 1899: "Now, how is it possible for an inspector to carry out his various and disagreeable duties to the highest point of efficiency, when he knows that by the time his re-appointment comes on, he may be outvoted by some of the members of his authority for interference with their property or interests?"[111] Most were contracted for between one and three years; only in London was it common to make nonlapsing appointments.[112]

A suite of other problems might be mentioned in this vein. A consistent item on the agenda was unwieldy workloads. In his report for 1897, for instance, the MOH for Coventry lamented that just one inspector, an assistant, and a clerk dealt with over twelve thousand houses on some forty miles of road.[113] Other gripes concerned the absence of any requirement to appoint specialist inspectors. If it was common in cities to find specialist inspectors—a food inspector, for example—elsewhere quite the opposite was the case. A typical "dual office" in a rural district combined the role of inspector with town surveyor; and it might combine with one or more of the following: school board officer, vaccination officer, relieving officer, even captain of the fire brigade. Nor, until 1910, was there any requirement outside of London (after 1894) to appoint qualified inspectors. In rural districts it remained common to employ former shopkeepers who, according to one MOH, knew "absolutely nothing of what should be required of them."[114] "What is the object of the State establishing an Examination Board," asked another in 1899, "if local authorities are still to be permitted to make a Sanitary Inspector of any ignoramus?"[115]

The independence enjoyed by inspectors thus varied from place to place. In general, they shared with MOsH and poor law medical officers (PLMOs)—who endured their own struggles—a stratified professional structure composed of three groupings: an elite group of metropolitan inspectors who enjoyed relatively ideal conditions of employment; a group of provincial urban inspectors, employed full-time but without security of tenure; and a group of rural inspectors employed only part-time, or in conjunction with other offices, and again without security of tenure.[116] Inspectors rallied around these issues and they endorsed calls for a more technocratic Ministry of Health to replace the LGB. Equally, there was much that they disagreed about, including whether or not inspectors should wear uniforms and the desirability of appointing qualified inspectors. Still during the Edwardian period inspectors were arguing about the need for more hands-on training as opposed to "theoretical examination."[117] Relations among themselves could be just as difficult as those with parliament, the LGB, and councillors. And yet, the modernity of this lowly profession was made of just this: ongoing reflection on inspectors' failings and successes, as they sought to better their status as independent officers nonetheless dependent on the political will of parliament and local authorities. As we shall see, it was also evident in the day-to-day ethos of their work, as inspectors mixed and mingled with those they sought to serve: members of the public.

THE ETHOS OF INSPECTION

In theory, inspectors had all the bureaucratic authority they needed. If statute law was imprecise when it came to conditions of employment, it did at least prescribe extensive powers of entry. Between 6:00 A.M. and 9:00 P.M. in London, and 9:00 A.M. and 6:00 P.M. elsewhere, inspectors could gain access to any premises they saw fit. The only exceptions were CLHs and "infected premises," which could be entered at any time. A written document or certificate attesting to an inspector's identity had to be produced if requested; and should entry still be refused, an inspector could lay a complaint before a magistrate and obtain a warrant that authorized the use of force. Obstruction was punishable by a fine of up to five pounds.[118] Contemporaries were certainly impressed by the powers they enjoyed, which were sometimes thought of in terms of the state. In 1893, one London vestry clerk suggested that the "interference of the State with individual liberty" had reached "its furthest known limits in the powers conferred by legislation on [sanitary] inspectors." He added: "the Englishman's castle is his castle no longer, but rather the happy hunting ground of sanitary inspectors whose polite but firm 'Open Sesame' is not to be withstood even by the iron gates of the most secluded nunnery."[119]

In practice, however, inspectors operated within a crowded sphere of roaming, regulatory agents, some of which—to use a distinction that became current in the late Victorian period—were "official" and some "voluntary," and inspectors forged working relations with both.[120] In terms of the former, inspectors relied on the cooperation of the police. Like inspectors, police officers were empowered to obtain samples of suspected foodstuffs, and in cities such as Sheffield and Manchester they assumed sole responsibility for inspecting CLHs. At the same time, inspectors forged relations with voluntary agents such as domestic missionaries.[121] In their case, the inspiration was variants of evangelical Christianity, and activities included the distribution of biblical tracts and encouraging prayer. But they also dispatched advice on child rearing and domestic hygiene; and much like PLMOs and doctors, they were a useful source of information. "He [the nuisance inspector] should be on terms of intimate friendship with the Scripture-reader and city missionary, most valuable source of information," noted Bristol's MOH in 1871, speaking before the BMA. He "ought to be acquainted with the relieving officers of his district; and, when opportunity offers, he should endeavour to acquire the confidence and goodwill of members of our own profession."[122]

Support was also forthcoming from a medley of female-led sanitary visiting societies modeled on domestic missions. The first organization of this kind was the Ladies' National Association for the Diffusion of Sanitary Knowledge (LSA), founded in London in 1857 to deal with the "women's side" of public health.[123] In just a few years, branches had been set up across England, and it provided the inspiration for kindred organizations, such as the Manchester and Salford Ladies' Sanitary Reform Association, established in 1862. "Diffusion" entailed home visiting, the distribution of tracts, and the organization of mothers' meetings, all of which might be accompanied by prayers and Bible readings. The industry of the LSA was immense. Between 1857 and 1882, it published just short of one and a half million tracts advising on matters such as domestic ventilation, diet, and clothing.[124] During the late Victorian period, "health visiting," as it became styled, was actively co-opted by local authorities, making for mixed systems of official and voluntary agency. In 1890, Manchester council began subsidizing the wages of six of the then fourteen agents employed by the local Ladies' Sanitary Reform Association. By 1907, when they were undertaking over ten thousand house-to-house inspections a year, all the association's visitors were subsidized and supervised by the city council's infant life protection subcommittee.[125]

In the same period, voluntary health visitors were joined by official female inspectors, paid for from the municipal purse, and equipped with statutory powers of entry and abatement.[126] The first official appointments were made in 1892, in Nottingham and Kensington, London, and more followed: by 1904, there were twenty-eight female inspectors working in the capital and seventy-five in the provinces.[127] Yet, in all cases the role was modeled on health visiting, meaning that female officers were generally accorded only a restricted set of tasks in keeping with their gender. These included the inspection of laundries and workshops where women were employed; the inspection of female public conveniences and commercial kitchens; and domestic inspections, especially homes where there were newborn infants or cases of puerperal fever. This was no doubt about protecting the professional interests of male inspectors (the Sanitary Inspectors Association refused to admit female members); but it was also about ensuring that inspection systems comprised the right blend of pedagogic and pastoral dimensions when it came to women. First, so it was argued, there was a woman's instinctive eye for domestic economy and cleanliness. Secondly, there was the interpersonal dimension: the so-called natural understanding shared by women, especially with respect to child rearing. "To the poor mother who imperils the life of her child through ignorance in feeding only a woman can minister," noted an editorial in the *Sanitary Record*.[128]

The premium placed on interpersonal relations, however, was common to *all* forms of inspection, male or female, voluntary or official, local or central.[129] Although they might be associated with the state, sanitary inspectors were intensely self-conscious about their status as such. Most agreed that if inspection systems were to work at all, then the public had to be worked with, as an active ally and *subject* of governance, rather than as a passive, regulatory object. Certainly the job was disciplinary and regulatory; but it was also educational, and a matter of tact and persuasion. And what made inspectors exemplary modern officials was precisely the need to get the balance right. As councillors and inspectors pointed out, their considerable powers of entry and abatement were only effective when allied with a certain kind of diplomatic competence. "We are very far from wishing you to carry out any system of persecution," urged one member of Birmingham's sanitary committee in 1875, during a monthly meeting held at the town hall. "Very much will depend upon you," he informed his audience of inspectors, and "upon the spirit of conciliation you adopt to secure the cooperation of the inhabitants."[130]

The self-consciousness of inspectors as such was partly informed by considerations of national character, and in particular the English regard for the sanctity of the home. The performance of a minor but crucial ceremony—knocking on the door of the inspected, and then doffing one's hat—was understood in these terms. Manners mattered. There was no place for what one handbook described as "rude or supercilious officialism."[131] As the MOH Alexander Wynter Blyth explained to an audience of inspectors in 1892: "Whether the large powers of entry into the Englishman's castle can be beneficially increased will depend upon the conduct of inspectors. . . . Of all nations, the English are the most tenacious of the principle of the privacy of the home; and this principle is outraged if an official enters without knocking, without permission, and with hat-covered head."[132] Further subtleties of conduct were required once the front door had been passed. The very act of examination—the questions asked; the comments passed; the gazes deployed—demanded great poise. Information had to be gathered with a delicate precision: the examination had to be thorough, but without giving the impression of snooping. An inspector was to look, but not look too much; to inquire, but not be inquisitorial. "The duty of seeking out nuisances should be performed with great discretion," encouraged one inspection manual, "so that whilst nothing important may escape his attention, he shall not be too prying or too much of a busybody."[133] A similar balance had to be struck in terms of an inspector's more general demeanor. A "blustering and overbearing manner," wrote one MOH in 1877, "tends to set people's backs up." "On the other hand, indecision and easy-going complaisance are faults quite as prejudicial."[134]

Inspection was indeed about deploying an inspectorial gaze; but this does not mean that it was characterized by anything like the anonymity evoked by accounts that talk in terms of a modern surveillance state.[135] In fact, the modernity of sanitary inspection resides in the subtleties of conduct noted above. In practice, it shared much with the ethos of voluntary bodies like the Charity Organization Society (established in 1869), which also combined bureaucratic modes of organization with a philanthropic emphasis on constructive interpersonal relations.[136] Firmness was crucial, but so too a capacity to place oneself "in sympathy" with members of the public. A sympathetic bearing was especially needful when inspectors visited houses where someone was gravely ill or had died, but it was to inform all of their visits. Many inspectors thought of themselves as "friends" and "advisers" of the public; others, more actively, as "missionaries of sanitation" and "apostles of cleanliness." For some, the job was an opportunity to "preach" the virtues of preventive measures such as smallpox vaccination, and public baths and personal hygiene.[137]

Crucially, this was not just about respecting public opinion for its own sake. Rather, working with the public as an ally and accomplice was a means of securing greater systemic and administrative efficiency. Those inspectors who attempted "to revolutionize suddenly and violently the whole of the bad habits of the people and the faulty construction of ancient houses," advised one MOH in 1897, would invariably end up engaged in expensive and potentially unsuccessful litigation.[138] The best inspectors relied only on preliminary notices. Three sentiments might be highlighted, all of which made inspection a shrewd art, at once bureaucratic and interpersonal: a conviction that in the interests of economy it was better to govern through encouragement and education; a general equation of legal coercion with administrative clumsiness; and a sense that people were capable of governing themselves, so long as they realized what was in their own best interests. The paradox that to intervene less was to intervene more was not lost on inspectors: "Let us [inspectors] cultivate patience and tact. Quiet and judicious persistence without self-assertion was the most powerful battering-ram."[139]

Pastoral and educational, official and bureaucratic: sanitary inspection combined various qualities, and not precluding those more commonly associated with philanthropic work and especially—and largely female— domestic visitation.[140] There are even affinities with the sphere of high politics. As Stuart Jones has described, by the late Victorian period the consensus was that the modern statesman had to work with rather than against the grain of public opinion, nurturing its progressive sentiments while taking care not to override its more conservative instincts.[141] The world of an inspector, of course, was far removed from that of a national statesman, and yet a similar kind of acumen was just as necessary. As "a body," boasted one inspector in 1898, "we have been just that distance in front of general opinion which our work necessitates, and which the sense of the community demands and will allow." A situation "approaching perfection" would be achieved when each individual had realized "his own duty in these matters by personal conviction"; and the means was not more legislation but education via visitation.[142]

PUBLIC COOPERATION AND RESISTANCE

The relation of inspectors to the public was thus internalized by inspectors themselves, both as a matter of professional comment and in terms their general demeanor and daily practice. Governing others was also a matter of governing the bureaucratic self: it was an interpersonal art and was no less modern for that. This seems to have paid off, given how much inspectors were able to accomplish. Clearly not all inspectors were demonized as unwelcome agents of "red-tapism." Some in fact seem to have enjoyed the respect of their local communities. In 1893, one of Burnley's inspectors died of typhoid contracted in the course of his duties. The local paper noted his "prominent position in the town," which had also included work for the fire service; membership of the Keighley Green Club; and his role as a music teacher at the local mechanics' institute.[143]

Sanitary inspectors also had to reckon with the public's right to act as an unofficial inspector. The 1848 Nuisances Removal Act empowered any "two or more inhabitant householders" to make a complaint in writing. Later, the 1875 Public Health Act specified that "any person aggrieved thereby" was entitled to report a nuisance.[144] Local authorities might remind the public of its rights in this respect, placing adverts in the local press soliciting information. In July 1869, Newcastle's corporation placed a "sanitary notice" on the front page of the *Newcastle Courant,* requesting that "information of all Common Nuisances in the Borough be forwarded to William Curry, Sanitary Office, Town Hall."[145] And the public was not averse to making complaints. In 1882, just over twenty-five hundred nuisances were reported by the public in Liverpool, about 3 percent of those reported by officials; in Manchester, during the six weeks leading up to mid-June, 1896, the city's sanitary department received an average of 33 complaints a week, compared to some 235 a week identified by inspectors.[146] In rural areas the input of the public might be especially pronounced. In Witney, Oxfordshire, the inspector received 98 complaints in 1893, compared to 352 identified on his own rounds.[147]

The input of the public could prove problematic, however, further complicating an already compromised system of bureaucracy. Complaints from tenants in particular required handling carefully. Under no circumstances was the tenant's name to be revealed to the landlord. Should this happen, not only might the tenant be given notice to quit, but it also meant that "in future, the inspector will have opposition from occupiers, instead of assistance."[148] Whether these complaints were of any use was another matter. It was widely acknowledged that complaints emanating from the public were just as likely to be specula-tive and based on hearsay, as they were to be accurate and useful. "No principle of action should be better established than this," explained one inspection manual:

> that he should never believe, much less act upon, any information until he has authenticated it by his own careful observation . . . and if there be reason to suspect any sinister influence, as ill-will, on the part of his informant, the surmise should also be noted. No part of his duty will require more caution than this, so that he may not be the dupe of ill-will or idle rumour, or be led into gossiping: whilst he should not repel those who would give him information.[149]

Inspectors thus had to be hard-headed and critical, treating any information given with at least some skepticism; *and* courteous and open to suggestion, for should they be too dismissive they risked offending members of the public and their entitlement to make complaints, some of which might be useful.

Another problem was hostility. One vocation an inspector would do well to emulate, suggested Taylor's *Handbook*, was that of a clergyman, not only that "he may preach the good tidings of sanitation," but "also that he may be able to patiently bear the abuse which he may sometimes receive for what is called his 'Prying Interference.'"[150] Resistance could also take the form of noncooperation. Cases were reported each year in which an inspector, on seeking to obtain a sample of food or milk for analysis, was flatly refused and ordered off the premises. Evasion was practiced. It was often remarked how vendors would keep an adulterated article in one receptacle for public sale, and a pure one in another for inspectors.[151] Tactics like this thus bred countertactics on the part of inspectors, who in some cases would rely on their assistants to buy a sample or a member of the public. This is one reason why some inspectors objected to wearing uniforms. It is "almost too obvious to require argument," noted one inspector, that "detective duties" of this sort "can be effectually performed only by a man out of uniform."[152]

Nor was it unheard of for the public to resort to physical intimidation. In 1900, for instance, one of Colchester's inspectors, fleeing an irate tenant, received a kick to the back while descending some stairs.[153] Some confrontational scenarios even gave rise to serious public disorder, as in 1898, during an inspection of a Saturday night market along Walworth Road in central London. The incident, which ended up in Lambeth Police Court, occurred after two inspectors attempted to seize some meat from a street stall. The vendor threatened the inspectors and struck one of them in the face; but not before a crowd of more than two hundred people had gathered.[154] Robust health was crucial given an inspector's exposure to diseased places and persons; likewise, given the possibility of a punch-up now and then. "It is necessary that he [the inspector] should have a fair amount of physical strength," noted one handbook, "for he is liable to be obstructed in the discharge of his duties, and should be at least able to hold his own."[155]

Widely regarded as hotspots of drunkenness, criminality, and disease, CLHs presented similar problems. The danger of assault was ever-present, which is why they were often visited in pairs by inspectors, or else placed under the responsibility of the police. Some lodging houses operated lookout systems, depriving inspections of a critical element of surprise. A report for the City of London, circulated in 1860, noted how difficult it was to ascertain the true number of lodgers in a given house: "for as he [the inspector] is well-known to the keepers of these places and is constantly watched for, preparation is made for his visit directly as he enters the localities in which the houses are situated."[156] In other houses the practice was simply to make a dash for it: "If there be a back door, it must be watched as well, lest the surplus sleepers be hurriedly awakened and expeditiously ejected before the door is open to the inspector at the front," noted a report on the LCC's lodging house inspectorate in 1898. Here too tactics of evasion provoked countertactics on the part of inspectors. The report went on: "A prolonged delay in the opening of the door usually means that some hasty readjustment is going on within, so to catch things 'on the hop,' as the lodgers put it, the inspector sometimes gets in through the window."[157]

More legitimate forms of resistance were pursued through the courts, commonly magistrates' courts. Orders of entry and notices of abatement were challenged in this way. Appeals of this sort invariably required that the relevant inspector take the stand, opening up a point of public scrutiny and interrogation. In one case, in 1906, an inspector was grilled by a magistrate over whether he was legally entitled to inspect a faulty drain while it was in the process of being fixed by the owner. The judge disputed the inspector's interpretation of the law and ruled in favor of the defense.[158] At the same time, court cases provided an opportunity for members of the public to have their say. During a case heard in 1892, the defendant, who was charged with obstructing entry, protested that "there was no smell" on his premises suggesting any kind of sanitary defect, adding that "he objected to people invading his house on the mere *ipse dixit* of an official, who in this instance had been somewhat rude in his claim and had behaved in a high-handed way."[159] The judge sided with the prosecution, but a legitimate legal fight had been staged.

As these cases suggest, recourse to legal action was no more stacked in favor of officials than it was members of the public, something borne out by further cases.[160] It is noteworthy that inspectors warned others against exaggeration in court cases and to lay the facts bare, even if they did tell in favor of the defendant.[161] Much like the political system, parliamentary and local, the legal system was by turns supportive and obstructive. Between 1895 and 1900, the LCC successfully prosecuted 147 lodging house keepers through magistrates' courts. Offenses included neglect of cleanliness and failure to separate single men and women at night.[162] Yet the same period also witnessed prolonged legal battles regarding the inspection of the down and out. In 1890, the LCC fought unsuccessfully to register a Salvation Army shelter as a "common lodging house." A further case was brought against The Harbour, as the shelter was known, in 1899 and was once more dismissed. On appeal, however, another judge, this time from the Queen's Bench Division of the High Court, ruled in favor of the LCC, overturning the original decision made in 1890.[163] In this instance the LCC scored a victory, but evidence suggests that it encountered setbacks only shortly afterward. A report published in 1909 noted that some fifteen to twenty metropolitan shelters remained exempt from inspection, and all because of another precedent set in 1905 at the Court of Appeal.[164]

Inspectors were thus ambivalent toward the legal profession and the legal system, just as they were toward politicians and the political system. On occasions, magistrates and High Court judges were praised for their reliability and common sense; on others, censured for their inconsistency. "One ruling today may prove a guide to the prosecutor, and another, the next day, will be a consolation to the cow-keeper," suggested one president of a sanitary inspectors' conference in 1911.[165] But whether good or bad, reasonable or not, judges could only interpret the law as it was given to them and the testimony they received; and this did not preclude receiving conflicting evidence from sanitary experts. In 1890, the owner of a slaughterhouse in Bradford appealed a decision by the local authority to close down his business, which involved calling on the testimony of Alfred Bostock Hill, then deputy MOH for Birmingham, who testified that all was well—much to the dismay of Bradford's MOH, who had suggested that all was not.[166] Similarly, in 1896, the otherwise respected metropolitan MOH for Marylebone, Alexander Wynter Blyth, testified against nuisance proceedings taken against a landlord in the neighboring district of Newington. The rancor was such that the Sanitary Inspectors Association notified the LGB regarding what it described as a "scandal."[167] Nor, finally, did inspectors always help themselves. In particular, procedural errors in the issuing of notices could lead to "technical victories" in favor of the defense. Ambiguities regarding the ownership and management of property, for instance, were not always clarified by inspectors, meaning that solicitors could later claim that a notice had been served on the wrong person.[168] In the bigger scheme of things, resort to court proceedings was rare; but clearly, when they were resorted to, they were capable of both frustrating and facilitating the cause of inspection.

CONCLUSION

Often analyzed as a generic feature of the modern state, bureaucracy is at once a specific task—specialized, but not necessarily expert; administrative, but especially concerned with rules and regulations—*and* capable of assuming various forms. Certainly sanitary inspection constitutes a singular instance. It was local for one thing, and developed as part of a modern intensification of administrative systems at this newly articulated level of governance. Equally, few other officials daily crossed the thresholds of private homes and businesses; and they were unique in deploying technologies such as scalpels and drain stoppers. They were no mere pen pushers. Nonetheless, it is easy to see why sanitary inspectors were regarded as meddlesome bureaucrats. They were hardly pervasive—they lacked the resources for this—but they did exercise a beady, regulatory eye wherever they went. Moreover, they possessed considerable powers of entry and abatement with respect to property, and they were immersed in paperwork, among other things clocking and recording infringements, and archiving them in increasingly elaborate municipal offices. A "sanitary terror," "faddy," and "grandmotherly": such was the verdict of some correspondents of the *Times* in 1897 with respect to inspectors and the laws they sought to enforce.[169]

The modernity of sanitary inspection, however, also resides in the way these powers were exercised as part of a diffuse field of governance that turned on both official-bureaucratic empowerment and public-political input and accountability. As we have seen in the previous two chapters, this dynamic underpinned the gestation of the public health system as a whole, as well as the provision of official statistics; but it was also at work at the local level, shaping the everyday actions of inspectors.

Three points might be emphasized. Firstly, sanitary inspectors were intensely self-conscious about their status as such and worked hard to enact quite the opposite persona during their rounds. "Officialism" was an anathema, partly because playing the friendly inspector—the nonofficial official—made for better, more efficient regulation. It involved, that is, a reworking and reanimation of the personal dimension, rather than its erasure or diminution. Second, their role was made possible by a variety of relations with other agents: MPs, councillors, judges, and further officials (LGB officials; MOsH and analysts; and police officers), as well as members of the public. These relations were more or less personal and regular, but they all played a role, making bureaucracy a shared and diffuse endeavor. Finally, these relations were highly contingent and variable, making for considerable variations of practice and status, and frustrating aspirations for "systematic" action, as statute had it. It was by no means a smooth or uniform process of bureaucratization. And this suggests a further feature, for these spatial-temporal variations were reflected on at the time as part of the professional culture that began to emerge in the 1870s. We might in fact speak of two processes: one external and properly bureaucratic, which involved regulating and reforming sanitary infringements on the part of the public; the other internal, which involved regulating and reforming their own status as officials.

As we have seen, much of this work concerned regulating not so much people as the infrastructures and things that governed their health and comfort. Foremost among these were technologies of domestic waste disposal. The next chapter considers the installation and reform of just these particular material elements. As we shall see, domestic drains and toilets were but one part of a hugely inventive and fractious process of technological system building.

CHAPTER 5

Matter in Its Right Place

Technology and the Building
of Waste Disposal Systems

The administrative systems discussed in the previous chapters were all distinguished by their novel scale and organizational ambition and complexity. The same modernity of scale, ambition, and complexity applies to the subject of this chapter: the advent of sewerage and domestic waste disposal systems for dealing with the growing volume of detritus and excreta that was the invariable accompaniment of a growing mass of human bodies. To be sure, managing dirt and removing waste was not the only meaning of "public health," which was also subject to more expansive visions of a state-medical sort. Nor are these systems the only example of the technological nature of public health reform, which extended from modest domestic ventilation mechanisms (e.g., airbricks and Tobin tubes) to large-scale water-supply systems—indeed, supply systems that were necessarily bound up with the waterborne sewerage schemes considered here.

The development of sewerage and waste disposal systems during the Victorian period remains remarkable nonetheless. In the early nineteenth century, managing waste was still largely a problem of *human* agency. Towns and their residents hired scavengers to remove the refuse dumped in laystalls, which was then tipped in outlying fields. Nightmen were employed to empty cesspools, the contents of which might be sold to farmers. Meanwhile, the deliberations of court leets, sewer commissioners, and magistrates remained crucial when it came to determining any remedial actions relating to mounds of filth and the repair of sewers, such as they were. None of this was displaced quickly, smoothly, or indeed entirely, as we shall see. Even so, by the early twentieth century the problem had been significantly reconstituted, so that it was also a matter of *technological* agency: or rather, the performance of millions of pipes, traps, and gratings; thousands of miles of subterranean sewer mains; outfall works and refuse destructors; and steam-powered pumping stations.

How did this come about? There are good reasons, of course, as to why sewerage and waste disposal systems feature in histories of the welfare state.[1] One is simply because they constituted a profound assault on sources of sickness and disease, especially the zymotic class, and more especially still what were dubbed "filth diseases": diarrhea, cholera, typhus, and typhoid. A second is because they were subject to central oversight by offices such as the GBH, LGAO, and LGB, and an accumulating body of statutory regulations. A final reason concerns their financing. Compared to the development of gas, water, and electricity infrastructures, there was less wrangling over the merits of public and private ownership.[2] Instead, sewerage systems and dust depots joined municipal parks, public baths, cemeteries, and isolation hospitals to rank among those facets of the local environment that were principally financed through central loans on the security of the rates. In 1900, the Liberal MP and former president of the LGB Sir Henry Hartley Fowler presented a paper to the Royal Statistical Society (formerly the SSL) detailing the history of municipal finance since 1800. It contained the striking figure that local authority debt for capital expenditure had increased from approximately £60 million in 1868 to over £262 million in 1898, some 10 percent of which related to sewerage schemes and 33 percent to municipal enterprises such as water and gas works, and electric lighting. But whereas "public opinion" now classified sewerage works among those "public obligations . . . towards which the whole community should contribute," this did not extend to municipal trading operations, which for Fowler at least failed to rank as "primary" responsibilities.[3]

The focus of this chapter, however, is not the assumption of a sense of collective responsibility, and how this was processed through the interaction of central and local authorities. Rather, the focus is on the *systems themselves,* and their peculiar contingencies and complexities of development. In particular, the chapter focuses on the options developed and abandoned, and the struggle to solve the problems created in the process of technologizing waste disposal. The novelty and enormity of what took place is manifest in the great accretion of discourse on the problem, which flourished as part of the modern administrative culture detailed in the last three chapters. Crucially, besides serving to historicize, statisticalize, and bureaucratize the progress that was and was not being made, this also served to place the problem on a translocal footing. Sustained scrutiny began with Chadwick's 1842 *Sanitary Report,* which was partly inspired by the work of the Paris-based hygienists Louis-René Villermé and Alexandre Parent-Duchâtelet.[4] The translocal nature of Chadwick's inquiry—which had included references to French practices—was then developed in the investigatory labors of the GBH and LGB, and a series of royal commissions and select committees. Between the 1840s and 1880s, sewage disposal alone was the subject of six select committee and seven royal commission reports. A further commission convened in 1898 published no less than nine reports. Throughout the principal field of reference was the national one and localized developments across Britain; but this did not preclude considering innovations from abroad.

Professional engineers of various institutional locations and associations were also part of the mix. Founded in 1818, the Institution of Civil Engineers (ICE) provided a home for some of the first sanitary engineers.[5] Among these was Joseph Bazalgette of the MCS and then the MBW, and Robert Rawlinson, who began as a GBH and then a LGAO inspector, before serving as chief engineer to the LGB. Of more importance was the emergence of a still neglected set of local agents, variously described as municipal engineers, town surveyors, and district engineers.[6] The first appointment was made in 1847 in Liverpool, where James Newlands assumed the post of borough engineer, and by the early 1870s their number and shared sense of purpose was sufficient to prompt the formation of the Association of Municipal and Sanitary Engineers and Surveyors (AMSES).[7] The inaugural meeting took place in 1873 under the auspices of the ICE and the leadership of Lewis Angell, AMSES's first president and borough engineer to West Ham.[8] By 1875, its membership had grown to 175, and in 1908 stood at over 1,200.[9] Early honorary members included Bazalgette and by the 1890s this status extended to six LGB inspectors and two European engineers, one the directeur des travaux of Paris, the other the ingénieur en chef of Brussels. The responsibilities of local engineers and surveyors included the maintenance of streets, the inspection of plans for new houses, and the supervision of engineering contracts; but the planning and management of sewerage and waste disposal systems were among their core responsibilities.

These, then, were the crucial technical officers, and indeed the problem was not without a couple of points of general orientation. All could agree that progress lay in technological solutions beyond cesspools, and the carts and shovels of scavengers and nightmen. Likewise, all subscribed, however tacitly, to the definition of dirt popularized by the Whig statesman Lord Palmerston in 1851, when he suggested that dirt was only "matter out of place," bad and pathogenic in one location but possibly useful in others.[10] Some even elevated the pithy formulation into the master principle of sanitary reform more generally. Speaking before the SIGB in 1881, the military surgeon and ventilation expert F. S. B. F. de Chaumont declared: "Now, although it may be said that after all there are no great fixed scientific principles here, such as the law of gravity or of chemical affinity, yet we may claim so far to have come to a general principle of some importance and that is this: that human ills from a sanitary point of view arise from the presence of matter in the wrong place."[11] At the very least it captured the basic premise that managing domestic waste and excreta was a twofold project which involved (a) removing it from where it was harmful and unnatural; and (b) ensuring that wherever it went next, it served either a useful purpose or was rendered harmless.

Yet, as we shall see, these were decidedly thin currents of consensus amid a hugely ambitious and disputatious culture of technological system building. This is partly because these currents developed within a field of governance that extended much beyond professionals and officials, and even councillors, landowners, and ratepayers, to embrace a group of agents so far overlooked in this study: namely, commercial actors, and in particular entrepreneurial inventors and sanitaryware manufacturers. But it is also, crucially, because technologizing the disposal of human waste created problems of its own, and most of all new sources of pollution in the form of sewage and sewer gas. It was anything but a linear process of problem solving, despite—or rather, *because of*—the transformative, historical powers now invested in technological systems.

Indeed, all this suggests another context in which this crucial aspect of public health should be considered. Not that of a proto-collectivist or centralized state; rather, the broader culture of engineering that emerged, and those other projects for which the Victorians are justly famous, such as the construction of railway and telegraphic networks, and municipal gas and electricity systems. Regardless of their ownership, these too evolved amid grandiose ambitions, failed projects, pragmatic compromises, and numerous disputes regarding the technical details of otherwise large-scale material systems (e.g., broad versus narrow gauge tracks; the merits of AC and DC electrical currents).[12] The chapter begins with the construction of sewerage systems, before detailing the problems they generated, and the alternatives that were pursued and entertained.

"CIRCULATION INSTEAD OF STAGNATION"

Victorian dirt was the subject of unprecedented disgust and despair, as multiple studies have detailed.[13] Clearly, during the 1830s and 1840s, some kind of threshold was passed that was as much sociological and moral as it was physical and epidemiological. The advent of the filth-obsessing genres of social investigation and slum reporting is testament to this.[14] Yet, at just the same moment, dirt became the stuff of modern, totalizing visions of system and human-technological progress; and this was no more so than for Chadwick. In 1844, amid escalating financial speculation surrounding the railways, he established the Towns Improvement Company to promote and sell integrated systems of water supply, drainage, and sewage disposal. Despite its prestigious array of directors, which included the Post Office reformer Rowland Hill, the company fizzled out and was effectively finished by 1847, having made unsuccessful pitches to towns such as Manchester, Bolton, and Bristol.[15] The advent of the MCS and GBH, however, provided new institutional platforms, the GBH especially—Chadwick was removed from the MCS in 1849—where the scheme was promoted as the "arterial-venous" or "tubular system."[16]

The most eloquent outline was provided by Chadwick's ally, F. O. Ward, whom we encountered in chapter 2, when he addressed the first International Congress of Hygiene, held in Brussels in 1852 (and he returned again to the congress in 1856 to give much the same address). Its "fundamental principle" was "circulation instead of stagnation," which in practice amounted to an all-embracing, steam-powered complex of pipes. In "one great movement" it transferred urban excreta to outlying agricultural fields and brought back pure rainwater from faraway hills. There were no cesspools or standpipes. Instead, a "self-acting" network of tubes linked homes and the countryside, simulating as it did so the natural efficiency of the body: small-bore pipes formed the "veins" and "arteries"; water the "blood"; and a liquid-pumping steam engine "the heart." "*Hygiene by steam power* is the logical extension and the necessary complement of *locomotion by steam power* which Europe has lately adopted," Ward concluded, referring to railway technology. [17] Crucially, the fact that excrement was recycled as agricultural fertilizer—

and so, eventually, as food—meant that nothing was wasted; or, as Chadwick had enthused in 1845, drawing on ancient mythology, the system "completed the circle" of Nature, realizing "the Egyptian type of eternity by bringing, as it were, the serpent's tail into the serpent's mouth."[18]

Such was the initial vision of a new order of technologized waste disposal characterized by circulatory speed and seamless connectivity. No foul gases escaped into homes or streets, just as water and waste remained in perpetual motion in ongoing cycles of collective replenishment. In chapter 2, we saw how Rumsey's uncompromising, agenda-setting vision of a national system of state medicine was only partly realized, passing as it did through a modern mix of MPs, ministers, professionals, and the deliberations of a royal commission. Just as uncompromising and agenda-setting, Chadwick's technological vision of system pursued a similarly contested and, ultimately, broken trajectory. This was not for want of sympathy with its general aspirations. Certainly at this point there was no aversion to sewage utilization, as we shall see. Likewise, the cesspools singled out by Ward as "pestilential" points of stagnation were roundly condemned. The so-called privy-midden system, for instance, which involved a rudimentary toilet attached to a cesspit or refuse heap (or midden), was attacked from all quarters as an insanitary relic of a barbarous, medieval past: Chadwick's *Sanitary Report* was damning, as was the evidence presented in the two reports of the Health of Towns Commission (1844–45). One "of the best tests of the progress a people have made in civilization is furnished by the manner in which they dispose of their excreta," noted a member of the London Epidemiological Society in 1853, before dwelling on "the evils arising from the cesspool system."[19]

Ward's promise of cleaner water, piped en masse, was also a widely shared ideal. Leakage from cesspools polluted drinking wells, and in cities such as London, Liverpool, and Bristol the growing use of water closets was causing problems of river pollution; and these problems were made all the more pressing given that these same rivers doubled as the source of supply for water companies. The term *sewer* originally meant "a fresh Water Trench, or little River"; but its meaning changed as landlords and tenants, with or without local sanction, began using and modifying sewers as a means of carrying away effluence.[20] Opinions were perhaps more mixed regarding the merits of "constant systems" of water supply versus "intermittent systems," which provided water only at set times. Even so, the constant service envisaged by Ward was not without supporters during the 1850s, when the work of private water companies was subject to unprecedented exposure.[21]

The problems with Chadwick's grand, circulating system of pipes were of a political, practical, and technical sort. Its reliance on "centralized" means of institutional diffusion made for resistance and suspicion at the local level, as we saw in chapter 2. The sheer technological scope of his system was also problematic. The question of water supply was indeed implicated in the question of sewerage systems. Yet engineers and local authorities preferred to treat them separately, if only because the matter was already being dealt with in this manner, whether through private or municipal means; and besides which, reforming existing water supplies was complicated enough, politically and technologically.[22] Finally, as Christopher Hamlin has demonstrated, there was little consensus among engineers regarding the details of the system: the obscure but all-important technical minutiae.[23]

The official line was outlined in a paper published by the GBH in July 1852 for the use of local authorities.[24] Besides advocating combined back drainage, which collected the drainage of several dwellings in a single channel to their rear, the paper also recommended the use of small-bore earthenware pipes, and the separation of domestic rain and waste waters from accumulations of rainwater and other surface liquids beyond the home and its environs (an early variant of what would become known as "separate systems"). It acknowledged the utility of large, egg-shaped brick sewers, of the sort pioneered during the preceding decade by John Roe, surveyor to the Holborn and Finsbury Commission of Sewers. But although an improvement on flat-bottomed sewers—largely because egg-shaped sewers allowed for a better flow of sewage by virtue of their ovoid shape—they were no match for the use of circular pipes. Or so the GBH claimed. Pipes were cheaper and more durable; afforded faster flows of sewage; less amenable to rat infestation; and self-cleansing, thus dispensing with the need for human maintenance.[25]

The majority of engineers begged to differ, giving rise to what was dubbed the "pipe-and-brick sewers war." Not all GBH officials were as strident as Chadwick, however. In November 1852, Rawlinson, then one of the GBH's engineering inspectors, gave an address to the ICE entitled "On the Drainage of Towns." The question of pipe and brick sewers was not the only thing he discussed; and though he praised pipes, he also dwelled on the advantages of bricks. It was essentially a matter of trial and error, he suggested: "Earthenware pipes cannot, however, be beneficially used as sewers, beyond certain limits, which can only be settled by practice."[26] Still, his cautious advocacy of pipes was enough to rile some sections of the audience, which included Bazalgette (as well as Toulmin Smith, incidentally, who spoke against pipes). By this point the tubular system had been installed in a handful of towns, including Croydon, Rugby, and Tottenham, and some of the discussants pointed to the shortcomings that had arisen: blockages, cracked pipes, and outbreaks of infectious disease. Others pointed to the dubious nature of the hydraulic experiments put forward to justify the superiority of pipes.[27] Others still argued that while pipes were good for some purposes, especially immediate house drainage, brick sewers were better for others, especially main sewers. Rawlinson concurred: "an indiscriminate application of the pipe-sewer system could not be maintained." In fact, he "was not wedded to any system."[28]

Rawlinson's paper captured the general consensus that would develop in subsequent decades, as elements of the GBH's initial vision were by turns rejected and reworked. Both pipe and brick sewers had their uses, where appropriate, just as each was liable to blockage. "It was a generally received opinion at one time that all brick sewers were sewers of deposit, and that pipe sewers were self-cleansing, but upon this point there can be no greater mistake," noted Baldwin Latham in his 1873 text *Sanitary Engineering*, the first comprehensive manual on the subject: "Pipe sewers may become sewers of deposit, and brick sewers may be made self-cleansing."[29] In any case, even in GBH-sanctioned towns the practice had been to mix the two. The system installed in Carlisle in 1854–55 comprised nine thousand yards of brick sewers and over fourteen thousand yards of earthenware pipes.[30] Other places simply ignored the advice of the GBH. In 1851, Bristol obtained powers under the 1848 Public Health Act, and although it was encouraged to use pipes by the GBH inspector Henry Austin, the town council pressed ahead with its original brick-based scheme for Clifton, where eleven miles of sewers were laid between 1855 and 1857.[31]

In the decades that followed, Chadwick continued to pipe up about his pipe system, doing so until his death in 1890.[32] And Chadwick's "dogma," as some put it, was entirely in keeping with what remained a remarkably inventive and contentious field of technological system building. Professional deliberation and central-official guidance provided a steer of sorts. What emerged in fact was kind of normalizing pragmatism, based on the prescription that general norms of construction, from broad principles of practice to minor technical standards, should be adapted as best they could to suit invariably peculiar local circumstances. Yet there were limits even to this, for the options were multiple and the sewerage systems of unprecedented complexity. Three areas of innovation might be highlighted: separating and combining; flows and flushes; and levels and lifting.

Separating and Combining

One point of codification was precisely the set of local variables that had to be taken into account in order to ensure that any given system had the required capacity. As detailed in official documents and professional guidebooks such as H. P. Boulnois's *Municipal and Sanitary Engineers' Handbook* (1883), these variables typically included the following: amount of rainfall; present and prospective population; the supply of water; the number and type of toilet appliances (see below); and the geological character of the district. In the case of rainfall, there was nothing that could be done about the amount that fell from the skies; but a choice could be made about whether or not to collect it in the same sewers that dealt with domestic sewage and subsoil water (and perhaps manufacturing refuse as well), thereby giving rise to "combined" and "separate systems."

By far the most extensive combined system was London's Main Drainage Scheme, built under the superintendence of Bazalgette and the MBW. Work began in 1859 and was finally complete in 1875 (see figure 11). In 1861, the *Observer* dubbed it "the most extensive and wonderful work of modern times," and so it proved, combining pipes for immediate house drainage; brick-built main and branch sewers; intercepting and outfall sewers; as well as storm overflows.[33] As Bazalgette noted during an address to the ICE in 1865, one consideration had been whether rainfall "should be dealt with by a separate system of sewers."[34] The point of contrast was Paris, where a separate system of sorts had developed since the 1830s that involved the disposal of rain and surface water in large brick-built sewers, but the manual collection of human "night-soil." By contrast, British engineers wanted to technologize the collection of *both;* and in the end, separation on this scale was judged "impracticable," for it would have involved a double set of drains to every house and a second series of sewers in every street. Instead, the system was designed to accommodate an average rainfall of ¼ inch every twenty-four hours. Meanwhile, given that catering for all possible rainfalls would have been too expensive (on account of the size of the sewers required), Bazalgette installed overflow weirs at the junctions of

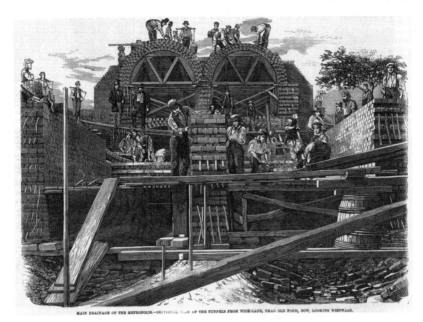

MAIN DRAINAGE OF THE METROPOLIS.—SECTIONAL VIEW OF THE TUNNELS FROM WICK-LANE, NEAR OLD FORD, BOW, LOOKING WESTWARD.

FIGURE 11. A section of London's Main Drainage Scheme in the process of construction in 1859. This particular section was in Wick Lane, Bow. Source: "Main drainage of the metropolis," *Illustrated London News*, August 27, 1859, 203. © The Bodleian Libraries, The University of Oxford.

the main and intercepting sewers, which acted "as safety-valves in times of storm."[35] Otherwise the principal destination was the outfall sewers, which carried London's sewage to Barking north of the Thames and to Crossness in the south, both on the outskirts of the city. In 1865, by which point most of the scheme had been completed, the system comprised thirteen hundred miles of main sewers and eighty-two miles of intercepting sewers.[36]

Following Bazalgette's intervention, combination emerged as the dominant preference and it was the one recommended by the LGB in 1878, when it published a series of suggestions authored by Rawlinson for use by local authorities.[37] Yet, if not quite the pipe-and-brick sewers war of the 1850s, combination was by no means hegemonic. This was partly for practical reasons and making do with what was available. The scheme carried out by Leicester's corporation during the early 1850s left intact some of the original natural sewers for the disposal of surface water, while constructing a second system of "deep sewers" for the collection of excreta.[38] As late as the Edwardian period, Doncaster was mixing the two: "The sewerage is on the combined system but as far as possible natural water courses have been utilized to take surface water," noted its borough surveyor in 1909.[39] Equally, from the 1870s, separation was championed as an alternative method and was not without practitioners among borough engineers.[40] During the 1880s, for instance, Angell—by then a former president of AMSES—constructed separate systems in Maidstone and West Ham. Other engineers followed suit, including in Reading, Slough, Wimbledon, and Southampton.[41] As was argued, given the reduced volume of sewage, one benefit of separation was that there could be greater recourse to cheap, small-bore pipes, making for a partial resurrection of Chadwick's preferences.[42]

Flows and Flushes

Chadwick's fault had been to urge the indiscriminate use of pipes, which he thought would prove "self-cleansing." Like other Victorian technological enthusiasts, Chadwick seems to have been mesmerized by the possibility of superefficient, self-acting systems.[43] The ideal persisted: "All Engineers endeavour to design both main sewers and branch sewers so as to be what is called 'self-cleansing,'" noted Salford's borough engineer in 1902.[44] Equally, while bricks were now part of the equation, engineers continued to strive for optimum velocities. Latham's *Sanitary Engineering* summarized the experience of engineers from England, France, and Germany. Among other things, he applied the formulas of Julius Ludwig Weisbach's *Lehrbuch der Ingenieur und Maschinenmechanik* (1845) to present a series of hydraulic tables regarding the precise relations of size, fall, volume, and velocity of circular and egg-shaped sewers.[45] Three feet per second, Latham argued, was about necessary in order to secure as much self-cleansing as possible. Manufacturers played their part. Although lead- and glass-glazed pipes were endorsed by engineers, salt-glazed pipes were judged to be of superior self-cleansing qualities. In 1846, Henry Doulton, then an acquaintance of Chadwick and his coterie, pioneered the production of salt-glazed pipes at his factory in Lambeth. Further factories followed at St. Helens in 1847 and at Dudley in 1848, and by the 1870s Doulton was one of a handful of companies, also including Armitage and Twyford, mass-producing salt-glazed sanitary ware and selling it around the world.[46]

The difference was that these efforts were now allied with those premised on the assumption that total self-cleansing was unachievable in practice; or rather, on the impossibility of securing entirely maintenance-free systems on account of breakages, blockages, and accumulations of silt.[47] In contrast to Parisian sewers, which featured banquettes and were uniformly large, no efforts were made to facilitate internal manual cleansing: as early as the 1860s it was noted that English engineers preferred to avoid any features which might compromise the optimal ovoid shape of brick-built sewers.[48] Instead a practice that Roe had first dwelled upon in the mid-1840s emerged as the dominant solution: flushing.[49] The installation of flushing gates was one variant, which involved stopping up and then releasing a flow of sewage, when and where required; another was the use of flushing tanks which moved on trunnions, collecting sewage water and then releasing it once a certain tipping point had been reached. Another still was manual hosing, which worked via the most signal manifestation of these self-cleansing limitations: maintenance and inspection manholes. By the 1880s, for instance, Croydon's system was home to forty flushing tanks, as well as eighty-five manholes that doubled as hose-based flushing stations.[50]

Levels and Lifting

A final set of considerations concerned the geography and geological morphology of any given district. The rule of thumb was that any engineer should be "Nature's journeyman," as Rawlinson put it in 1852, respecting the peaks and troughs of the landscape and the proximity of rivers and shorelines. More simply, gravity and what nature had to offer had to be exploited as best as possible. Sewerage systems were thus built as a series of "levels," "zones," and "sections." The most impressive example is once again London, where the Main Drainage Scheme comprised two principal works, one north of the Thames and one south, coupled with high-, middle-, and low-level main sewers within each, which drained into a set of intercepting sewers, before flowing to the outfalls. Similar, if much less extensive, patchworks developed elsewhere. By the mid-1870s, Bristol's system comprised six district sections, which together contained roughly forty-three miles of sewers: Clifton high level district (built in 1855–57); Bedminster (1855–58); Clifton low level (1858–59); St. Philip's (1858–61); the Frome intercepting district (1860–66); and the Avon intercepting district (1871–74).[51] Another example is Leicester, where the sewerage system was first reformed during the 1850s, and then again in the 1880s and early 1890s. Designed by the borough engineer, Joseph Gordon, the scheme was based on two principal works, one west and one east of the river

Soar. The former comprised five high-, middle- and low-level zones, and the latter two, one high and one low, whilst each zone was served by a main sewer that flowed into one of the two outfalls situated either side of the Soar.[52]

Harnessing gravity, however, also meant overcoming it in places with the aid of technology, before it could be mobilized once more. So-called gravitation schemes combined both nature and technological artifice in this respect; or in terms of the latter, recourse to steam-powered pumping. The key innovations were made by the engineer Thomas Wicksteed in the late 1830s, when he adapted a mining pump, known as the Cornish engine, for use in the water supply of the East London Waterworks Company.[53] The idea of using a similar technology for sewage disposal first came to him in 1841 while working as a consultant to the city of Berlin. It later featured in Chadwick's plans, which relied on "hygiene by steam power"; but it was the MBW's Main Drainage Scheme that was the first to make extensive use of what became known as "pumping stations." There were four altogether: Deptford (built in 1859–62); Crossness (1862–65); Abbey Mills (1865–68); and Pimlico (1870–74). The stations lifted sewage from lower-level sewers to a point where they could join either higher-level sewers or the outfall sewers directly. Of the four, the most powerful was Abbey Mills. Dubbed "the Cathedral of Sewage," the four-story structure housed eight rotative beam engines of 142 horsepower each, which between them were capable of lifting some fifteen thousand cubic feet of sewage per minute to a height of thirty-six feet (see figure 12).

Pumping stations became the technology of choice, though none matched the scale of those used in London. Built during the late 1860s, Portsmouth's system, which comprised one high- and one low-level main sewer, relied on a single station composed of two twenty-five-horsepower beam engines.[54] Opened in 1891 as part of Leicester's reformed system, the Beaumont Leys Pumping Station housed four engines, which helped to deliver the town's excremental effluence to a neighboring sewage farm.[55] As elsewhere, the options were many, however, and in 1878 Isaac Shone, then mayor of Wrexham in north Wales, presented to the SIGB what would become the principal alternative to steam-powered pumping.[56] Recommended for towns situated on low-lying or unusually level ground, the Shone system relied on pneumatic power, which was compressed at a central hub, and then delivered via pipes to subterranean "ejector" chambers that collected the sewage. Once full, each ejector automatically lifted the sewage a foot or more so

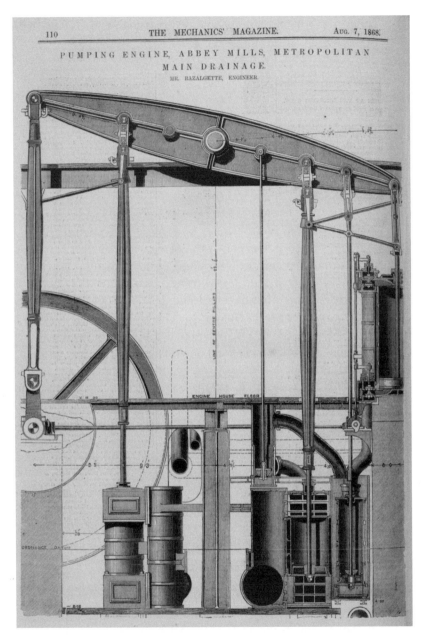

FIGURE 12. A cross-section of the rotative beam engines housed in Abbey Mills Pumping Station. Source: *Mechanics' Magazine*, August 7, 1868, 110. © The Bodleian Libraries, The University of Oxford.

that it could join a higher sewer. Shone was a visionary in the Chadwic-kian mould and he also promoted a more total variant of his system, essentially a pneumatic separate scheme composed of small-bore pipes; but as with Chadwick's arterial-venous system, the skeptics were many and most engineers preferred to rely on Shone-style ejectors only at particular points and places. Besides the Houses of Parliament, where a Shone-style, "hydro-pneumatic system" was installed in 1887, other locations included Eastbourne and Southampton, where ejectors were used in short, low-lying stretches of sewer mains. In fact, the only sig-nificant place that seems to have implemented in full the Shone system was the tide-locked city of Rangoon in British Burma, where some twenty-two "ejector districts" were built between 1888 and 1890.[57]

Such were the principal points of innovation via which human waste was gradually incorporated into the functioning of infrastructural systems of unprecedented complexity and scale. It was a triumph neither of artifice nor of nature, of course, but of both, combined, in a process of system building that mobilized technological (e.g., beam engines and bricks), natural (rainfall and rivers), and human (labor and money) resources. It is a process that might be understood in terms of growing specialization. Certainly the emergence of sanitary engineering as a modern domain of professionalized expertise provided a space where technical developments from home and abroad could be discussed, refined, and implemented. Yet, besides grappling with novel technologies and peculiar geographies, engineers also had to work with multiple other human agents, in particu-lar contractors and their workmen, central officials, and councillors and landowners. As with the building of gas, railway, and telegraphic net-works, the gestation of sewerage systems remained entangled in a dense field of conflicting interests and perspectives.

London's scheme, for instance, was roughly ten years in the making, before it began in earnest under Bazalgette's leadership. His first plans of 1856 were vetoed by the first commissioner of works, Sir Benjamin Hall, who objected to the siting of the outfalls. Only after 1858 was the first commissioner's power of veto withdrawn, essentially giving Bazalgette free rein. Even then contracts had to be drawn up—some twenty-seven in all—and approved by members of the MBW, before being put to ten-der; and problems arose during the course of construction. Besides hav-ing to negotiate the installation of new railway lines—including a fledg-ling London Underground system—prices fluctuated beyond original estimates; contractors went bust; and navvies went on strike. Examples might be multiplied.[58] The LGB sanctioned hundreds of loans every year for sewerage schemes. Yet the sanction of the LGB was not always forthcoming, should one of its inspectors have disagreed with a proposed plan; and the plan itself may have been subject to dispute among councillors and neighboring local authorities. In 1875, a public inquiry was held into plans formulated by Surbiton's improvement commission for a combined sewerage district that encompassed no less than thirty other authorities. Conflicting testimony was received by the chair of the inquiry, the LGB inspector Lieutenant-Colonel Cox, who in the end recommended more limited combinations of five or six local authorities, which is largely what happened.[59]

Protests on the part of councillors and ratepayers were by no means illegitimate. Quite the contrary: struggle of this sort was built into the very structure of England's broadly liberal system of modern center-local relations. The 1875 Public Health Act, for instance, prescribed that sewerage plans had to be published in the local press and served as public notices three months before their projected commencement. Subject to any objections or complications, an LGB inquiry could take place; and they frequently did. The case of Surbiton is one among many: in 1876 alone, more than one hundred inquiries were staged regarding issues such as the formation of sewerage districts, the scale and scope of particular projects, and the compulsory purchase of land.[60]

There were, evidently, various factors in play, from the cost of building new works to local property interests, and even the sheer hassle of engaging in reform. At the same time, however, the water-carriage systems then in the process of being introduced also *created problems of their own*. Put another way, it was not entirely clear that waterborne sewerage systems really did amount to "progress," that all-important and pervasive modern-historical reference point. Grappling with these and other problems ultimately found technological expression at the level of the domestic toilet, as we shall see; but first to the two problems with which—necessarily, technologically, systemically—water closets were connected: sewer gas and the disposal of sewage.

"THE DARKNESS OF DRAINS"

"Present experience shows," noted Latham in his *Sanitary Engineering*, "that there is something in the air of sewers that is dangerous to health."[61] Quite what this "something" amounted to was never quite resolved; but the basic charge that sewerage systems had created a danger in the form of "sewer gas" was widely endorsed. The problem was not entirely new. In 1847, in the course of giving evidence to a royal commission on metropolitan sanitation, Roe condemned existing flat-bottomed brick sewers as "elongated cesspools," fit only for spreading foul air and disease.[62] The distinguishing feature of sewer gas was the scale and complexity of the water-carriage systems that generated it. Of particular importance was the fact that houses were now connected—quite directly, where a connection was made—to expansive networks that carried the waste of thousands of other dwellings. Only a soil pipe stood between the interior of a house and a continual flow of other people's waterborne excreta. As Michelle Allen has argued, whereas the cesspool system was an image of stagnation and disconnection, the waterborne sewerage system was an image of circulation and connection; and both were frightening.[63] "You may abolish cesspits, 'the source of zymotic disease,' from the neighbourhood of your houses by proper sewerage," noted the author of *A Lay Lecture on Sanitary Matters,* "but unless you are guarded against the return into your dwellings of the gases of decomposition from the sewers, you may be worse off than before."[64]

The problem was first brought to professional notice in the early 1850s in a series of reports on an outbreak of "fever" in Croydon, recently sewered under the superintendence of the GBH. One cause among others was a lack of ventilation in the pipes, which meant that there was no escape for foul gases other than through water traps that led directly into houses.[65] The first sustained investigation followed in 1858, when Henry Letheby, MOH to the City of London—and later adversary of the GRO—published a *Report . . . on Sewage and Sewer Gases.*[66] Public attention stirred more slowly, flaring up now and then at the local level during the 1860s; but it assumed national proportions in late 1871, when the Prince of Wales contracted typhoid at Londesborough Lodge, Scarborough, owing, so it was claimed, to defective drainage and sewer gas. "As to risk of fire, in almost every house there are many elements of danger," noted the *Times* in December. "So much for fire," it went on, before turning to the subject of sewer gas: "It is a more terrible . . . and far more insidious danger which now occupies the foreground of public anxiety. It is the pestilence that walketh in darkness— that is to say, in the darkness of drains, traps, pipes, close fittings, abstruse mechanisms, out of reach and out of sight altogether."[67] The winter of 1871–72 represents the high point of public alarm regarding the danger of sewer gas; but it was now established as a matter of ongoing concern, and especially on the part of the middle classes, for it was they who could most afford the new waterborne technologies and the water they required. In 1876, the *Times* once again urged vigilance in order "to keep the enemy at bay." "Each house" in London, it dramatized, was now exposed "to the attacks of the sewage of the whole town."[68] One family's sewer gas was now another's, at least potentially, courtesy of having been technologically networked.

Ultimately, bacteriological research in the 1880s and 1890s brought into question the capacity of sewer gas to cause zymotic diseases, suggesting that the microbial life of sewers was more complex and, in atmospheric terms at least, more salubrious than had hitherto been recognized. MOsH and engineers begged to differ, pointing to the epidemiological evidence that had accrued since the 1860s that suggested a link with infectious diseases such as diphtheria and, most of all, typhoid.[69] Yet these intricate disputes, which at root were methodological, did not matter much in practice. In terms of its chemical composition, all professionals could agree that sewer gas *might* contain sufficient sulfureted hydrogen, carbonic acid, methane, and ammonia to induce some kind of poisoning; and even the bacteriological skeptics acknowledged that sewer gas *might* play a role in "predisposing" the body to attacks of disease. Just as importantly, the public was convinced that it constituted a danger, and it was certainly objectionable from a sensory point of view. It was also a systemic problem, to the extent that it was intrinsic to the functioning of sewerage systems. It was, in short, a perfect nuisance: unsavory, discomforting, and a pervasive and potential threat to health.

It was not, then, a question of eradicating the problem, but of managing and mitigating it as best as possible in the interests of safety and civility. Two key points of regulation emerged (we shall return to water closets below). One was the house and its immediate drainage. Beginning in the 1840s, building bylaws began specifying details such as the fall and form of soil pipes; but it was only with the LGB's model set of bylaws, published in 1877, that arrangements were prescribed that specifically targeted sewer gas.[70] In particular, they specified the use of water traps at the point where house drains connected with sewer mains; and the installation of ventilation mechanisms, one at the point where the drains met the sewer, in the form of a disconnection chamber or grated opening, and another where it joined the house, in the form of a shaft leading up the side of the house to the gable.[71]

The LGB's bylaws became a key point of reference. By 1882, over fifteen hundred local authorities had laws of their own, as approved in Whitehall.[72] Adoption, of course, was by no means synonymous with enforcement. Connections had to be made between house drains and sewer mains, and this could prove sluggish: it took Reading's borough engineer over six years—from 1876 to 1882—to secure the connection of roughly six thousand houses.[73] Equally, a variety of agents much beyond municipal engineers converged on these intricate arrangements, specifying how standards could be met and improved, or else identifying where they had been, or might be, infringed. As we saw in chapter 4, sanitary inspectors chased up details of this sort. Meanwhile, a profusion of handbooks pitched at plumbers and the building trade emerged, among others William Eassie's *Healthy Houses* (1872) and W. H. Corfield's *Dwelling Houses* (1880). They were principally about detailing optimal arrangements of pipes, drains, traps, and shafts, but they also sought to guide their readers through a busy marketplace of products. "There are traps and traps, just as there are watches and watches," noted Eassie's *Healthy Houses,* before discussing the merits of over fifty trapping arrangements in relation to sinks, toilets, and drains.[74] A pamphlet on sewer gas published in 1877 detailed three of these: Weaver's ventilating trap; Bavin's dip trap; and the Registered Interceptor sewer-air trap.[75]

Once installed, none of these elements—pipes, drains, traps, and shafts—necessarily cohered in a systematic fashion. First published in 1878, for instance, T. Pridgin Teale's *Dangers to Health* depicted a range of common defects, including unsyphoned traps, misaligned joints, leaky pipes, and rat-infested floors (see figure 13). The work of sanitary inspectors attests to the prevalence of breakages and blockages, which may or may not have been the product of slipshod "jerry-building." Practices of maintenance and inspection were and would remain crucial. Still more problematic, however, was the other point of anxiety: sewer mains, and in particular their means of ventilation as they coursed beneath streets on their way to the outfalls. The idea was straightforward enough: to relieve pressure on a local system as a whole, so that domestic mechanisms were not the only means of diffusing sewer gas; and to allow for the introduction of fresh air. It was problematic because the solution itself posed problems, at least potentially. The 1875 Public Health Act stated that sewers should be subject to ventilation while also insisting that they should "be kept, so as not to be a nuisance or injurious to health." But as was argued, the former prescription threatened the latter, simply because ventilation meant releasing foul-smelling sewer gas into streets. As one engineer put it in 1882, "as a means for securing that every person passing by shall breathe the

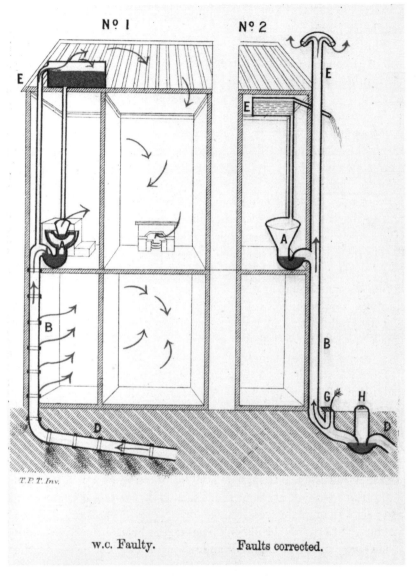

greatest possible amount of poisonous gas, this arrangement [sewer ventilation] is almost perfect."[76]

Ventilation assumed various forms as borough engineers wrestled with this conundrum. The surveys undertaken at the time highlighted three principal methods.[77] One was the installation of shafts leading upward from a sewer to the surface of a roadway, or so-called open or surface ventilation. There were two types: modified manholes incorporating an adjacent shaft, and grated openings. Between 1873 and 1878, Liverpool's engineer installed over seventeen hundred grated shafts along eighty-one miles of the city's sewerage system.[78] In each case there was resort to charcoal on account of its deodorizing qualities. Pioneered by Rawlinson in 1856, the provision within manhole shafts of baskets containing charcoal pellets was widely adopted, as was the use of charcoal trays attached to the underside of grates. Another method first tried by Bazalgette in the mid-1850s, was to install pipes linking the crown of a sewer to nearby factory and workshop chimneys: by 1887, Leicester's borough engineer had managed to erect fifty-two such fittings.[79] The third was ventilation via street lighting. The most elaborate mechanism was the Holman-Keeling sewer gas destructor, first marketed in 1886, which involved the installation of miniature gas burners at the base of similarly gas-powered lamps.

From the start it was a process of trial and error, and each method had its advocates and detractors. A further complication was the atmospheric peculiarities of sewers, which meant it was difficult to generalize about solutions: "every sewer, every section of a sewer," noted Ramsgate's engineer in 1878, "has its own climate; not only in the nature of the gases and the humidity of the air, but in the temperature and the current."[80] In 1897, Birmingham's MOH, Alfred Bostock Hill, pointed to problems with *all* of the methods then in use, noting how sewer gas and related complaints constituted one of his profession's "greatest troubles."[81] Certainly the most popular method was surface ventilation. It had the approval of the LGB and it was also the cheapest and most straightforward; but it was also the most problematic. As early as the 1870s engineers has been abandoning the method owing to public complaints of nuisances, and the practice of closing open ventilators on these grounds gathered pace around the turn of the century.[82] In 1902, Grimsby's borough engineer sent questionnaires to fifty-one local authorities on the subject; of these some thirty-five had abandoned, or were in the process of abandoning, surface ventilation. Instead attention shifted back to two other points in the system: better flushing mechanisms within sewers (see above), and the improvement of chimney and gable shafts running up the sides of houses.[83] A consensus was thus forming by 1900; but as Leicester's borough engineer acknowledged in 1901—himself an advocate of "shaft" as opposed to "open systems"—it remained a most "difficult and perplexing question," and he encouraged more research on the subject.[84]

"THE SEWAGE QUESTION"

Sewer gas was thus one unintended problem generated by the construction of large-scale, waterborne sewerage systems. The other key problem was the very material substance from which these gases emanated: namely "sewage," a term that first emerged in the 1830s.[85] Distinct from the excrement that emptied into cesspools, as well as the rainwater that coursed along natural sewers, this novel substance combined both, plus some other ingredients: household slops, miscellaneous surface waters, and in places industrial effluence. Sewage was an unruly substance in all kinds of ways, besides the gases it created. For one thing, its precise composition varied from town to town, making it difficult to speak of any sort of universal sewage matter. Variables included the size and social makeup of the population; the extent and nature of industrial activities; the quality and quantity of water supply; and average amounts of rainfall. Quite what to do with sewage once it reached an outfall was another matter. By the 1860s, it had become known as "the sewage question," amid routine affirmations of its status as an issue of national importance. "It will be universally conceded that the great national question of the day is the Utilization of Sewage," noted one pamphlet published in 1869.[86] By this point, as noted above, the problem of sewage disposal had already been explored in numerous official and parliamentary investigations; and many more would follow, mixing with a similarly prodigious production of professional comment.

Some expressed bemusement at precisely this: the sheer range of schemes up for grabs in a debate that spilled much beyond the confines of professional associations and official inquiries, entering into council chambers, law courts, and the daily pages of the national and local press. "To attend a meeting of Sewage Doctors, and hear them wrangle and explode each other's doctrines is enough to bewilder any unscientific auditor," noted one self-styled "plain man" in 1872.[87] Yet the stakes were incredibly high, certainly as they were posed during the midcentury. Relieving towns of their miscellaneous dirt promised at least two things. First, it promised some kind of improvement in the moral and physical condition of the working classes, who were otherwise blighted by a careless intimacy with cesspool-based filth. Second, it promised to mitigate river pollution. "Pollution" was variously defined and part of the problem was pinpointing precisely the environmental damage that was being inflicted. It was not until the early 1870s when a workable standard of river purity was officially recommended, and then only after much acrimony.[88] But most were agreed that something had to be done, especially in towns, where factories were relying on watercourses and rivers to dispose of effluence; and/or where water closets had been installed without reforming existing sewer systems that drained into rivers. The Great Stink of London in 1858 is notorious, but other cities were similarly afflicted. In 1840, for instance, the river Aire that flowed through Leeds was described as "a reservoir of poison."[89] The ingredients included refuse from cesspools and water closets, and waste from factories and slaughterhouses, making for a mix of excreta, industrial dyes, chemical soaps, and dead animals.

Sewerage systems and sewage management, however, promised much more besides cleaner rivers and improved death rates and popular habits. They also promised food and a kind of natural efficiency of resource utilization. The premise was simple enough: that sewage, especially human excreta, could function as crop fertilizer, thereby affirming the circular efficiency of nature, where nothing was wasted in a closed system of reciprocal replenishment. As the architectural journal the *Builder* neatly put it in 1875: "The round of Nature is ever a perfect circle. Food makes the muck-heap and the muck-heap makes food."[90] The practice of recycling in this fashion was long established, dating back to the medieval period, and it was still going strong in Europe at the start of the Victorian period: the first report of the Health of Towns Commission (1844) cited evidence from Edinburgh's Craigentinny Meadows and Milan, Italy, where excreta was channeled and applied to outlying fields.[91] Further validation was forthcoming from the emergent discipline of agricultural chemistry, including the much-cited work of the German pioneer Justus von Liebig, which confirmed that human excreta contained much of what was required for plant and crop growth, in particular nitrogenous compounds (especially ammonia), potash, and phosphates. It all seemed to make perfect sense: as the *Builder* further explained, "some great law of nature" was at work, so that "it has been made not only advantageous for us to remove our refuse to the fields, but positively detrimental to our health, and disgusting to our senses, to keep it in the neighbourhood of our houses."[92]

A final twist was the possible economic benefits to be had. In the 1840s British farmers had begun relying on Peruvian guano, essentially solidified bird droppings, and one benefit of putting homemade sewage to agricultural use, so it was argued, would be to enhance national self-sufficiency. Indeed, others suggested sewage utilization put paid to pessimistic Malthusian visions of a structural antagonism between population growth and its means of subsistence; others still, that it struck a blow against the thermodynamic "doctrine of the 'Dissipation of Energy.'"[93] More commonly, advocates simply affirmed how much money was at stake, amid a flurry of numbers detailing the excremental output of the average Englishman and Britain's acreage of underutilized farmland. Calculating the monetary value was tricky, however, since while sewage furnished the right chemical elements (nitrogen, phosphorus) and compounds (potassium chloride), they were mixed in with a mass of unwanted material, principally water. Estimates varied, though most were substantial, fluctuating in the case of London between an annual value of £1 million and upward of £4 million during the early 1860s. Figures at the upper end were sometimes mocked, but the basic premise that sewage represented an untapped source of wealth was widely endorsed. In 1865, one enthusiast noted the progress that had been made by Bazalgette's system and looked forward to the "pellucid river" that would result. Still more satisfaction could be had by thinking of what lay at the outfalls at Barking and Crossness: "a new jewel," as the author put it, "for the civic crown of old LONDINIUM—a mine of gold."[94]

It was thus a compelling mixture of moral, sanitary, and commercial considerations that presided over the first experiments in sewage farming, coupled with utopian visions of plenty and an impulse toward a totally efficient, systematic use of resources. This same impulse had informed Chadwick's arterial-venous system and it inspired a profusion of projects in subsequent decades. In 1876, the LGB undertook a survey of existing methods, listing for the years 1856 to 1875 a total of 417 different sewage treatment patents. Meanwhile, over thirty private companies were established, seeking contracts with local authorities.[95] Two broad systems might be highlighted, both of which were designed to detoxify and utilize sewage, before allowing it to pass into rivers. The first, *irrigation,* was the method endorsed by the GBH and some of the first official inquiries, including the Royal Commission on the Sewage of

Towns (1857–65) and the Select Committee on the Sewage of the Metropolis and Large Towns (1864). For the most part, irrigation involved the use of collecting tanks and the application of sewage over a field via either pipes and hoses, or networks of open conduits. The latter variant came to predominate and was experimented with in various places, including Rugby, Aldershot, and Croydon; and still further variants emerged during the 1870s, such as "intermittent downward filtration," whereby sewage was applied alternately to particular parcels of land. The second principal method, *precipitation,* turned on the application of chemicals to sewage held in tanks, where the valuable constituents were induced to form a seam of sludge, which could then be prepared and sold off as manure. First pioneered in Manchester in 1844, the technique was later adopted in places such as Leicester and Coventry, where the chemical ingredients typically included lime, alum, and iron salts.[96]

The 1876 Rivers Pollution Act provided a statutory push to schemes of this sort by banning the admission of crude, untreated sewage into rivers and streams. Further local initiatives were thus adopted during the late Victorian period, building on what had been achieved by the mid-1870s: in 1878, Rawlinson noted that twenty-three towns and districts had adopted precipitation methods; twenty-four, intermittent filtration; and eighty-seven, broad irrigation.[97] But what, precisely, had been achieved—how much progress really had been made? Assessments were forthcoming on a regular basis, which included résumés of foreign practices. In 1876, the LGB inquired into schemes in Paris, Brussels, and Berlin; a conference organized by the Society of Arts in 1878 even solicited information regarding the systems used in the Chinese cities of Peking and Foochow.[98] The evidence from home was at best mixed. In 1872, Letheby produced a survey which provided a devastating critique of irrigation methods, highlighting their failure to realize a profit and, above all, the nuisance they posed. "The ground, in fact, was everywhere sodden and stinking," he wrote of Aldershot's farm, having detailed how "the great bulk of sewage" was running over the land into a nearby stream, with nothing in the way of purification.[99] Letheby's preference was for precipitation; and yet precipitation was not without its critics, and by the early 1890s this too was being written off as an expensive failure. As another survey concluded in 1892, the sludge it generated made for bad manure, containing on average only one-sixth of the valuable matter contained in sewage, while the effluent water it left behind remained highly impure.[100]

The LGB attempted to diffuse norms of good practice, for instance regarding the amount of land required in relation to the population from which the sewage derived. Yet, as the LGB itself acknowledged, it was difficult to be prescriptive given the number of variables in play, in particular the method used and the quality of sewage.[101] In any case, obtaining the land could prove a struggle, given the assertion of riparian rights on the part of landowners. In 1855, Birmingham's borough surveyor proposed a scheme of irrigation based at Saltley, just east of the center, where the city's nascent sewerage system drained into the river Tame. Then, in 1858, having yet to be developed, local landowner and Tory MP Charles Adderley obtained a court injunction on the grounds of the river pollution that had resulted on his estate in Warwickshire. Irrigation experiments followed; options were explored; private acts were pursued and rejected; further court injunctions were obtained; and it was not until 1875 when Saltley Farm (roughly 270 acres) was fully up and running, though it was soon supplemented in 1881 by a farm in Castle Bromwich (over 800 acres).[102] Examples might be multiplied.[103] In 1868, the aristocratic owner of Esholt Hall, an estate bordering the river Aire roughly four miles below Bradford, obtained an injunction from the Court of Chancery preventing the town's corporation from constructing any further sewers with an outfall into the river Beck (which then flowed into the Aire). In 1872, the council agreed to precipitate the sewage, entering into a contract with the Peat Engineering and Sewage Filtration Company; but the scheme was a financial failure, forcing the council to take charge, and switch from peat charcoal filtration to the use of lime and coke breeze filtration.[104]

Legal disputes and financial failures continued into the late Victorian period, as towns and cities variously refined their methods, took control of private enterprises, or belatedly imposed some form of treatment. Between 1894 and 1903, the journal the *Surveyor and Municipal and County Engineer* detailed more than fifty disputes entertained at various points within the legal system, from county courts to various divisions of the High Court.[105] It was grist to the mill of skeptics, whose voices had been heard since the 1860s, when a handful of chemists and engineers had suggested that in most cases sewage contained too much water to render utilization either profitable or desirable. Various crops were tried, but experience showed that only rye grass and in places cabbage and mangold wurzel really prospered in sewage-ridden soil. Farmers spoke up now and then to ridicule the utopian fantasies which, quite rightly, they sensed inspired some of the projects.[106]

Profit and utilization versus purification at ratepayer expense: the sewage question was sometimes posed in this bald fashion, and by the mid-1870s opinions were beginning to harden in favor of the latter. "The fact is, sewage is of great theoretical value, but not a commercial value," declared one speaker at a meeting of AMSES in 1874, urging his fellow engineering professionals to opt only for "such expense as is necessary for purification . . . and get rid of the sewage in the cheapest way."[107] Advocates of utilization died hard, however. In 1884, a royal commission on London's sewage disposal distinguished between six different schemes, which included relocating the outfalls lower down the Thames. It disregarded broad irrigation on the grounds of the amount of land required and the cost and legal difficulties in getting hold of it; but as critics of the royal commission noted, the example of Berlin, home to Europe's biggest sewage farms by this point, extending over ten thousand acres, suggested the success of such schemes.[108] In the end, the commission endorsed land filtration supplemented by precipitation, amid decidedly less speculation regarding the monetary value of sewage.

It is no surprise that coastal towns opted to dump their sewage in the sea, or that some major cities decided to opt for alternative systems that avoided the large-scale production of sewage, as we shall see. During the 1890s, however, a solution was found in the "biological agency" of bacteria. Bacteria, of course, had always been purifying sewage somewhere, facilitating a process of nitrification, whereby ammonia was converted into nitrate. The mid-Victorians largely understood this as a chemical process of oxidation, and it was only during the 1870s and 1880s when researchers in France, Germany, Britain, and the United States began to appreciate the role of micro-organisms. A new premise thus emerged, namely that successful sewage treatment turned on the active facilitation of the agency of bacteria.[109] The technical details were subject to experimentation and there were those who remained wedded to methods of land filtration; but the basic premise was gradually accepted. In 1898, a Royal Commission on Sewage Disposal was convened, and in 1908 its fifth report concluded: "There is no essential difference between the two processes [land treatment and artificial filters] . . . for in each case the purification, so far as it is not mechanical, is chiefly effected by means of micro-organisms."[110]

Crudely, two sets of practices were pioneered.[111] One of these was designed to concentrate the work of anaerobic bacteria, principally using large tanks that shut out air and light. Key innovations included the "cultivation tank" designed by the engineer W. D. Scott-Moncrieff at Ashtead, Surrey, where sewage was admitted from below before passing upward over a bed of stones; the "septic tank," pioneered by Donald Cameron, Exeter's borough surveyor in 1895, which collected sewage and allowed it to stand; and the German-made Imhoff tank, patented in 1906, essentially an improved, two-story variant of Cameron's invention. The other set of practices developed out of experiments in land filtration, and were designed to cultivate the work of aerobic bacteria. Crucial here was the research undertaken by the Lawrence Station in the state of Massachusetts, and by William Dibdin at Barking Creek during his time as chief chemist of the MBW and then the LCC. The former led to the development of the "trickling filter," while Dibdin pioneered the "contact bed," each variants of a method that turned upon the passage of sewage through two or three aerating filter beds composed of materials of varying granularity, such as coke breeze, clinker, and sand. In England, the first major experiments were inaugurated in 1896 by Dibdin at Sutton, Surrey, which quickly became a translocal model of emulation. Dubbed "the Mecca of sanitary engineers," the so-called Sutton system was visited by 305 deputations in 1898 alone, principally from Britain, but including interested parties from India, New Zealand, Belgium, and Austria.[112] Further experiments followed at Sutton and elsewhere; but as one engineering handbook noted in 1902, the method had "revolutionized" waste disposal practices, and it was eventually endorsed by the LGB.[113]

At last, then, by the early twentieth century, a new consensus was beginning to emerge based on the amplification and management of microbiological processes. The ideal of utilization, which had been dominant in the 1860s and 1870s, was now retreating to the margins of professional opinion. An element of clarity had been injected into the sewage question, and it was much needed. Perhaps in towns and cities it might have been clear that *something* had to be done; yet quite what this should be was decidedly less so. It was not easy being a local councillor in these circumstances. Even professionals sympathized. "The difficulties which present themselves to an average representative of the people . . . are many and weighty," noted Halifax's public analyst in 1897:

> He is called upon to go in for an undertaking of enormous cost; he has no guarantee that it will be an unqualified success when finished, especially in face of the numerous failures he has heard of; he does not understand the details of competing systems, which require a combination of engineer and chemist to weigh them up; and he is further disturbed by the knowledge that when everything has been done that reasonable beings might expect, the effluent from the

sewage works, which he has watched growing with so much anxiety, may not be regarded as satisfactory by the ruling powers [the LGB].[114]

And yet the sewage question, for all its own considerable intricacies, was still more complex, for it was impossible to disentangle from some of the other technological considerations examined so far. A crucial argument in favor of separate systems, for instance, was that they minimized the amount of rainfall allowed to mix with domestic waste, thereby making for more predictable, manageable amounts of sewage further along the systemic line at the outfall. Equally, a particular council might choose not to generate waterborne sewage in the first place and to opt instead for alternatives to the water closet. And there were many alternative systems, as we shall now see.

TOILETRY TECHNOLOGIES

Sewage disposal doubled as a moral problem, to the extent that it raised questions about the overall design of nature—or "Nature"—which for most was designed by a more or less distant God.[115] Of all the points in any given waste disposal system, however, it was the toilet that was charged with reforming personal habits. It is here where we find a lonely point of long-standing consensus: simply that the toilet should be a private technology. It was the urban poor who suffered most in this respect. The location of privies varied, as did housing arrangements more generally, which included cellar dwellings and partitioned town houses; but the most common arrangement was the inward-looking, horseshoe-shaped "court," where one or two communal privies—as well as a standpipe for water—were situated near to the entrance.[116] Intense public scrutiny began in the 1830s: if the Manchester Statistical Society was the first to detail ratios of inhabitants to beds, which it did in a landmark survey conducted between 1834 and 1838, then it was Leeds town council that was the first to detail ratios of inhabitants to privy middens.[117] In 1839, it revealed that in one of the city's poorest wards there were but two "offices" serving more than four hundred inhabitants; in another only one privy midden to fifty persons.[118] It was only the beginning, of course: the moral and physical problem of court-based promiscuity became an item of recurrent description in the Victorian period, as officials, journalists, and civic activists (clergymen and doctors especially) evoked gruesome scenes of pent-up bodies and a miscellaneous mess of surface liquids and solids.

The extra provision of toiletry technologies was thus conceived as part of a broader assault on the overcrowded and filth-ridden state of working-class districts, especially back-to-back courts. There was no question of seeking to democratize the kind of convenience that was now a common feature of upper- and middle-class dwellings, where at least two toilets—one for the family and one for the servants—could be found, each forming a discrete space within the confines of a large domestic interior. Even so, as early as the 1840s, one toilet per dwelling was generally thought of as a minimum requirement, at least where it was possible to erect new houses from scratch. Few, at any rate, disputed the assumption that, besides improving health, toilets had a role to play in civilizing the poor.

Privatizing defecation en masse proceeded sluggishly, as part of a broader set of struggles concerning the resolution of what, by the 1880s, was being dubbed the "housing problem."[119] In the absence of any substantive capital input from either philanthropic associations or councils, it was largely left to bylaws and ad hoc regulatory initiatives to do the work. Early efforts included the simple expedient of furnishing lockable doors: in 1842, Leeds corporation introduced regulations relating to new back-to-back courts, which were to provide one privy per five households, coupled with a corresponding distribution of keys.[120] Similarly, in 1869, Manchester city's health committee commenced a program of renovation which included roofing over existing privies, refitting doors, and attaching locks.[121] Building bylaws further encouraged privatized practices. The regional variations that emerged have been documented at length, ranging from the two-story flats of Tyneside to the "two-up, two-down" terraces of the Midlands and the Northwest; but as Martin Daunton has detailed, there was a broad shift towards enclosed, self-sufficient dwellings and the greater provision of toilets.[122] In 1864, Liverpool prohibited the building of back-to-back courts, paving the way to the construction of terraced houses with a toilet situated in the backyard; and other towns followed suit, including Nottingham in 1874 and Birmingham in 1876. Elsewhere, modified back-to-back arrangements emerged, notably in Leeds, where, in the absence of a backyard, toilets were placed in basements. The LGB's model bylaws provided some official input. Whether situated inside or outside, any toilet had to be housed within a structure that incorporated a "window of at least two feet by one foot" and that provided "adequate means of constant ventilation by at least one air-brick."[123]

The persistence of inner-city courts and slum property meant there were still pockets of crowded communal facilities in the Edwardian period (and beyond): in 1904, for instance, it was revealed that in the center of Manchester a block of forty back-to-back houses shared only six closets.[124] In the meantime, however, the number of toiletry systems on offer had undergone a bewildering expansion. The official line was that water closets constituted the best option. In 1852, the GBH recommended the water closet as a key component of its tubular system, and the technology was subsequently endorsed by the MDPC, the Rivers Pollution Commission (1868–74), and the LGB. The rationale was straightforward: water closets disposed of excreta in an expeditious fashion, removing what, in a domestic context, was a disgusting and potentially disease-inducing substance. Civility and health were both a matter of speed in this respect. As Latham put it in his *Sanitary Engineering,* a "good water-closet is the only appliance fit to be used within a house, for by it all matters are at once conveyed away, and cease to have the power of producing evil."[125] Bazalgette's London led the way, and by the mid-1870s there were over 700,000 in use serving a population of over 3.5 million. Wealthy towns in particular might be especially well served by this point: in 1876, Harrogate was home to roughly 1,500 houses and 1,620 water closets; Cheltenham 8,725 and 8,500, respectively.[126]

Opinions were decidedly more mixed beyond central offices. The problem was partly one of *interconnection,* and the fact that water closets relied on the successful functioning of the other parts of any given waterborne system, not least domestic drains, street sewers, and outfall works. And yet, as the previous sections have detailed, quite how to manage each point without creating further problems was far from clear. Equally, water closets demanded an adequate water supply; tenants or landlords who could afford the water they required; and a more careful, conscientious population, for they were decidedly more complex than privy middens. The result was a fractious debate which lasted from the 1860s through to the 1890s regarding the best kind of toiletry technology and accompanying system. In 1880, AMSES heard from one borough engineer who feared to broach the question of water-closet waste: "the subject as a system is a red rag, and has been thrashed threadbare."[127] For some, water closets indeed represented the very opposite of progress: a move backward rather than forward. "Of all our domestic institutions," noted one pamphlet published in 1884, "the water-closet system is the most extravagant, the most wasteful and the most dangerous to human life."[128] Entitled *The Difficult and Vexed Question of the Age,* the author objected to sewer gas and, above all, the generation of sewage. One kind of pollution had simply been replaced by another: a technologized, waterborne variant for a stagnating, cesspool-based variant.

The most sophisticated alternative was the Liernur system pioneered during the 1860s by the Dutch engineer of the same name. Much like Isaac Shone's later schemes, it relied on pneumatic power, and separated rainwater from household slops and excreta; but here houses were equipped with "air closets" connected to steam-powered, vacuum-sucking street reservoirs, which in turn pumped the excreta to "decanting stations," where it was deposited in barrels and delivered to outlying fields. Ultimately, despite finding favor in cities such as Amsterdam and Prague, the system failed to attract any business in England, and in 1876 it was dismissed by the LGB as a "costly toy."[129] This was not for want of trying. In 1867, one advocate published an extensive promotional treatise rubbishing the waterborne schemes of Chadwick and Bazalgette; and Liernur himself visited Liverpool in 1874, where he was interviewed by members of the city's health committee.[130] Nor indeed was it for want of wishful thinking: "We are evidently on the point of arriving at the conclusion that water-closets are too costly and too dangerous to be any longer tolerated," noted one enthused Liernurean convert in the same year.[131]

At the other end of the scale of technological complexity was the earth closet, first patented by the Dorsetshire vicar Henry Moule in 1860. In essence, it involved updating the much-derided cesspool, and placing it on a more environmentally sustainable basis; or in practice, collecting excrement in a moveable pan or brick-built vault and covering it with dried earth dispensed from a container; and then applying the resulting manure to small plots of land or selling it to farmers. Variants emerged as commercial manufacturers reworked the basic design, including Moule's own Patent Earth Closet Company, and later models featured handle-activated earth dispensers.[132] It was principally used in small towns and villages. Letheby's survey of 1872 noted that in Lancaster some ninety earth closets were in place, serving roughly 450 houses. Otherwise they were adopted by disciplinary institutions, such as workhouses and barracks: indeed, they became the technology of choice for Britain's armed forces serving in the Raj, where they were first introduced in 1865.[133] Critics made the point that Moule's closet was unsuited to urban areas, where there was a lack of readily available earth. Proponents countered by advocating the intervention of private enterprise to make the system feasible in towns and affirming the "natural" efficiency of returning excrement to the soil, unsullied by the addition of water. Most advocates gave up on the prospect of seeing them used in towns, but they were still being promoted for use in rural areas in the 1890s.[134]

The same modern desire informed the very different systems of Liernur and Moule: namely, that it was possible to combine human habits and material technologies so that nothing was wasted in perfectly profitable, systematic cycles of use and reuse—the same totalizing urge that had earlier animated Chadwick's vision. In theory, there was no such thing as "dirt," only matter forever assuming new and useful forms. Like others at the time, Liernur's system promised an end to Malthusian struggles. Moule even suggested that the sale of manure would yield sufficient profits to abolish local taxation.[135] For the majority of engineers, MOsH, and councillors, however, the real battle was between water-closet systems and a clutch of "conservancy systems," similar to Moule's closets, but relying on substances other than earth and the work of municipal collection teams and refuse works (see final section). These, too, were an intermediate solution between the cesspool and the water closet, at least in terms of the concentration of waste matter and the speed of removal.

One variant was the practice of applying ash to a small cesspool, or ashpit, lined with cement or flag stones, and shared by two to six privies. Ash was a readily available by-product of domestic coal fires, and ashpit closets were installed both in existing courts and new builds. A variant was introduced in Manchester during the 1860s, where the ash was administered via an attached bin and shoot; shared by two privies, the ashpit was then emptied every three months. In Hull, where collection was weekly, a miniature brick receptacle was situated beneath the toilet seat and the ash was applied using a hand-held scoop. Ashpit closets were still being installed in northeastern towns in the 1890s: as late as 1913, Gateshead was home to roughly eighteen thousand ashpits compared to eighteen hundred privy middens and five thousand water closets.[136]

More popular was the use of pail closets, which were not without precedent abroad. In 1850, the GBH published a report on Paris's cesspool system, where use was made of moveable tanks and barrels.[137] The Parisian example seems to have been disregarded; but certainly the first experiments in England drew on French practices, in particular a method pioneered by Pierre Nicholas Goux, a landowner based near Paris, which involved using small wooden tubs lined with absorbent

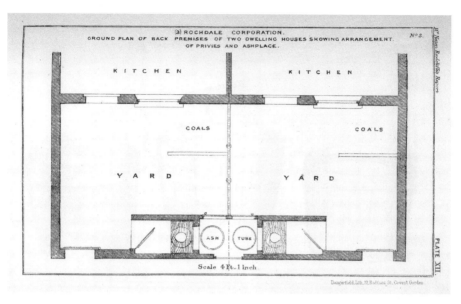

FIGURE 14. Ground plan of the Rochdale pail-closet system. (See figure 15 caption for the source.) © The Bodleian Libraries, The University of Oxford.

materials, such as sawdust or dry peat. Goux's absorbent closet system was patented in 1868 and trialed in Rochdale in the same year, where the tubs were subject to weekly removal. But while weekly removal was judged a success, Rochdale's corporation abandoned the use of Goux's absorbent lining, opting instead to provide two pails per house, one for excreta, the other for house refuse. Each tub was made of a paraffin cask cut in two and provided with handles and airtight covers; only Halifax persisted with Goux's method, where it was introduced in 1869 (see figures 14 and 15).[138]

Variants of the so-called Rochdale system were adopted in a number of manufacturing towns in the Midlands and the North, including Nottingham, Leicester, Blackburn, and Warrington, and exclusively in working-class districts. "This appears to be the principle," noted one borough engineer: "the rich man should have the water-closet, the poor man the pail."[139] In 1873, Birmingham began a process of conversion, and by 1877 there were over twenty thousand pail closets compared to roughly seventy-five hundred water closets, nineteen thousand ashpits, and twenty-seven thousand unreformed privy middens; more followed, as pail closets became the dominant technology in the early 1880s.[140] Manchester was quicker still. In 1871, the council opted for iron pails,

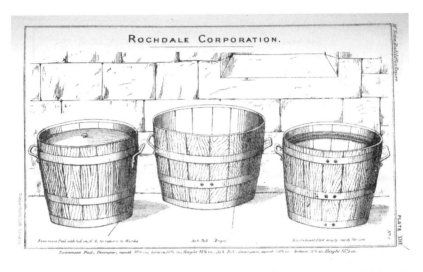

FIGURE 15. A Rochdale ash tub; and on either side an excrement pail with lid (left) and without (right). Source: *Reports of the Medical Officer of the Privy Council and Local Government Board*, new series, no. 2, C. 1066 (1874), 236. © The Bodleian Libraries, The University of Oxford.

coupled here with the addition of ash in the interests of deodorization; and by 1879 the number stood at fifty-two thousand.[141] Overall, by the 1890s, more than thirty urban centers had some form of "dry" provision: one estimate made in 1895 suggested that in fifteen of these, home to some 2.6 million inhabitants, there were roughly 230,000 pail closets compared to 135,000 water closets and 90,000 privy middens.[142]

It seems the majority of local engineers adopted a pragmatic approach. The first official survey of dry methods, which was carried out by the MDPC in 1869, weighed up the pros and cons of pail closets, something that formed a staple feature of subsequent assessments.[143] Most could agree that pail closets were an improvement on midden systems and cesspools, principally because they allowed for the regular removal of excreta. Death rates at least were quoted to this effect. Meanwhile, there was some agreement that much depended on local circumstances, including adequate water supplies and the proximity of rivers to receive sewage. In 1878, Rochdale's borough engineer, Thomas Hewson, spoke before AMSES, where he was forced to defend the town's pail system. "The question to a large extent hinged on the supply of water and the condition of the sewer outfall works," argued Warrington's engineer in the discussion that followed. Hewson agreed: "It was all very well for gentlemen, who were the representatives of towns where there were large tidal rivers, to speak of the nastiness of the pail system, but let them go into the North of England where town upon town was land-locked, and the operatives heaped and pent." In the circumstances it constituted a definite advance on midden systems.[144]

Equally, it was difficult being pragmatic, for if the considerations were at once multiple and place-specific, then the proposed solutions were at once many and contested; and in the 1860s and 1870s these (contested) solutions were growing in number. Manchester is a case in point.[145] In June 1869, the city's town clerk, Joseph Heron, was called to give evidence to the Royal Sanitary Commission, where he explained the council's reluctance to expand the city's modest system of natural and artificial sewers that drained into the river Irwell. The pollution was bad enough and would only be made worse by sewage farming ("irriga-tion"), for which, in any case, there was no readily available land.[146] Heron was speaking in the wake of a heated debate that had taken place only months earlier within the MSSA. Contributions were heard in favor of water closets, but the majority were opposed. In one review, entitled "Principal Systems Proposed or Adopted," which included the systems of Moule and Liernur, the MOH for Salford concluded in favor of move-able boxes. The danger of sewer gas was his principal objection to water closets: "No trapping will thoroughly overcome this evil."[147] Another contributor, in a paper entitled *The High Death Rate: An Answer to the Question, What Is to Be Done?* argued that a "greater objection" remained in the form of river pollution, a point he embellished by high-lighting the failure of existing schemes of sewage recycling.[148]

Conversely, a number of engineers and MOsH toed a hard line, opposing pail closets regardless of local circumstances. Angell, as presi-dent of AMSES, denounced them "as completely as possible," simply because they allowed excreta to remain on household premises.[149] Yet, besides the problems posed by sewage, the pro-water-closet case was hampered by the closets themselves. Pioneered during the late eight-eenth century, two principal models dominated during the first half of the nineteenth: the pan closet and the valve closet. Both drew on over-head cisterns and were complex devices.[150] Pan closets consisted of an earthenware basin attached to a shallow copper pan containing water. Once activated by a handle, the pan dropped its contents into a lower cast-iron receptacle, which was attached to the drains via a so-called D-trap and soil pipe. Valve closets were still more elaborate, consisting of a bowl with an opening at the bottom sealed by a valve, which opened into a pipe leading to an S-shaped siphon trap. When flushing took place, the combined action of a handle, lever, wires, and counterweights temporarily removed the valve while admitting water from the cistern. Of the two, the cheapest and most popular was the pan closet, but it was also the most defective. Like the valve closet, it was difficult to repair (in both cases the traps were installed beneath floors); added to which was the tendency of the D-trap to clog. The GBH was among the early critics, and the number grew substantially during the 1870s, amid the growing anxieties surrounding sewer gas noted above. "The 'puffs' of bad smells which such apparatus [pan closets] send up, after they have been fixed for some time, are enough to make one wish for the old-established privy again," noted the manufacturer S. Stevens Hellyer in his best-selling *The Plumber and Sanitary Houses*, first published in 1877.[151] Advocates of dry technologies had pointed to these defects; and in the case of pan closets, water-carriage enthusiasts only could agree. Such was the degree of consensus that the notorious D-trap arrangement was banned by the LGB's model bylaws.

Commercial agents proved both a hindrance and a help in this respect. On the one hand, defective models such as the pan closet continued to be marketed into the late nineteenth century, as manufacturers exploited middle-class demand for familiar technologies. On the other, it was the very same manufacturers that were responsible for the improvements that took place, as they fought for trade in an increasingly crowded and global marketplace. Excluding U.S. innovations, between 1872 and 1914 over 150 patents were secured for different models of water closet, which included improved valve closets.[152] Ultimately, the model that would come to dominate in the twentieth century was the wash-down closet that combined a basin and a trap in a single piece of glazed earthenware, leading to an S-shaped curve. It entered the market in the 1880s and in essence was a combination of two earlier innovations: valveless, single-piece hopper closets, comprising a funnel-like pan attached to a water-sealed trap; and similarly valveless wash-out closets, where a shallow pool of water in the main bowl was separated by a lip from an S-shaped trap below. Wash-down closets, such Humpherson and Co.'s Beaufort model (1885) and Twyford's Deluge (1887), were not an immediate success, and it would not be until the interwar period when they became the dominant appliance; but by the 1890s they were being widely praised as the best on the market. In 1896, one of Manchester's senior sanitary inspectors addressed a meeting of colleagues and councillors with a talk called "Drainage and

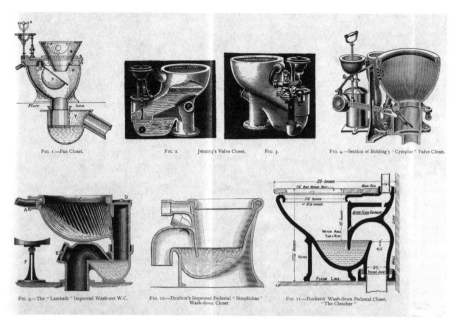

FIGURE 16. A selection of some of the principal water closets in use at the turn of the century, beginning with the pan-closet model, top left, passing clockwise through two valve-closets, two wash-down, and one wash-out. Source: Colonel E. C. S. Moore, *Sanitary Engineering: A Practical Treatise on the Collection, Removal and Final Disposal of Sewage*, 2nd ed. (London: B. T. Batsford, 1901), 316–17. © The Bodleian Libraries, The University of Oxford.

Plumbing: Past, Present and Future." He began with valve and pan closets ("diabolical infernal machines"), and ended with the wash-down model, which he described as "the most perfect closet of the present day": it was simple, cheap, and guaranteed a reliable, scouring flush (see figure 16).[153]

Pan, hopper, valve, and wash-out closets: all of these and more jostled for attention prior to the ascendancy of the wash-down model, and further variants included those installed in working-class districts. As even advocates acknowledged, the relative complexity of water-closet technologies made them more vulnerable to negligence. "In the crowded districts of a large town," noted one MOH in 1877, "the ordinary form of water-closets [valve-closets] have proved a failure, partly on account of the complicated character of the contrivances for flushing, but chiefly on account of the carelessness and filthy habits of the poorer classes."[154] This was part of the rationale for placing water closets in a backyard, where any blockages or leaks would cause less damage to health and property; but it also spurred the redesign of closets and various local experiments. Relatively simple, valveless hopper closets pioneered during the 1840s had been designed to overcome this; and further variants were endorsed by the GBH in 1852, along with other pared-down technologies.[155] Other arrangements simplified still further, even doing away with the need for manual flushing. In the 1860s Liverpool's council experimented with the use of trough closets, which consisted of a series of partitioned units placed over a sloping, water-charged channel, at the end of which was a plug (administered by a refuse collector) that allowed the contents to be emptied into the city's sewerage system. By 1869 more than two thousand were in use in the city's crowded courts.[156] A more popular variant was the slop-closet system, patented in 1874 by Salford's borough engineer, Alfred Fowler (later president of AMSES), which also did away with the need for a water-mains connection. Instead, it mobilized domestic slops and rainwater, which were drained toward a stoneware pan, or tipper basin, situated beneath a closet in the backyard. Once full, the pan tipped over, sending a flush of water along a pipe that washed the excreta through a trap. Variants of the slop closet were especially popular in northern towns such as Salford, Blackburn, Bradford, and Newcastle (see figure 17). In 1891, a report commissioned by the LGB to investigate their merits noted that some forty-three hundred were in use in Burnley, out of a total of nineteen thousand closets and privies.[157]

Variations of technology thus increased rather than diminished during the latter decades of the century, and were at their peak in the 1890s, when conservancy systems had become an established—if class-specific—alternative to waterborne systems, and most of all in northern towns. It was at this point, however, when professional opinion began to turn decisively against conservancy systems, including among MOsH, who up to this point seem only to have provided reluctant endorsements. Leading officers such as Alfred Bostock Hill (Birmingham), Philip Boobbyer (Nottingham), and John Tatham (Manchester) published evidence showing a higher incidence of zymotic diseases, and especially typhoid, in pail-closet districts compared to those with water closets.[158] Opinions among engineers were also beginning to turn. The "North of England generally is much behind the times in regard to the question of the satisfactory removal of excreta," stated one primer on refuse disposal published in 1898 by William Maxwell, assistant engineer to London's Leyton district. He looked forward to the point when pails and the like

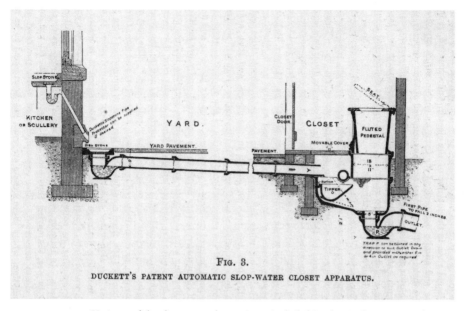

FIGURE 17. Variants of the slop water-closet system included Duckett's closet, pictured here, and another one pioneered in the railway town of Crewe. Source: William H. Maxwell, *The Removal and Disposal of Town Refuse* (London: Sanitary Publishing Company, 1898), 62. © The Bodleian Libraries, The University of Oxford.

would be "remembered only as curious bits of ancient history."[159] During the 1860s and 1870s, conservancy systems had seemed otherwise: a means of progress given the circumstances, and the expense and problems associated with water-closet systems. "Water-carriage is now, without exception, regarded as the *best,* and in fact the only, system that can be adopted for large (or even moderate sized) towns, ensuring, as it does, greater health, cleanliness, and convenience to the inhabitants accommodated," Maxwell went on, though not before noting the "good deal of controversy" the problem had generated.[160]

Only in the interwar period did water closets become the standard technology among England's working classes. This coincided with a broader expansion of sewerage and water-supply systems, both within urban areas and beyond, in rural districts. As before, getting connected took time and was partly complicated by the resistance of landlords. In Manchester, for instance, the decision by the Tory-led council in 1892 to convert to water-carriage provision for all classes was opposed by the Manchester, Salford and District Property Association on account of the costs involved. The dispute rumbled on into the early twentieth century, despite the council agreeing in 1901 to provide subsidies at two pounds ten shillings per closet.[161] Nonetheless, a technological-systemic threshold had been passed by roughly 1900. Even if circumstances might dictate otherwise here and there, all professionals could now agree that, in principle, water closets were the way forward.

REFUSE MANAGEMENT

The final node in any domestic waste disposal system was the local dust depot or refuse works under the charge of either a borough engineer or, in major cities, one of a new class of cleansing superintendents that began to emerge in the 1870s. The advent of municipal control meant the eclipse of the dust contractors and farmers that had previously been enlisted to scavenge dwellings and streets. Most towns and cities made the switch in the 1870s and 1880s, with only a handful holding out for longer: it was not until 1892, for instance, when Bristol corporation took full charge of the city's refuse disposal, opening a depot in the same year.[162] All depots dealt with "house refuse," a new substance made possible by its differentiation from excreta; but they also managed what statute law began to distinguish as "trade" and "street refuse." It was no less of a logistical challenge than dealing with growing volumes of excreta. Combined, the amounts were enormous: in 1887, Liverpool generated some 238,711 tons of refuse; in 1890, it was estimated that London's annual total topped 2,200,000 cubic yards.[163] Much as with sewage, the composition of house refuse was meticulously detailed and standard ingredients included breeze (cinders and ash); hard core (bottles, bones, crockery, and metal pots); and soft core (animal and vegetable matter, paper, and textiles). Quite what happened at the refuse depot depended on the choices made elsewhere in any local system. In 1888, one of the LGB's engineering inspectors, Thomas Codrington, published a survey that distinguished between works employed in water-closet towns, and those in ashpit and pail-closet towns, where excreta had to be dealt with as well.[164] Yet, the persistence of privy middens in water-closet towns meant that all depots had to deal with excrement, however modest the amount; and all towns were home to streets and thoroughfares littered with horse dung.

Collecting refuse was the least troublesome aspect: a question of combining hardy men and horse-drawn carts—and shovels, where necessary. In 1881, Exeter's borough engineer published one of the first specialist texts on the subject, *Dirty Dustbins and Sloppy Streets,* which distinguished between three systems: house-to-house visitation, which entailed knocking at doors; the emptying of large, wooden public bins into which tenants emptied their own; and the more popular signal system, which involved alerting residents by ringing a bell or one of the scavengers crying, "Dust oh!"[165] It was dirty work, but it was helped by the regulation of waste receptacles. The ashpits noted in the previous section furnished a repository for house refuse, and bylaws duly prescribed standards of construction: the LGB's model set of 1877 prescribed that no new ashpit should hold more than six cubic feet of rubbish.[166] The alternatives were many in water-closeted homes, including hooped wooden tubs and baskets lined with tin. The state of the art at the end of the century was the dustbin made of galvanized iron: bylaws issued by the LCC in 1893 insisted that all domestic dustbins had to be made of metal, provided with an airtight cover, and provide for no more than two cubic feet of refuse.[167]

The key problem was disposal. The options varied and not all of them involved sophisticated technological fixes. Quite the contrary: land-tipping was widely practiced and served as the default option for most local authorities. In 1902, it was noted that more than eight hundred authorities in England land-tipped the majority of their refuse, including major cities such as Sheffield, which at this point annually tipped somewhere in the region of a hundred thousand tons.[168] A further variant was to dispose of it at sea, should a town be suitably located. In Liverpool, two steam barges were employed, which in 1887 dumped over eighty-nine thousand tons of refuse some eleven miles beyond the bar of the river Mersey.[169] Equally, towns continued to recycle the refuse they collected, albeit on a grander scale. In cities, most dust depots were situated near a wharf on a river or a canal, where the waste, once manually sorted, could be transported by barge; otherwise it was carried away again in horse-drawn carts. Generally, where a market could be found, breeze went to brick makers; hard core to road contractors; and soft core to market gardeners and farmers.

Besides the number of people served, the scale and sophistication of these operations was also determined by the kind of matter collected. In particular, towns with a significant number of pail closets required some means of turning bucket-bound sludge into something useful: or more precisely, of manufacturing saleable substances for use in agriculture—the "dry" analog of farming the sewage generated by water-closet systems. It is fitting that it was in the industrial center of Manchester where the country's largest municipal manufactory of this sort emerged. In

1878, the corporation supplemented its existing Water Street depot, situated by the city's gas works, with a new six-acre complex known as the Holt Town Works. The main building comprised three floors, the bottom of which contained eighteen steam-powered "concentrators," where the excreta from pails was collected, raised to about boiling point, and reduced to a fine fertilizing powder. It was then transferred to the top floor, adjacent to a branch line of the Lancashire and Yorkshire Railway, where it was bagged and loaded onto trains for dispatch around the country. Meanwhile, the Water Street depot generated old-fashioned manure, which was sent by rail and boat to a thousand-acre site at Carrington Moss, southwest of the city center, where it was put to agricultural use.[170] By 1886, the city council was employing over 500 men and footing the bill for 275 horses, 100 railway wagons, and 100 collection carts.[171]

Of the two methods, recycling and tipping, it was the latter that was the most obviously offensive. Besides wasting matter that might be put to better use, tipping entailed land tips, and so rats, flies, and unwholesome smells that drifted over neighboring properties; and if sea-tipping was judged more sanitary in this respect, it came with its own risks. In the 1890s, Liverpool's refuse washed up now and then on the North Wales coast.[172] The defense was that tipping was the only practical means of disposing of growing volumes of refuse, but for some it was a "primitive," nuisance-generating throwback. "Tipping has been rightly styled a wretched relic of antiquity," noted one engineer in 1901, "a miserable link with the insanitary past."[173] Ironically, however, it was another method which also claimed a long historical pedigree that emerged as the principal site of technological innovation: destroying by fire, or "refuse destruction." The first destructor technology was pioneered in 1874 by Alfred Fryer of the engineering company, Manlove and Alliott, based in Nottingham. Variants of Fryer's model typically consisted of a block of back-to-back furnaces or cells (see figure 18). Refuse was tipped into a cell through a shoot, from where it was raked over a hearth and firebars, before being pushed into the furnace proper. Doors were attached for the extraction of clinker (a stony residue) at the firebar stage, as well as the insertion of items such as infected mattresses and condemned meat. Finally, each cell contained a main flue, which joined with others, before passing to a chimney of anything between eighty and two hundred feet high.

In 1876, Manchester's Water Street depot became the first municipal works to incorporate a Fryer destructor in what quickly developed into

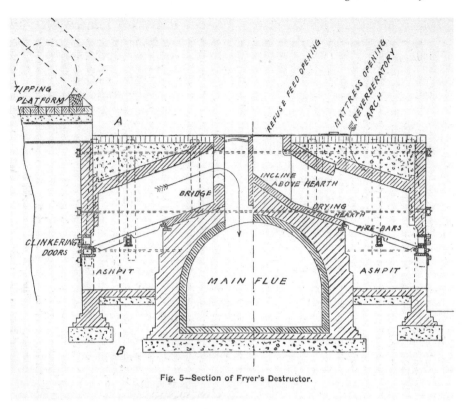

Fig. 5—Section of Fryer's Destructor.

FIGURE 18. A cross-section of Fryer's destructor. Source: William H. Maxwell, *The Removal and Disposal of Town Refuse* (London: Sanitary Publishing Company, 1898), 91. © The Bodleian Libraries, The University of Oxford.

a crowded marketplace of models, each distinguished by the temperatures at which they operated (upward of two thousand degrees Fahrenheit by 1900), and the design and integration of their components. Healey's destructor (patented in 1880), Warner's Perfectus (1888), and Hart and Royle's Acme (1892) were among the dozen or so on offer at the turn of the century.[174] The virtues of destructors were many: they reduced the load that had to be tipped in a speedy fashion; eliminated much of the manual sorting of refuse, which some considered disgusting; and were relatively cheap compared to the costs of generating manure, the demand for which, in any case, was variable. "No one will dispute the fact that destructors properly worked are a great improvement on the existing alternative systems of dust disposal," stated the *BMJ* in 1893, arguing that the days when tipping and filling in land might be considered acceptable had passed.[175] At this point, some forty sanitary authorities had adopted destructors; just ten years later in 1903 they were in use in 180 towns and cities.

Destructors were thus part of the settlement of waste-disposal technologies that was taking shape at the start of the Edwardian period. Their rise was certainly rapid, if not without dispute, professional and popular. This was mainly on account of the chimney-funneled smoke they generated. "Such fires, though doing something to lessen the evil [of tipping], are nuisances in themselves," noted the MOH for Leeds in 1895 in what was a widespread source of criticism.[176] The problem had been noted from the start—by design, they involved generating smoke— and further innovations included the Fume Cremator patented by Ealing's borough engineer, Charles Jones, in 1885, which provided a secondary furnace situated between the cells and the chimney. But none of this did anything to quell anxiety on the part of ratepayers, prompting special meetings, LGB inquiries, and fact-finding missions on the part of councillors.[177] In 1894, residents of Birmingham's Saltley ward convened a public meeting to protest against a proposed destructor in their vicinity, which, it was argued, would only add to the array of municipally-owned nuisances that sapped the enjoyment and value of property: a gas works, a sewage farm, and a smallpox hospital.[178] In this case, the protest worked; elsewhere it served only to delay. Earlier, in 1892, local opposition in Birkenhead had prompted a three-day LGB inquiry into the building of two destructor sites. The town clerk, MOH, and the cleansing superintendents of Bolton and Salford testified in favor; the Birkenhead Brewery Company, borough hospital, and a handful of councillors argued against. Ultimately, the LGB inspector agreed to a loan of roughly five thousand pounds. Work eventually began at one of the sites in 1896, though not before a fifteen-strong team of councillors had visited destructors in Dewsbury, Oldham, and Bath.[179]

The appeal of destructors extended beyond their ability to destroy growing volumes of household waste in an expeditious fashion. Crucially, they were also technologies of "utilization," and were not without some of the enthusiasm that had earlier attended practices of sewage recycling. All depots sought to recycle the clinker destructors generated, which was normally put to use in road building. More ambitiously, efficiencies were sought by incorporating boilers into the architecture of the cells, so that the heat could be harnessed for the production of steam power, which could then be put to other purposes. One option pioneered during the mid-1880s in Ealing and Southampton was to combine refuse and sewage works. In Ealing, the steam power was used to drive the pre-cipitating machines that mixed lime and clay with the town's excreta; in Southampton, it was used to power two Shone-style ejectors.[180] By 1904, thirty-eight towns had erected destructors in conjunction with sewage works, principally for the provision of power to pumping stations. The more popular alternative was to combine refuse works with the provision of electricity (see figure 19). Ealing was once more among the pioneers, doing so in 1893, and just ten years later there were sixty combined works of this sort. As advocates acknowledged, destructors could hardly supply all the energy needed to power electricity stations, but they helped to reduce the rates and were a source of municipal economy. In July 1897, the physicist Lord Kelvin was among the dignitaries assembled to celebrate the opening of Shoreditch's combined works. "The Vestry achieves a double object in its municipal electric installation," noted the *Sanitary Record*. "It secures the absolute destruction of refuse teeming with all the elements of decay and disease, and in the process of that destruction abstracts an energy whence issues the electric spark."[181]

Yet, for all the ingenuity of technological refinement and municipal utilization, refuse destruction enjoyed only a relatively brief moment of promotion; or at least relative to water closets and sewage-treatment works, which were now—and would remain—in the ascendant. During the interwar period, tipping returned as the method of choice, albeit in the reworked form of "controlled tipping" pioneered in Bradford.[182] The reasons were many: the increasing volume of house refuse that had to be administered; the difficulties of disposing of clinker; and ongoing complaints about the air pollution caused by destructors. Still, during the 1890s and first years of the twentieth century, it was principally on account of the development of destructors that Britain was judged a world leader in refuse management. One handbook published in 1901 noted their adoption in Chicago, Berlin, Bombay, Melbourne, and Per-nambuco.[183] Curious engineers from abroad made their way to Britain on this account: remarkably, in 1897, the surveyor to the Australian city of Sydney made the long journey by ship to consult more than thirty local authorities in pursuit of the best destructor design.[184] "It will be noticed that I have not made any references to Continental or Amer-ican authorities in my paper," noted Salford's cleansing superintendent in 1902, speaking before the RSI on the subject of refuse disposal. "This is so, not because I refuse to learn from outsiders but because I believe in this matter we are not one bit behind the authorities beyond the seas."[185]

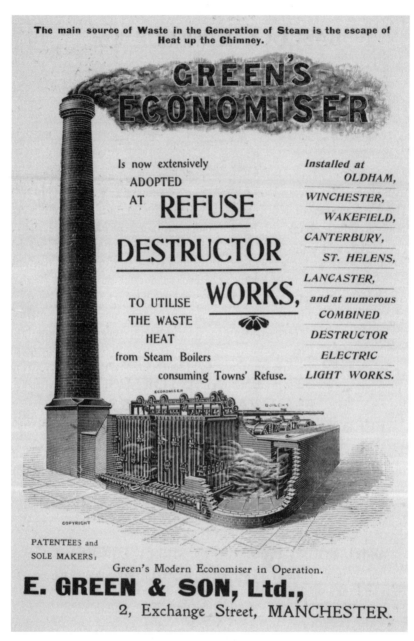

FIGURE 19. Still further efficiencies were sought by recycling the heat generated by the boilers themselves, including the use of "economizers," such as the one advertised here. Source: Francis Goodrich, *The Economic Disposal of Towns' Refuse* (London: P.S. King, 1901), 341. © The Bodleian Libraries, The University of Oxford.

CONCLUSION

Three points might be made in conclusion. The first is the most obvious: simply that Victorian and Edwardian public health, for all the frustrated work of assembling and coordinating administrative systems, was also about assembling and coordinating technological systems. It is impossible to dissociate the two, of course. Waste disposal systems were localized achievements, but they developed as part of a modern form of governance where technological choices on the part of local authorities were figured out in concert with the agency of central officials and engineering and surveying professionals, all of whom drew on—and disputed—a common pool of technical knowledge that transcended any given locality.

The second point is that these systemic qualities are obscured by thinking in terms of a bigger and more expansive state. This is partly because of the crucial role played by entrepreneurial and commercial agents; but most of all because waste disposal entailed harnessing the powers of technology. Perhaps there was, as chapter 1 described, growing reference to a more anonymous and abstract state. Yet clearly, in practice, governing involved quite the opposite: the advent of a novel world of multiple, maddening technical details and components, none of which escaped obsessive critique, refinement, and commercial promotion. This is not to suggest that we should therefore speak of the triumph of technological over human agency. Although the disposal of domestic waste was technologized, and in ways that were truly unprecedented in terms of their scale and complexity, these networks had to be designed and installed, and then operated and maintained. More accurately, then, we should speak of the advent of increasingly ramified and diffuse human-technological relations. The same is true of the similarly expansive gas, water, railway, telegraphic, and electricity systems that emerged at the same time.

The third and final point is that waste disposal systems developed in a contingent and contested fashion. In the end, of course, the water closet triumphed; but there were various types of water closet and, more importantly, water-carriage systems generated problems of their own, thereby prompting new solutions. It was indeed a systemic problem in the sense that the viability of particular parts and points was dependent on the viability of others in any given system; and it took until the Edwardian period to arrive at some kind of settlement as to what amounted to "progress" (save for refuse destructors). Equally, the project of putting matter in its right place was not without grandiose visions of system and aspirations toward a total environmental-technological solution. Chadwick and his allies were the first to sense this possibility, and they were followed by others who sensed much the same. What transpired was altogether more compromised and messy, as we have seen, and the pipe-and-brick sewers war of the 1850s but the first of many skirmishes. Even so, these aspirations were in the mix, vying for attention and realization. At the very least they attest to the modern sense of historical—if also, in this case, human-technological—possibility that informed the resolution of a very material and organizational challenge: namely, what to do with the growing volumes of excreta and refuse that was the invariable accompaniment of pronounced demographic growth and concentration.

Meanwhile, as we shall now see, a different kind of infrastructure was taking shape that was also designed to meet this challenge: localized systems for notifying, isolating, and disinfecting infected persons.

CHAPTER 6

Stamping Out

Logistics, Risk, and Infectious Diseases

Curiously, perhaps, one place where historians have located the power of an increasingly distant, centralized, and bureaucratic modern state is in the performance of intimate acts of bodily interference. The two best-known examples are smallpox vaccination and a series of Contagious Diseases Acts (CDAs) passed in the 1860s.[1] Both emerged as part of the development of a more state-medicalized, "person-centered" conception of public health; and both were designed to prevent what was referred to as the "danger" and "risk" of the spread of infectious diseases. Today, we might say that a "danger" is something known to be such—as dangerous, harmful, injurious—and that a "risk" lies in the possibility or chance of being exposed to a danger, which might be more or less certain.[2] The Victorians often conflated the two; but the assumption, certainly, was that they could be controlled and even eradicated with the help of the state. In 1840, vaccination was provided for free at public (poor law) expense, and then made compulsory in 1853 for infants up to three months of age. Further acts of 1867 and 1871 tightened the statutory framework, among other things extending the provisions to children under the age of fourteen. In the meantime, the CDAs introduced a system of forcibly detaining prostitutes to protect against the spread of venereal disease in the armed forces. By the early 1870s, it was in use in eighteen naval and garrison towns. Vaccination generally entailed the application of a lymph-loaded lancet to the upper arm, where the flesh was scored and crossed. The CDAs enabled doctors to inspect women suspected of prostitution.

These were compulsory measures, backed up by the authority of statute law, parliament, and the courts, which is why it makes sense to speak of state power. Yet the modernity of these measures also lies in their organizational complexity—the immense bureaucratic-legal intricacies; the struggle to ensure systematic administration—and the way they were assembled and resisted through a diffuse field of governance that turned upon both professional-bureaucratic empowerment and public-political input and accountability.[3] Did these systems work? Even this basic consideration was hotly disputed, amid dense exchanges of statistical and anecdotal evidence. Their political morality was also meticulously picked apart. In the case of vaccination, MPs and pressure groups invoked the rights of parents and English traditions of liberty. In the case of the CDAs, resistance was still more moralized, not least the charge that "the Government" was effectively sanctioning—because it was sanitizing—the "evil" of prostitution. The broad defense was that these measures were about securing safety, and that liberty had its limits when it jeopardized the containment of infectious diseases. To quote John Simon's pan-European survey of smallpox prophylaxis published in 1857, these were measures "undertaken by the State for the security of the public" against sickness and, ultimately, death.[4] But the resistance was not without consequence. In 1883, the CDAs were repealed and in 1886 abolished. In 1897, following a mammoth royal commission inquiry, exemptions to vaccination were allowed on the grounds of "conscientious objection"—a term that would enjoy a new lease of life in the context of conscription during the First World War.

This chapter examines a kindred set of measures for governing the dangers and risks of infectious diseases, three tactics in particular: notification, isolation, and disinfection. Combined, they were known as "stamping out," a term popularized during the cattle plague epizootic of 1865–67. Stamping-out systems coalesced just as the measures noted above were variously reformed and rejected, eventually forming something like a national preventive strategy that was practiced both inland and portside. As we shall see, much like smallpox vaccination, stamping out was about redefining "liberty" as safety, and as freedom from the danger of *other* infected people. It was also of a piece with Rumsey's totalizing vision of state medicine, where historical progress was equated with professional empowerment, and the exertion of an all-encompassing administrative mastery over life-sapping forces. Indeed, as it was imagined at the time, stamping out was about "waging war" on an array of infectious diseases, and closing down as quickly as possible epidemiological risks and potential points of "attack."

The most aggressive vision was provided by the Bristolian doctor and fever theorist William Budd, when, speaking before the NAPSS in 1869, he called for the following: "the earliest intimation of occurrences of infectious diseases"; the universal provision of local disinfection depots and specialist isolation hospitals; powers to compel the hospitalization of diseased persons and to prevent infected children from attending school; and measures for suppressing the movement of vagrants. Only the state, he argued, in the form of compulsory laws of national scope, could guarantee the kind of action that was at once necessary and legitimate, not the work of what he distinguished as "volunteers," "individual effort," and "municipalities": "Take, by way of illustration, this one trait. A man has an infectious disease in his house. The neglect of certain known precautions on his part may become the cause of disease and death to you and me. Such a striking and terrible characteristic not only places infection at once within the sphere of State action, but claims this action by the highest of all titles which a citizen can prefer to the protection of a government."[5] This was not true of constitutional afflictions such as gout, which was a properly individual affliction; but in the case of infectious diseases, all-out war was required: "By beating down these plagues, wherever they appear, by crushing them in their small beginnings, by pursuing them into their strongholds, and rooting them out, by making every advantage gained the ground of new reprisals, by carrying on incessant, implacable, internecine war against them, as against our direct enemies, which in sober truth they are—we should soon see a great falling off in the number of their victims, and gradually pave the way to their extermination." "No doubt such an idea will seem in the highest degree utopian," he noted, before reminding his audience of the growing powers of man to manipulate nature—to "subdue the most Titanic forces of the universe to his will"—and the progress that had been made in understanding the transmission of infectious diseases.[6]

Ambitious, technocratic professionals such as Budd would remain disappointed. In the end, only notification was made compulsory, and then as late as 1889 in London, and 1899 elsewhere. To be sure, the state functioned as a crucial referent in terms of contesting different "spheres" of responsibility, and posing questions of compulsion; and there was some of this. Yet, as will be argued here, neither the gestation nor the practice of stamping out is best captured by thinking in terms of a growing modern state. Crucially, if by no means uniquely, stamping-out systems were put together as part of the modern settlement of center-local relations detailed in chapter 2, and were the contingent product of complex mixtures of resistance and cooperation among multiple agents, from LGB officials and MOsH to councillors and doctors.

Likewise, it was much less about building an interventionist state, than it was coordinating localized counterstrikes against the mounting logistical-demographic—and, by extension, epidemiological—pressures that shaped Victorian public health reform; or in this case, the relative intensity with which human bodies mixed and moved around. As the GRO detailed, by 1851 just over 50 percent of the population was living in "towns," which it defined as settlements of more than two thousand people. By 1911, the figure stood at roughly 80 percent. Meanwhile, following the advent of universal elementary education in the 1870s, children of all classes were packed into schools. In 1900, it was a population in excess of 4.5 million.[7] And it was a problem made all the more unruly by increasing popular mobility—the growing use of cab and omnibus services, and railways and ocean-crossing steam-ships—and in cities at least, the advent of more anonymous forms of society.

In this respect, the military metaphors are much more suggestive of what happened in practice, and the place of stamping out within the broader reconfiguration of the spatial and temporal dynamics of English public health. Two features might be emphasized. The first is that stamping-out systems were designed to be ready and waiting to pounce on the "enemy." To be sure, the particular elements—notification, isolation, and disinfection—can all be discerned in the responses to cholera, but these were temporary measures. By contrast, stamping-out systems were distinguished by their permanence and their organizational presence even in the absence of crises—indeed, they were precisely about preventing crises and closing down risks as quickly as possible. Like the GRO's registration system and systems of inspection, they institutionalized a bureaucratic capacity to know and to act on an ongoing basis. The second feature is that while stamping out was understood as a means of securing progress and an epochal struggle against infectious diseases, it also entailed *compressing* the interrelations of time and space, and positing each as homogeneous variables that had to be mastered administratively. As we shall see, it involved assembling systems which could (a) act with speed when it came to locating afflictions; and (b) then divide and disinfect bodies and spaces. It was partly a logistical art, and for all the growing specificity with which the transmission of different zymotic diseases was understood, stamping out also entailed a certain kind of risk-averse, preventive indiscrimination.

The chapter begins with responses to cholera. It then turns to the further reforming threads that slowly, if haphazardly, crystalized as stamping out and that would eventually emerge in an international context as the "English system."

TEMPORARY MEASURES

Cholera has maintained its status as the "shock disease" of the nineteenth century. If hardly the biggest killer, it was novel, foreign ("exotic"), and brutal. Originating in the Indian subcontinent, cholera first arrived in 1831 for a year-long stay, and it visited again in 1848–49, 1853–54, and 1866, when it claimed some sixty-two thousand, twenty-three thousand, and then fourteen thousand lives. Hereafter Britain remained largely cholera-free, if also cholera-vigilant, and with good reason. For besides the threat of further epidemics stemming from mainland Europe, cholera was ruthless. Not all those afflicted died from it, and the symptoms were familiar from indigenous cholera nostras; but what was distinguished as "malignant" or "Asiatic cholera" was altogether more violent.[8] After the first symptoms, the body was convulsed with abdominal spasms, vomiting, and gushing evacuations, and then, perhaps, nervous collapse and death; and all within a matter of twenty-four hours.

What has diminished is the status of cholera as a driver of modern public health reform, and rightly so in some respects. On the one hand, the practices put in place recalled those deployed in the early modern period against plague: namely, portside quarantine, whereby the healthy and sick alike were detained at appointed maritime stations; and a kind of "catch-all" approach inland, which included hospitalizing the sick, removing nuisances, disinfecting houses, and speedier burial of the dead. On the other, the confusion cholera provoked was immense. For "extreme" Christian evangelicals, to use Boyd Hilton's designation, cholera was not even primarily a public health problem.[9] Rather, it was a sign of profound spiritual crisis, having been sent by a wrathful God as physical punishment and moral prod. What was really required was some penitential prophylaxis for the soul—hence a national Day of Fasting in 1832, and a Day of Thanksgiving in 1849 once the worst was over. Meanwhile, amid a struggle to wrest interpretive control from clergy and laymen, medical professionals failed to reach any consensus regarding the genesis and transmission of cholera. There was some movement, perhaps, during the 1850s toward the idea that it was caused by a specific "germ" in insanitary circumstances, making for a kind·of midpoint between strict "anticontagionist" (more environmental) and "contagionist" (more person-centered) approaches. It was the sensible option given the jumble of theories. In 1849, the *Times* distinguished between seven: zymotic; animalcular; a "cognate fungus theory"; telluric; electric; ozonic; and a "specific volatile poison" theory.[10] In 1867, one metropolitan MOH distinguished between nine. He provided much the same account as the *Times* had published, except that it also included John Snow's now famous theory regarding the "effects of impure water," which featured last on the list.[11]

Doubtless cholera functioned as a site of confusion, and of the reactivation of inherited practices and providential reasoning. Furthermore, the administrative responses were of a temporary character, a matter of pulling together in the midst of crisis and then relaxing once the danger had passed. One could even argue that the responses to cholera were more early modern than modern. Yet, in other respects, cholera was strikingly modern. First, cholera was posed as a problem of international commerce, connectivity, and cooperation. This built on arguments that had been developing since the late eighteenth century in relation to plague and yellow fever, just as the term *international* was coined; but it was cholera that was the first disease to provoke efforts at this novel level of governance, giving rise to International Sanitary Conferences (ISCs).[12] Initially proposed by the French in 1834, and then in the mid-1840s by the British, the first meeting took place in Paris in 1851, where it was hoped less draconian and more "uniform systems of Quarantine Regulation" would result, to quote British diplomatic dispatches.[13] Another ISC was held in 1859. Both were dominated by European powers and the danger of cholera.[14] Nothing came of these meetings, but they marked the opening up of a new front in the reform of quarantine and the battle against globe-trotting diseases.

Second, it was cholera that prompted the first articulation of "central" and "local" authorities in Britain, and the formation of some kind of specialist institutional supervision. Recently empowered by the 1825 Quarantine Act, the Privy Council in concert with the Board of Trade retained control of portside measures; but in June 1831 the Council set up an advisory board composed of medical, military, and customs officials. In November, it was replaced with a Central Board of Health

(CBH) charged with issuing domestic regulations. A similar committee had been convened in 1805 to deal with yellow fever in Gibraltar and its possible transmission to Britain. The difference in 1831 lay in the desire to develop a *national* system of protection inland and to secure the cooperation of what were now styled as "local boards of health"; or as the principal clerk of the Privy Council had it, to institute "a general and combined system of sanative regulation, which in case of necessity may be acted upon throughout the country."[15] Roughly twelve hundred local boards were formed in 1831–32, which generally brought together parish-based (clergymen), county-based (magistrates), and borough personnel (councillors), plus a smattering of doctors. After the Whig reforms of the 1830s, the principal authorities were boards of guardians and municipal corporations, acting under the central direction of the GBH (in 1848–49 and 1853–54), and then the MDPC (1866).

Finally, cholera was subject to unprecedented informational capture. There was certainly frustration to begin with. Although the CBH issued updates of deaths, it did so only on the basis of what local boards saw fit to supply; and efforts on this front might be ignored. In 1832, the CBH issued forms that local boards were supposed to fill out once the epidemic had passed, detailing cases and deaths. A meager forty-five were returned.[16] By the time of later epidemics, however, the GRO was in place, furnishing weekly updates, which were then reiterated in the press. After the epidemic, the GRO—much like the GBH and MDPC, which drew on its data—was able to present a series of bulky reports detailing variations of cholera cases at home and abroad. Maps were also generated. In 1831, the *Lancet* published what has been described as the map that "launched the idea of global health," which depicted cholera's deadly march through Asia, Europe, and Africa in a single cartographic snapshot.[17] It was the first of many: in 1850, the GBH's five-hundred-page report on the 1848–49 epidemic opened with a map detailing the "places and dates of attack," beginning with Cabool (Kabul) in 1845, and ending some twenty "points" later in Hamburg and Edinburgh in 1848 (see figure 20).

Evidently, none of this did anything to quell confusion, popular or professional; arguably, it only stoked it. But it was in this modern institutional and informational environment that inherited practices were reworked, contested, and reformed. The most striking development was the decline of quarantine. In late 1830, as news reached London that cholera was in Moscow, the Privy Council ordered quarantine for ships arriving from Russia. Further orders were issued as cholera made

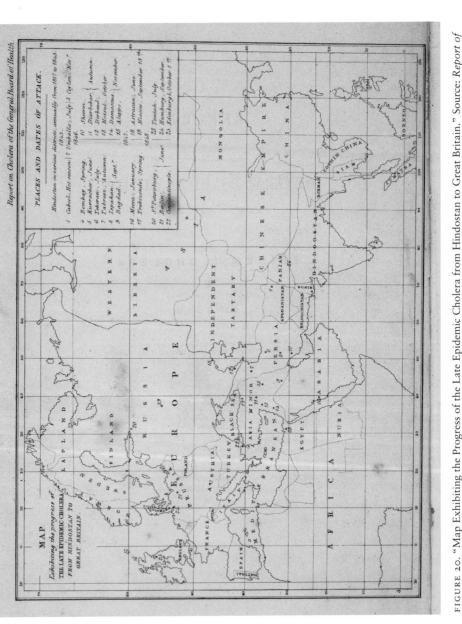

FIGURE 20. "Map Exhibiting the Progress of the Late Epidemic Cholera from Hindostan to Great Britain." Source: *Report of the General Board of Health on the Epidemic of Cholera of 1848 and 1849*, No. 1273 (1850), opp. title page. © The Bodleian Libraries, The University of Oxford.

inroads ashore, including two relating to ships sailing from northeastern ports to other domestic ports. The measures met with resistance—
ship owners petitioned parliament; MPs complained; release fees were
amended by the Board of Trade—and were eventually lifted in 1833;
but by this point more than twenty-five hundred ships had been quarantined.[18] It was the last substantive flourish of quarantine measures in
Britain. Although ordered in 1848 and 1866, they were repealed once it
became apparent that cholera had struck inland. Indeed, it seems that
between 1848 and 1866 only seventy-eight ships were quarantined for
all diseases, and now for only days, rather than the three weeks formally allowed under the 1825 act.[19]

It was a reflection of the growing antipathy toward quarantine.[20] The
tension between national security and the demands of international commerce was already a point of reference in the 1830s, and this became
more pronounced at midcentury, just as free trade emerged as an articulate ideology, both within and beyond parliament. Figures were quoted
regarding the loss of commercial revenues; anecdotes were recalled of the
inconvenience caused to travelers. Humanitarian concerns were also in
play, given that quarantine endangered the lives of those travelers and
sailors who might not be sick. The more compelling argument was simply
that quarantine had failed in the past and continued to fail abroad,
whether in relation to cholera, plague, or yellow fever; and that this failure was partly on account of the growing density of international trade
and travel. It culminated in the radical anti-quarantinism of Chadwick's
GBH, which accumulated a mass of official literature on the subject, citing examples from around the world. The GBH, however, was no advocate of laissez-faire. Rather, it encouraged a set of tactics that were at once
more sanitary and person-centered. In place of the crude lines of exclusion entailed by quarantine, it suggested something more flexible and
nuanced—indeed, more interventionist in some respects: that is, improved
onboard sanitation; medical inspections, thereby enabling distinctions to
be drawn between particular persons, rather than ships per se and their
ports of departure; and the management of the afflicted as discrete points
of danger, whether onboard or offshore.[21] In 1848, the GBH issued regulations to all merchant shipping companies urging better cabin ventilation; the quick identification of any "looseness of bowels," followed by a
dose of laudanum; and, should any sailor actually contract cholera, his
immediate isolation in a bed armed with a hot-water bottle.[22]

Responses inland, by contrast, followed much more in the groove of the
old. Various means of disinfection were applied, from the tried-and-tested

burning of household goods and limewashing to the fumigation of houses using chlorine gas. Efforts were made to secure some kind of ad hoc hospital accommodation, or what were still being dubbed "pest-houses," echoing early modern parlance. In 1831–32, local boards of health resorted to a variety of buildings, from bricked-off sections of workhouses to disused, dilapidated houses.[23] Military-style arrangements were also used: in 1849, Plymouth's poor law union erected a number of large tarpaulin tents outside the city center to house a cholera hospital.[24] But there were also some significant innovations. The prevention of nuisances was prioritized after the first epidemic. In 1846, as reports arrived that cholera was making tracks in Europe, parliament passed the first (if temporary) Nuisances Removal and Diseases Prevention Act, which set out procedures for the abatement of nuisances when certified by two medical practitioners. When cholera arrived in 1848, a new act was passed which dropped the need for medical adjudication while enabling the appointment of local inspectors.[25] It was renewed in 1849 and mobilized once more in 1853–54. This was bound up with another novelty. Whereas household quarantine had formed a crucial feature of early modern responses to plague, this was now abandoned in favor of more exacting systems of house-to-house inspection in search of victims and those with developing symptoms, who could then be managed and medicated either at home or in some kind of hospital. To this extent, new forms of prophylactic combat were enacted inland that were also both more sanitary and person-specific. No more was it a matter of appointing watchmen to stand guard outside stricken houses by way of ensuring that all inhabitants remained padlocked and "shutt up" inside.[26]

None of this was implemented without a struggle, which began to assume a modern form and intensity. The center prescribed and reacted, prodded and publicized. Regulations were issued and renewed (e.g., three CBH circulars in late 1831; seven GBH notifications in 1848–49); officials were dispatched when and where necessary to encourage good practice (e.g., in 1832, the CBH dispatched sixteen inspectors to the provinces as the crisis deepened; in 1866, the MDPC sent four inspectors and two engineers to London's hard-hit East End). Meanwhile, local authorities both repelled and amplified these directions. Variations of response were partly determined by the incidence of cholera, but even where it did arrive there might be resistance. In Newcastle, in late 1831, there was even opposition on the part of the town council to proclaiming that cholera had arrived at all, as the CBH suspected it had, for fear that it would interrupt trade and deprive workers of wages.[27] On-site chivvying by central officials was ignored. In July 1849, one of the GBH's inspectors visited Hull for a second time, shortly after the first cases had been reported. He met with local boards of guardians, who agreed to a plan of action; but he had to return again in September after learning that nothing had been done, despite further casualties: no houses of refuge had been set up; no system of house-to-house visitation had been implemented; and only a few nuisances had been removed.[28] During August and September, the GBH began issuing special orders in the metropolis in an attempt to enforce its national regulations. In response, the parish of St. Saviours, Southwark, refused to close its overcrowded burial yard; the guardians of Whitechapel and St. Pancras declined to appoint extra inspectors; and though the Bethnal Green union eventually appointed one medical visitor and one nuisance inspector, no provisions were made for special dispensaries or a cholera hospital. Court cases followed, none of them successful for the GBH.[29]

Stories like this might be multiplied for all four epidemics. Just as multiple, however, are stories of administrative urgency and remarkable diligence on the part of local authorities. *Urgent:* the term captures the spatial-temporal density of the measures enacted, and the informational connections that brought them together to form localized systems of emergency surveillance and care. In November 1831 a Special Board of Health was convened in Manchester, where in the end some seven hundred lives perished. It carried out in full the recommendations suggested by the CBH, meeting at least weekly, often daily. The city was divided into fourteen districts; to each was appointed a druggist, dispensing medicines, and an inspector, drawn from the clergy or other professions, who carried out daily visits. Three thousand pamphlets were distributed advising on matters of diet and cleanliness; a specialist squad of twenty scavengers was hired to deal with nuisances; three cholera hospitals were set up; and a special site was arranged for the burial of corpses, where they were topped with quicklime once interred.[30]

Later responses of a similar intensity might be attributed to growing professional leadership. In London, efforts in 1853–54 were roundly condemned by the GBH. In contrast, in 1866, at which point MOsH had been appointed throughout the capital, all districts were primed and readied before cholera arrived. Hospitals were prepared; extra inspectors employed; disinfectants stockpiled; handbills dispatched. And when it did arrive the efforts were immense: in Whitechapel alone more than thirty-seven thousand houses were visited from July through to September.[31] Yet, where professional leadership was lacking, civic initiative was more than capable of compensating. Earlier in Oxford, in 1854, after the first cases had been reported in August, an emergency committee was formed, composed of poor law guardians, street commissioners, and aldermen, which then met daily in the town hall. Fifteen medical attendants were enlisted, each responsible for one of five districts and one of eight dispensaries. All attendants had to make daily reports of cases. Houses were disinfected; the clothes and bedding of cholera victims were burned or buried. A team of messengers was employed to call on nurses, and to distribute hot-water bottles and beef tea. Finally, a military-style "field of observation" was established outside of Jericho, where different miniature hospitals catered for suspect cases, actual cases, and convalescents. Three hundred died in the end.[32]

Practices of surveillance, isolation and disinfection were thus already being combined as elements of emergency prophylaxis. None of this was as yet provided for on a permanent basis, however, and they lacked a clear institutional base at the local level. In towns and cities responsibility was often shared between poor law and municipal authorities. Quarantine also remained a live issue, despite its decline in practice. This was partly because the Privy Council retained powers under the 1825 act; and partly because it remained a widespread practice abroad, including among British imperial possessions: between 1845 and 1854, some three thousand ships were quarantined at Gibraltar, and over nine thousand in Malta.[33] Quite what should replace it was still a matter of debate at the highest levels of officialdom. In 1858, prompted by fears that the Privy Council would impose quarantine following an outbreak of plague on the Barbary Coast, the NAPSS formed a subcommittee on the matter. Eventually the mass of evidence it collected extended to ports as far flung as Papeete (Tahiti) and Rio de Janiero. Its final report, which was submitted to the Board of Trade in 1861, developed the alternative system the GBH had earlier urged, concluding with a plea "to amend . . . not to abolish the existing machinery of action": namely, better onboard sanitation; rigorous medical inspection on arrival; and the immediate release of healthy seafarers combined with the hospitalization of the sick.[34]

Equally, quarantine had its defenders, and not just in the Board of Trade. Notably Simon, as head of the MDPC, was not wholly opposed to quarantine, even citing successful instances on the islands of Sicily and Dominica in his annual report of 1867.[35] His major statement on the matter had been laid out in the previous year's report, where he made the argument that, given the present state of knowledge regarding cholera—that it could spread via an individual's evacuations; that just one individual could trigger an outbreak in insanitary areas—quarantine made absolute sense. The crux was whether or not it could be effectively implemented, which Simon suggested it could not: "Only in proportion as a community lives apart from the great highways and emporia of commerce, or is ready and able to treat its commerce as a subordinate political interest, only in such proportion can quarantine be made effectual for protecting it." To which he added: "and the fulfilment of such conditions ['of national seclusion'] by England would involve fundamental changes in the most established habits of the country." In short, it was simply not practical, given England's commercial interests and international connections.[36]

Instead, he urged that "foreign contagions" such as cholera ought to be considered as part of "our ordinary home-bred contagions," in particular typhoid, smallpox, diphtheria, and scarlet fever. All should be subject to the same kind of regulations, enacted, not by the "general executive of the country," but "by the vigour of local authorities": "Subject to the condition that proper hospital-accommodation can be offered, the authority ought to be able to enforce, in regard of any dangerous contagious disease, that the sufferer should not be in circumstances which promote the spread of the disease to the general population."[37] Perhaps the 1825 Quarantine Act might be applied locally, Simon speculated. Regardless, it was time to regulate infectious diseases beyond cholera. This was in March; in August, as cholera arrived once more, the 1866 Sanitary Act was enacted, which besides further expanding the scope of nuisance regulations also empowered the building of isolation hospitals by local sanitary authorities.

NOTIFICATION SYSTEMS

This was a novel recommendation at the time, and in the 1890s, Simon's 1866 report was credited with having kick-started a "distinct epoch" in the history of English public health.[38] What he had done, certainly, was capture something of the way in which things would develop, two aspects in particular: first, a normalization of measures put in place during exceptional cholera outbreaks, so that local authorities—and in particular those constituted as sanitary authorities—were in a *permanent* state of alert, ready and waiting; and second, an expansion in the number of diseases that were provided for in this way. Put another way, he had at least mooted the integration of infectious disease control into

England's emerging system of modern, bureaucratized prevention. Yet, the roots of what emerged are decidedly knotty, and there were pockets of more recent innovations, besides the measures put in place to combat cholera. In the late 1840s, Simon himself, as the City of London's first MOH, had improvised a system of enhanced sanitary inspection that drew on the weekly mortality records of local registrars, as well as those of PLMOs in relation to cases of sickness.[39] Acts passed in 1851 and 1853 compelled CLH keepers to "give immediate notice" of any cases of "fever and infectious or contagious disease." Also worthy of note are the measures enacted in the wake of the rinderpest epizootic of the mid-1860s. The 1866 Cattle Diseases Prevention Act enforced the slaughter of infected cattle, restrictions on the movement of healthy livestock, and stringent measures of disinfection in all cases.

More importantly, the details of what emerged did so as part of the contested realization of state medicine described in chapter 2. Crucial among these was instituting some kind of system of ongoing surveillance, or what became known as the "notification of infectious diseases." The key protagonists are easy to identify: MOsH. Some one hundred strong in the 1860s, their number increased dramatically when their appointment was made compulsory in 1872. As early as 1876, the LGB had vetted the appointment of just over eight hundred; by 1901, the number had doubled to over sixteen hundred.[40] Expansion was accompanied by professionalization—the initial London-based association of MOsH was made national in 1873; a journal, *Public Health*, began in 1888; university-based qualifications were introduced—and, much like their subordinate colleagues, sanitary inspectors, MOsH styled themselves as disinterested servants of the public. "Whatever his political bent may be, he must strictly avoid making any public parade of it," stated one summary of the role penned by Reading's MOH: "it is absolutely essential that he should banish any suspicion of political bias from all his official proceedings."[41] Yet, while MOsH affirmed their official autonomy and the disinterested nature of their expertise—this, after all, was what defined them as such—practicing this expertise entailed quite the opposite, much as it did for inspectors: its messy entanglement, that is, in political disputes and decision-making processes. For besides struggles for status and security of tenure, and so parliamentary lobbying, the powers they enjoyed were a product of compromise and of long, frustrated gestation. Likewise, enacting these powers required resources, interfered with property and privacy, and entailed forming relations with various other agents, councillors and doctors among them.

Notification is a case in point, for it represented a remaking of what began as a desire to institute something altogether more total and systematic: a national register of sickness. As early as 1844, and then in his 1856 *Essays,* Rumsey called for the registration of sickness and the national coordination of data generated by PLMOs, hospitals and dispensaries, and friendly societies. The aim was to supplement the GRO's statistics on mortality as a means of measuring salubrity; to enable more focused remedial efforts at the local level; and to furnish more data for research purposes.[42] Support was forthcoming from the London Epidemiological Society and Benjamin Ward Richardson's *Journal of Public Health and Sanitary Review,* which in 1858 editorialized in favor of a registrar-general of disease.[43] Such calls even gave rise to a handful of experiments, notably in Manchester, where in 1860 the MSSA began coordinating voluntary and official sources of information regarding sickness (from poor law institutions, charities, and hospitals) and the weather (from the Salford Observatory). In 1870, one of its core members, the physician Arthur Ransome, reflected that during an outbreak of typhus in 1865 the speed and accuracy of the system had helped to quell public alarm and ensure the quick isolation of infected cotton operatives.[44]

Meanwhile, the NAPSS, the BMA—which in 1865 had set up a special committee on the subject—and statisticians from the GRO continued to champion the measure, pressing it before the Royal Sanitary Commission and parliament, and in deputations to the Poor Law Board and then the LGB.[45] Quite how such a national system might be organized was disputed, but it was partly promoted as a kind of early warning system, akin to a storm-forecasting service for ships (and in fact the Meteorological Office, earlier founded in 1854, had recently commenced such a system in 1860).[46] "Registration of deaths represents the wrecks which strew the shore," noted the MP and sanitary activist Lyon Playfair in 1874, speaking before the NAPSS, "while that of sickness would tell us of the coming storms and enable us to trim our vessels to meet them." "Till we have such a system of disease-registration, public health cannot be administered with full intelligence."[47]

This particular strand of state medicine would remain frustrated, and calls for a comprehensive system of sickness registration persisted to the end of the century.[48] The campaign was not without consequence, however, for in the late 1860s calls began to emerge for the compulsory registration of a more restricted set of diseases in the interests of preventing their diffusion, regardless of any statistical benefits that might accrue. In 1868, the surgeon Sir James Young Simpson offered a *Proposal to*

Stamp Out Small-Pox and Other Contagious Diseases, which urged measures of compulsory notification on the part of householders and doctors.[49] A year later, speaking before the NAPSS, the MOH for Paddington and public baths enthusiast, William Hardwicke, called for "systematic action" that concerned only "returns of all contagious diseases," or what he called "zymotic," "preventible diseases." "This record would not only suffice for most practical sanitary purposes but would render less urgent the need of a general registration of diseases," he argued, before recommending that doctors ought to be compelled to supply information, should they attend someone with an infectious disease.[50] Other professionals, including Budd, quoted above, made much the same argument.

Parliament was hardly inactive in the years that followed, passing the 1872 and 1875 public health acts. Yet, on the question of compulsory registration and what was increasingly distinguished as "notification," neither Liberal nor Tory governments were prepared to introduce a general bill. In the end, amid ongoing crises, including two smallpox epidemics in 1870–72 and 1876–78, a set of local authorities pressed ahead in a regionalized burst of activism. Between 1876 and 1881, some twenty-three towns passed local improvement acts containing clauses enforcing some kind of notification, beginning with Huddersfield and Bolton. Each authority emulated the other in what were dubbed "local experiments." All were in the North of England, save for Norwich and Reading, and two Scottish authorities, Edinburgh and Greenock. The key factor it seems was the enthusiasm of local MOsH: in 1875 and 1877, the Northwestern branch of the Society of MOsH petitioned the president of the LGB urging compulsory notification.[51] Not that all authorities proceeded in the same fashion.[52] One difference was the range of diseases subject to notification. Cholera, smallpox, scarlet fever, diphtheria, typhoid, and typhus were targeted in almost all the towns; measles and erysipelas in just a handful; whooping cough in only one. Another was the level of fines inflicted for failure to report, which ranged from two pounds at Barrow-in-Furness to ten pounds at Birkenhead.

In this way, pockets of institutionalized surveillance emerged that were shaped and enabled via the broader settlement of center-local relations, and the regulated liberty afforded to England's sanitary authorities. The measures themselves, however, also raised questions about liberty, if here at the *personal* rather than local level. Crudely put, did these measures infringe personal liberty or secure it, to the extent that freedom required health? The question was asked from the start. In terms of notification per se, most professionals could agree that to intervene in this fashion was legitimate. Public safety was at stake and speed was everything: the quicker one acted, the less risk there was that others would become infected. Analogies were made with the protection afforded by fire services and police forces. If it was about balancing liberties, then here it was necessary to come down on the side of "society," rather than on the side of the "individual." In 1876, Gloucestershire's MOH developed this point, arguing "that society has the same right to interfere with the liberty of the subject in seeking to carry out this object [notification], which it is admitted to have in repressing murder, robbery and other acts which are confessedly prejudicial to its welfare."[53]

Decidedly more intricate was the question of which agents, precisely, should notify MOsH and how they should do it.[54] Inspectors were formally obliged to do so, and in 1879 the LGB issued orders imposing the duty on newly appointed PLMOs and school medical officers. By contrast, the responsibility of those positioned beyond the official core of local public health systems, in particular householders and doctors, was much disputed, giving rise to a complex politics of paperwork. Four principal systems were practiced from the mid-1870s. The two extremes were notification by the householder only, as in Greenock, and by the doctor only, as in Edinburgh. The more popular systems combined both agents: by the doctor indirectly, whereby he filled out a form which it was then the duty of the householder to forward (e.g., in Bradford); and by both the householder directly and the doctor directly, or what became known as the "dual system" (e.g., in Leicester).

The merits of each were discussed extensively, but it was the compulsion of medical practitioners that stirred the most resistance. In 1878, the Bolton Medical Society protested against the practice of notification, demanding its amendment or abolition by the town council. In 1879, Leicester's doctors petitioned parliament against the notification clauses of a corporate bill passing through committee stage.[55] Later, as awareness grew among the medical profession, protest kicked in from the start. In Liverpool, the city's Medical Institution mobilized against a local bill proposed in 1881. The following year the council's health committee collected favorable evidence from neighboring local authorities; in response, the Medical Institution undertook its own survey, authored by one of the leading agitators, Robert Hamilton, which was damning of existing schemes. The *Sanitary Record* complained that Hamilton's "ponderous blue book" was biased and that the facts were unclear.[56] In the end, the measure was dropped. Similarly, in Bath the city council commissioned a report on the matter, which found in favor of a system of indirect notification. Local practitioners quickly rallied, disputed the report, and lobbied the city's sanitary committee. The protest worked: a plan to enforce notification via an LGB provisional order was defeated by eight votes to three in the council chamber.[57]

The payment of fees was supposed to provide some relief, yet the arguments against notification were many, including that it was an inducement to conceal cases, and that it would lead to needless friction between MOsH and doctors. And matters of professional principle were at stake, regardless of any misgivings about how such measures had worked, or might work, in practice. Crucial among these was that compulsory notification represented a breach of trust between a practitioner and his private patient, which some presented as a "sacred bond." Doctors feared being turned into "spies" and "agents of the State." The physician "ought, by his conduct, to show that he deserved the confidence of his patient. Would he have that confidence if he acted as the tool of the Government?" asked one doctor in 1882.[58] Notification was fine in principle, perhaps; but in order to negotiate these client-based sensitivities, a suitably subtle system was required. The BMA's position was that indirect notification was best, and that the information should be communicated verbally rather than in writing.[59]

The response to such demands was mixed. There were loud voices of dissent among MOsH, notably Croydon's respected officer, Alfred Carpenter. A critic since the mid-1870s, he was especially concerned about criminalizing doctors, and the awkward scenarios that might arise were the matter to go to court. How, under the dual system, could a doctor testify against his patient for non-notification if he himself was also legally obliged to do so, he asked during a set-piece debate at the 1884 International Health Exhibition? Carpenter was in favor of indirect notification, but as a matter of moral not legal obligation.[60] The majority of MOsH, and indeed some doctors, wondered what all the fuss was about. Doctors, after all, were already required to register the cause of death and, ultimately, in the case of infectious diseases, private health *was* public health; or rather, might and frequently did become so. It followed, as one advocate put it in 1882, that "private interest must give way before public necessity," and the dual system was the most secure means of ensuring notification.[61]

It was these arguments that prevailed. Despite lobbying by the BMA, the dual system was endorsed by a select committee that met in 1882 charged with reviewing existing local acts, thereby emerging as a "model clause"; and by the end of the 1880s, of the fifty English authorities that had adopted notification, most did so in a dual fashion.[62] It was also the method that found its way into statute, when, in 1889, parliament passed the Infectious Disease (Notification) Act, which was steered through by the Tory president of the LGB, Charles Ritchie. The only concession was that beyond London the act was permissive. It was eventually made compulsory by a further act in 1899, and by then it was a matter of tidying up, for the 1889 act was readily adopted. By late 1889, it had been adopted in over three hundred sanitary districts; and by 1892, in more than a thousand, meaning that over 80 percent of the population of England and Wales was covered by the act.[63] It makes for a rare instance of relatively rapid local-political mobilization in favor of compulsory measures. As the *Morning Post* commented in November 1889, although MPs had prophesized reluctance on the part of sanitary authorities, quite the opposite was the case: the eagerness was "astonishing."[64]

Slowly, then, if with something of a bang in the end, a key element of stamping out was institutionalized at the local level throughout England: a system of surveillance premised on practicing "liberty" as freedom from the danger of infected others. As with the work of the GRO and sanitary inspectors, it required the generation of immense amounts of paperwork. In London, for instance, during the ten years 1889–99, almost 410,000 cases were notified, most relating to children suffering from scarlet fever (206,000) and diphtheria (99,000).[65] Like those used by inspectors, the certificates required bare statements of clocked particulars: name, age, residence, disease, and date. Some authorities such as Newcastle's even provided different colored forms: scarlet paper for scarlet fever, mauve for typhus, white for diphtheria.[66] Once received, whether by post or by hand, they were archived in local sanitary offices and used as the basis for on-site visits by MOsH and inspectors. In Huddersfield, the master source was dubbed the "Zymotic book," which served as the repository for all notification-related activities and inquiries.[67]

Invariably, perhaps, none of this worked as it should. The key weakness was that the dual system was in fact more of a mono system. Doctors quickly fell into line and court cases were few: in Derby, which introduced a dual system in 1879, only three prosecutions were made in eight years; in 1898, one MOH described court cases as "rare."[68] MOsH sometimes complained of misdiagnosis, but this was excused on the grounds that it was better to be safe than sorry. At worst it meant a wasted follow-up visit and notification fee. By contrast, members of the public were much more problematic, despite efforts to publicize measures using handbills and posters. The poor especially were unreliable and could not always afford to call on a qualified doctor; and although PLMOs could be relied upon, they encountered only the neediest. "What ordinarily happens is something like this," began the president of the Home Counties branch of the Society of MOsH in 1897, after suggesting that the problems were located mainly among the "working and lower middle classes": "A child has, say, a mild attack of scarlet fever; it is kept at home for a few days; perhaps the mother goes to a chemist, gets a bottle or two of medicine, is told as probably as not 'Oh! It has got the measles, I dare say; keep it warm, it will be alright in a few days.' The rash disappears and the child goes back to school . . . and the mischief has been done, and the result is a crop of fresh cases amongst its classmates and playfellows."[69] The problem of "non-notification" and "missed cases" was thus a recurrent source of frustration for MOsH, who urged more draconian sanctions. This was hardly the kind of resistance—organized, rallied, and principled—that in places frustrated smallpox vaccination. Rather, it was resistance as diagnostic ignorance, or even, perhaps, wishful thinking that an infection would somehow pass; and as MOsH conceded, there was little to be done when someone pleaded ignorance. Here too fines and legal proceedings were only occasional.[70] Official threats were made and handbills reissued, but it was evidently a struggle when it came to turning members of the public into agents of their own surveillance. It seems a key source of early warning went missing as a matter of course.

BUILDING HOSPITALS

Still, if not quite the systematic system desired by MOsH, notification represented a triumph for security and the management of risk. Crucially, it was institutionalized, so that local authorities were now in an ongoing state of alert. Permanent provision had been made for possible danger. A similar kind of institutionalization occurred in the case of smallpox hospitals and fever hospitals—also known as isolation hospitals and sanatoria—the key architectural element of stamping out. There were some precursors on this front, such as the "houses of recovery" that had emerged in the early nineteenth century in Manchester and Newcastle, and London's fever and smallpox hospitals erected in 1848–49.[71] Fever wards also featured as part of general hospitals. It was only during the 1860s, however, as part of the emerging MOH-led push for notification, when hospitals for infectious diseases began to emerge as discrete objects of translocal scrutiny and promotion. The expansion that took place was remarkable, given that most were paid for using local authority funds, as councillors opted to take advantage of a series of parliamentary statutes that either consolidated existing provisions (such as those contained in the 1866 Sanitary Act) or extended them, notably the 1875 Public Health Act and the 1893 Isolation Hospitals Act. In the 1860s, specialized institutions were rare, restricted to only major towns, even if fever wards had become common. By 1914, there were no less than 755 municipal or county-based fever hospitals, plus 363 smallpox hospitals.[72] Just as strikingly, stricken persons could now be compelled to enter them.[73]

In some quarters, all this was considered decidedly un-English, provoking the same kind of rhetoric that attended opposition to smallpox vaccination and the CDAs. In 1882, an editorial in the then liberal-radical *Pall Mall Gazette,* entitled "The New Despotism," suggested that compulsory isolation smacked of the kind of arbitrary powers employed on the continent, both past (the Spanish Inquisition) and present (Russian antiterrorist laws). "All these restraints and restrictions and interferences with the liberty of the subject may keep people alive a little longer, but they bid fair to make life itself not worth living," it dramatized, before invoking "the irksome strait waistcoat of martinet sanitarianism."[74] Others made explicit the connection with vaccination and the CDAs, and much more besides. During the early 1880s, the Vigilance Association for the Defence of Personal Rights lobbied parliament and the LGB against measures of notification, arguing that they were yet another encroachment on the historic rights of the English to live free of tyranny. "Look at the whole tide and tenor of modern legislation," stated the anti-CDAs and antivaccination campaigner, Charles Bell Taylor, at the annual meeting of the Vigilance Association in 1885, having quoted Edmund Burke: "Compulsory vaccination . . . Compulsory re-vaccination . . . Compulsory registration of births; Compulsory registration of still births; Compulsory registration of disease; Compulsory notification of infectious diseases; Compulsory isolation of sick people; Compulsory violation of women [the CDAs]; Compulsory education—it is all compulsion, none needed and none efficacious." The state, he argued, had no right to force people to be healthy: "Who will protect us from our protectors?"[75]

Certainly some MOsH sympathized with these arguments; and yet MOsH also presented themselves as the guardians of liberty, developing the arguments noted above in favor of notification. Two points were made: that measures such as notification and isolation helped to secure a more positive variant of liberty, namely liberty as health; and that these measures protected those who were not infected from the danger of those who were. "To take precautions against the spread of smallpox or cholera is surely as legitimate and justifiable as against felony," argued Bolton's MOH, John Livy, in the pages of the *BMJ* in 1882. "There is not much individual liberty left to a man laid prostrate from typhus. . . . To restore him to health is to restore his lapsed liberty," to which he added: "we must not permit free trade in disease."[76] This was the other key point: "Was it right when infectious disease occurred in one family that the other families should be exposed to a terrible danger in order to conserve the liberty of an individual?" asked T. Orme Dudfield, MOH for Kensington, in 1884: "The liberty of an individual to spread disease!"[77] GRO statistics were quoted regarding the lives lost to infectious diseases, and it did not pass unnoticed that freedom meant all kinds of things. "The word liberty," Livy noted, "is perhaps the most abused term in our language."

Ultimately, on matters of broad principle, MOsH won the argument, as MPs and ministers opted to define "liberty" as security in statute. And yet, only in optional statute; and as with notification, the provision of specialist hospital facilities involved working through England's modern system of center-local relations, defined as this was by a broadly liberal ethos of diplomatic interaction and oversight. The details mattered—of design, size, situation, and so on—and the building process mobilized an array of agents just as complex as that which attended the gestation of sewerage systems examined in the previous chapter. In particular, LGB officials, MOsH, borough surveyors, and private architects kept an eye on emerging variations of practice, both at home and abroad, while seeking to promote general standards of construction. In architectural terms, the key innovation was a French import known as the "pavilion system." Pioneered in hospitals in Bordeaux and Paris, it was promoted in Britain by the likes of Florence Nightingale and the architect, George Godwin, during the midcentury.[78] The key elements were one- or two-story ward blocks placed at right angles to a single, connecting corridor; ward pavilions separated by lawns and gardens; and thorough cross-ventilation within wards using opposing rows of tall windows.

Pavilion wards became one of the most distinctive features of all hospitals built after the midcentury, and this included fever and smallpox hospitals. A variety of both began to emerge in the 1860s, as the LGB

inspector Richard Thorne Thorne detailed in a national survey published in 1882.[79] They ranged from large, brick-built structures in towns
to temporary cottages and iron sheds in villages. At the same time, as
permanent structures became more common, official efforts were made
not so much to standardize arrangements as to encourage the flexible,
place-specific application of architectural norms: the same kind of normalizing pragmatism evident in the case of sewerage systems. In 1871,
the MDPC issued the first memorandum on the subject, detailing both
permanent arrangements and temporary ones, which included military-
style tents.[80] The memo was published again in 1876 and 1882; but
further memoranda issued to local authorities focused on permanent,
pavilion-style buildings for use in towns and villages, and all according
to the norm of one bed per thousand inhabitants. Between 1888 and
1908, four model sets were drawn up with the help of the LGB's in-
house architect, each containing four plans, A to D, which catered for
between two and twelve patients. The most popular, it seems, was plan
C, serving twelve, which comprised two wards of six beds situated
between a nurses' duty room (see figure 21).[81]

These models were crucial since it was the LGB that sanctioned
the loans that were required. Other facets of the localized-centralized
gestation of hospitals included on-site LGB inspections, meetings in
Whitehall with councillors, and local authorities inspecting the work of
others. In 1885, Sunderland's health committee agreed to replace the
town's house of recovery (erected in 1822) with a state-of-the-art isolation hospital. Deputations were organized to Sheffield, Manchester,
Bradford, and Darlington; tenders were vetted by the borough engineer;
a public inquiry was held in 1886 by the LGB, which eventually
approved the committee's plan; in 1887, the hospital was built, providing for forty-two patients.[82] Similarly dense processes informed the
development of all hospitals, from the very small, catering for as few as
four patients, to the very large in cities, catering for upward of one hundred. The largest emerged in London under the authority of the Metropolitan Asylums Board (MAB), which was established in 1867 to provide for the integrated management and hospitalization of the capital's
sick poor.[83] Building began in the late 1860s with a set of hospitals distributed strategically throughout the capital at Hampstead (the North-
western Hospital, opened in 1870), Stockwell (the Southwestern Hospital, 1871), and Homerton (the Eastern Hospital, 1871). By 1899, the
MAB had built ten hospitals, providing over 4,600 beds. The biggest
was Park Hospital in Lewisham, which catered for some 548 patients.[84]

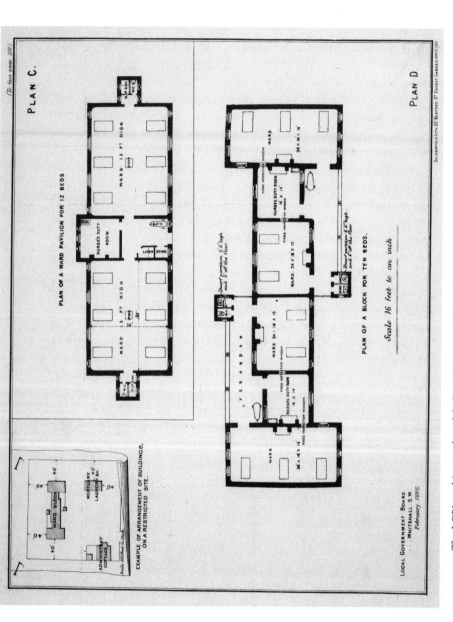

FIGURE 21. The LGB's architectural models C and D, as specified in the late 1880s and 1890s. Source: *Seventeenth Annual Report of the Local Government Board, 1887–88: Supplement Containing the Report of the Medical Officer for 1887,* C.5526-I (1888), 200–201. © The Bodleian Libraries, The University of Oxford.

Of course, cooperation prevailed over obstruction—more and more hospitals were built, after all—but in all cases it was an intricate process. The LGB might withhold its support on financial or architectural grounds. Even once the decision to build a hospital had been agreed among councillors, any project still had "the gauntlet of the Local Government Board to run, with all its meshes of red-tapism," to quote the *Leicester Chronicle* in 1899, as it celebrated the laying of a foundation stone for a new 160-bed hospital.[85] An additional problem was securing relations *between* local authorities. The 1893 act empowered the formation of joint hospital boards composed of district authorities under the auspices of county councils; and forging these agreements could make for a fraught process, as different authorities disputed their precise financial contribution and sought to withdraw; or else lobbied to join emerging agreements. In 1904, the Oakwell Joint Hospital Board opened a twenty-six-bed hospital at Birstall, Yorkshire. The scheme, however, had first been mooted in 1894 by the local MOH, and in 1896 an order was obtained from the LGB constituting a joint board composed of the urban authorities of Birstall, Birkenshaw, and Drighlington. As various sites were explored—and rejected, owing to unwilling landowners—the LGB approved the addition of Gomersal council in 1898 and Gildersome council in 1899. An initial loan agreement with the LGB was rejected by councillors on account of the rate increases it would entail; plans were amended; new loan arrangements sought; in 1902, the LGB gave the go-ahead.[86]

Negotiation, compromise, frustration: hospitals were made of this, just as much as bricks and mortar. MOsH argued for more systematic action and comprehensive coverage: that more might be built, more quickly, and to a higher and more uniform standard. Legal ambiguities were detailed at length. There was debate, for instance, about whether to charge a fee to patients, since the 1875 Public Health Act was unclear on the matter. Most chose not to, largely on the grounds that hospitals were there to safeguard the community and not just stricken individuals.[87] Meanwhile, councillors bemoaned the costs, and with some justification given that hospitals were only required occasionally. The LGB's standard ratio of one bed per thousand inhabitants was judged about right in terms of balancing cost and need, given that it was "too high for ordinary times and too small for epidemic times," as one MOH put it.[88] Nor was it deemed practical to isolate every kind of zymotic disease. There was debate among MOsH about how to deal with measles. It was not part of the statutory schedule of notifiable diseases; but it could be added to local schemes if agreed by councillors. Notifying and isolating measles, however, was never widely practiced, partly because it was most infectious in its "pre-eruptive state," meaning that most of the epidemiological damage was done before diagnosis could take place; and partly because outbreaks were normally so extensive that any hospital accommodation would prove insufficient.[89] Only a small number of authorities opted to isolate measles cases: some eighty-eight by 1894, dropping to seventy-six in 1903.[90]

Another point of contention was the risk posed to nearby residents by the concentration of infected persons. This was most pronounced in the case of smallpox hospitals, principally because smallpox, of all the zymotic diseases, had long been considered among the most contagious—albeit variously, ranging from degrees of spatial-aerial proximity to direct contact—and it could be incredibly disfiguring, facially and physically. Especially fierce ratepayer opposition took place in London, where it played a role in forcing the MAB to revert to shipping hulks moored far along the Thames. Opposition led by an elderly Sir Rowland Hill (of Post Office fame) resulted in two law suits in 1878 and 1879, which claimed that the MAB's smallpox facilities in Hampstead constituted a nuisance. Further entanglements with the legal system followed, some of which passed through the Court of Appeal and the House of Lords, before the case was settled out of court in 1883.[91] Three ships were still being used at the turn of the century: the *Atlas* (opened in 1881), the *Endymion* (1881) and the *Castalia* (1884), which together provided over three hundred beds.[92] Only in 1904 were they decommissioned, following the opening of the MAB's Joyce Green Hospital in Long Reach, Dartford. Beyond London, the most cited case was heard at the High Court in 1893, where Withington urban authority sought to obtain an injunction preventing Manchester council from erecting a smallpox hospital on some land it owned, which was then in use as a cemetery. The argument was that a hospital of this sort constituted an "offensive trade" under existing nuisance regulations; but the judge sided with the city council and threw out the claim, a decision upheld by a subsequent ruling at the Court of Appeal.[93]

These were not isolated cases. In 1912, an LGB survey summarized that there were two consistent points of objection among local residents: first, that hospitals for infectious diseases posed a danger to those living nearby; and second, that hospitals depreciated the monetary value of neighboring land.[94] It is tempting to regard this as a manifestation of middle-class "nimbyism," and to some extent it was: the 1912 survey also noted the "sentimental objection" that hospitals were an eyesore. But as LGB officials and MOsH conceded, hospitals *did* pose a danger. In the case of smallpox in particular, all professionals conceded that concentrating victims in hospitals posed a risk to neighboring communities. The problem was explored at unprecedented length in a royal commission inquiry held in 1881–82 into London's smallpox and fever hospitals, and it was affirmed thereafter.[95] More importantly, MOsH also conceded that there was the danger of "cross-infection" *within* hospitals, whether between patients, or between patients and staff. This too was a long-standing problem, but it intensified with the advent of specialist isolation provision, when the interrelations of scarlet fever and diphtheria became a particular cause of concern. As John Eyler has detailed, the debate that developed proved inconclusive: statistics poured forth on both sides, but no decisive knockout blow was delivered either way.[96] Even so, a small minority of MOsH were quite prepared to suggest that isolation hospitals generated just as many problems as they solved.

STAMPING OUT IN PRACTICE

The counterargument against these criticisms was simple, and indeed inscribed in their very expansion: namely, that these problems were not intrinsic to isolation hospitals. Rather, they were *risks,* necessary risks perhaps; but equally, risks worth taking and risks that could be managed. This, after all, was the very premise of stamping out. It is certainly the case that growing levels of epidemiological and etiological precision made for confidence in this respect. Bacteriology, for instance, transformed the therapeutics and diagnosis of diphtheria during the 1890s with the development of an antitoxic serum and swab testing, both innovations stemming from research in France and Germany. Municipal and university-based laboratories became a key part of the systems that developed.[97] Likewise, germ theories prompted a more specific grasp of the pathways and vectors peculiar to different infectious diseases, meaning that spatial and hygienic tactics might be tailored accordingly. The 1912 LGB survey quoted above summarized the broad consensus as it had developed over the previous twenty years, noting eight means of transmission and ranking each according to their "striking distance."[98] These extended from physical contact (e.g., diphtheria), parasites (typhus), and expelled droplets from the mouth and nose (scarlet fever), to aerial convection (smallpox), and food and water (typhoid).

A related source of growing confidence lay in disinfection, which emerged as a discrete field of professionalized refinement and commercial innovation during the second half of the century. This by no means precluded its integration with general measures of cleanliness. Still at the turn of the century the term *disinfection* possessed what was described as a "loose" or "generic" meaning, whereby it referred to any practice that rendered the spread of infection less likely.[99] These broad definitions, however, reflected growing specificity elsewhere. During the 1860s and 1870s, LGB officials, chemists, and manufacturers had begun to offer more restricted applications of the term, often relying on a threefold distinction between deodorants, which prevented only smells and effluvia; antiseptics, which sought to arrest or impede putrefaction; and true disinfectants, which killed germs and infective matter.[100] A further distinction was drawn between disinfection by heat and chemical disinfection, which together formed the focus of what some now promoted as a specialist subfield of sanitary science.[101]

The science of disinfection principally consisted of assessing the "germicidal efficiency" of any particular method or substance. The LGB was an early pioneer, conducting a series of laboratory experiments in 1884 on chemical and heat-dependent techniques.[102] It marked only the start of what would become an ongoing preoccupation, as MOsH and university-based researchers sought to navigate an expanding marketplace of technologies and products. In the case of chemical disinfectants, a number of existing techniques continued to prosper: limewashing, for instance, and the use of chlorine gas for fumigation. Midcentury products such as Burnett's fluid (derived from zinc chloride) and Condy's fluid (from potassium permanganate) also remained popular. The most notable development was the growing use of carbolic acid (phenol) and related products involving cresols, such as Jeyes fluid, Izal, and Lysol, a German import.[103] Similarly, in terms of heat, destruction by burning and immersion in boiling water continued to be practiced, but there was also resort to an abundance of specialist machines that began to emerge in the 1870s. All involved some kind of ovenlike arrangement into which household articles and clothing could be inserted. The key shift was from those that relied on dry heat, such as Ransome's disinfector, to those that relied on steam. The most popular models were Lyon's steam disinfector, the Equifex saturated steam disinfector, and Reck's disinfecting machine, an import from Denmark (see figure 22). The benefits of steam were many: it destroyed germs more quickly compared to dry heat; it was versatile and could be applied to furniture and mattresses;

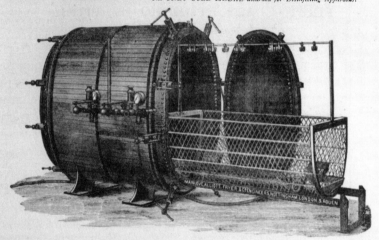
FIGURE 22. Lyon's steam disinfector, built by the same company responsible for manufacturing Fryer's destructor (see chapter 5). It also traveled around the world, as the advert boasts. The advert regularly featured in the journal *Public Health* during the late 1880s and early 1890s. Source: *Public Health* 2, no. 2 (1889–90): 48–49. © The Bodleian Libraries, The University of Oxford.

and in the case of fabrics, it steered clear of two extremes, scorching by dry heat and shrinkage by boiling (there was some regard for the integrity of private property).[104]

The laboratory was one space, however; the world beyond of jostling people and teeming things quite another. It was not just that "germs" could not be seen with the naked eye. There was also much that was difficult to verify with any degree of accuracy in situ, such as who or what a particular person had come into contact with; his or her levels of immunity; and the precise stage of incubation-infection. Not even swab testing for diphtheria was judged absolutely reliable: in Brighton, for instance, the MOH Arthur Newsholme insisted on three negative results before a patient could be deemed free from infection.[105] In practice, then, for all the science that helped to specify particular vectors, and the antiseptic and bactericidal agency of different disinfecting techniques, there was still a necessary—indeed defining—element of proactive, preventive indiscrimination; or what amounted to a kind of all-purpose hygienic vigilance that was deployed irrespective of the disease or person in question. As Michael Worboys has shown, both the "seed" (some kind of germlike agent) and the "soil" (the body and environment) remained crucial in terms of understanding the generation and diffusion of infectious diseases at the end of the Victorian period.[106] To this we might add, in administrative terms, a capacious risk-aversion that privileged urgency and action, whatever the case.

Disinfection was the most pervasive practice and we will turn to this in a moment; but the stamping-out systems that emerged also involved managing the location and movement of bodies. Three points might be highlighted: removing and excluding persons; transporting persons; and isolating persons.

Removing and Excluding Persons

Once a notification certificate had been received a visit was made by an inspector or MOH, or both, to the location of the infected person. As with inspection, tact and discretion were judged crucial if the system was to function smoothly.[107] MOsH were encouraged not to challenge the diagnosis of a doctor and to seek his approval in cases where removal to hospital was deemed necessary. Making these judgments ultimately rested with the MOH, and statute provided some guidance. In particular, the 1875 Public Health Act permitted removal in cases where the infected person was "lodged in a room occupied by more than one family," or in a

CLH, or onboard a ship. But the act also allowed for removal when a person was judged to be "without proper lodging or accommodation," which was altogether more ambiguous.[108] In these cases, the key consideration was whether a person could be isolated at home, and afforded sufficiently salubrious accommodation and attentive nursing. Other factors included whether there was spare capacity in a local hospital and the type of infection. It seems hospital isolation was urged in all cases of smallpox. By contrast, typhoid was judged more manageable at home than either scarlet fever or diphtheria. The result was variable levels of hospitalization according to place and infection: in 1899, for instance, of all the scarlet fever cases notified in London, roughly 74 percent were hospitalized; of diphtheria, 62 percent; and of typhoid, 41 percent.[109]

Another set of decisions centered on children attending elementary schools. General statutes provided no guidance on this front. Instead, beginning in 1882, national education codes prescribed that board school managers had to comply immediately with the wishes of a local authority, whether this meant excluding particular pupils or closing the premises.[110] These were considerable powers, partly because they interfered with the work of the education system, and partly because grant funding depended on levels of attendance. Nonetheless, the exclusion of a child—and perhaps his or her siblings as well—was ordered as a matter of course by MOsH, and by the early 1890s systems had emerged in cities such as Birmingham, Manchester, and London that relied on two kinds of supplementary notification: one authorizing the exclusion of a scholar; another his or her return, subject to inspection.[111] Closing a school was a different matter: as a memorandum issued by the LGB in 1890 made clear, it was a measure of last resort, only to be enacted in times of epidemic emergency.[112] Even then a MOH had to be convinced it would work, given that outside a school it was difficult to regulate the movement of children. As Maidstone's MOH suggested: "Practical experience convinces me that in the general way less risk is incurred by keeping children together under discipline and intelligent observation, than by sending them home to run loose upon the streets and out of sight and beyond the reach of discipline."[113] Closure was "an extreme measure," as the president of the British Institute of Public Health put it in 1894.[114] When it did take place, it was normally for severe outbreaks of scarlet fever, diphtheria, and measles, during which a school might be closed for anything between a single day and three months. In 1901, an outbreak of diphtheria prompted the closure of all of Colchester's elementary schools between mid-June and early September.[115]

In general, it seems MOsH enjoyed good relations with elementary schools, board and voluntary.[116] The same applies to relations with doctors and members of the public in cases where removal to hospital was sought. To be sure, doctors might contest an MOH's decision and there was occasional resort to inflicting fines and acting on the basis of a magistrate's order, as statute permitted. The local and professional press is dotted with instances of resistance, including scenes of mothers refusing to let go of their children, and inspectors and police constables breaking down doors.[117] Conversational persuasion seems to have been the principal countertactic, even if more creative solutions were pursued in places. In 1894, Southampton's MOH suggested that when faced with resistance the best response was to install sanitary inspectors outside the afflicted houses to take note of who was coming and going. The inhabitants soon relented, he boasted, and it resolved matters more quickly than going to court.[118] Even so, aggressive obstruction was rare, and it seems that most families complied without protest. Notably, in Leicester, a stronghold of antivaccination sentiment, whole families agreed to move into a hospital annex for two weeks when just one child or adult had been diagnosed with smallpox—the much-admired "Leicester system."[119] A regard for personal safety; official diplomacy; and the background menace of possible fines and court orders: a mixture of these elements made for a mostly compliant public.

Transporting Persons

Another focus of regulatory activity was the delivery of infected persons to hospital. The use of hired, horse-drawn cabs had long created anxiety, especially in cities where increased mobility and public anonymity meant that it was difficult to know the identity, still less the health, of a previous occupant. It made for a recurrent item of comment in the national and local press, where reference was made to "pest-vehicles" and "perambulating fever nests," all of which tapped into broader concerns about the dangers of commuting with unknowns. This was not simply a matter of press-fueled panic: journals such as the *Lancet* and the *BMJ* commented upon the risks generated by the unregulated traffic of infected persons, and the problem was explored at length in the 1882 royal commission on London's fever and smallpox hospitals noted above.[120]

Two strategies emerged during the 1860s. One was to criminalize the act of using "public conveyances" by anyone suffering from a "dangerous infectious disorder." First specified in the 1866 Sanitary Act, where it featured as part of a broader assault on the public exposure of infection, it was confirmed in subsequent statutes, such as the 1875 Public Health Act and the 1891 Public Health (London) Act. Indeed, the latter act specifically targeted cab drivers for knowingly accepting the custom of infectious persons.[121] Prosecutions were rare, however, and this is partly because regulations were relaxed in times of emergency; and partly because of a second strategy, namely empowering local authorities to provide their *own* means of conveyance, another feature of the 1866 act and subsequent statutes. During the 1870s, these became known as "ambulances," which as contemporaries explained—and indeed celebrated, as part of "the spread of the ambulance movement in civil life"—represented a relocation of military-style discipline and technology.[122] The term *ambulance* initially referred to a "hospital in miniature, attached to an army and following its movements"; but this was slowly displaced by more civilian applications, where it referred to the speedy and safe dispatch of infected and injured persons and associated vehicles.[123]

Thorne Thorne's 1882 LGB survey of existing hospitals detailed a variety of ambulance vehicles, ranging from simple stretchers on wheels drawn by hand to purpose-built omnibuses drawn by horse. The most popular type was a converted four-wheel cab, or "brougham."[124] By 1900, purpose-built ambulances had become common, comprising stretchers, seating space for a nurse, shock-absorbent rubber wheels, and a speaking tube to communicate with the driver (see figure 23). It was part of a remarkable flourishing of civilian ambulance systems, many of which looked to U.S. cities such as New York and Chicago for models of good practice.[125] Further components included the diffusion of first-aid expertise and the incorporation of new technologies to enhance the logistics. In particular, the telephone, a technology pioneered in the United States during the 1870s, was put to use by way of coordinating the dispatch of horse-drawn ambulances located at hospitals, police headquarters, and fire stations.[126]

Logistical-demographic pressures were most intense in London, and it was here, under the auspices of the MAB, where the most elaborate ambulance system emerged, comprising land and river services. The former began in 1881, when an ambulance station was established in East London; by 1900, there were six stations, each attached to a MAB hospital, and employing more than three hundred people in total. The river service, which catered for only smallpox victims, began in 1884, and was based around five steamers and three wharves, North (Blackwall),

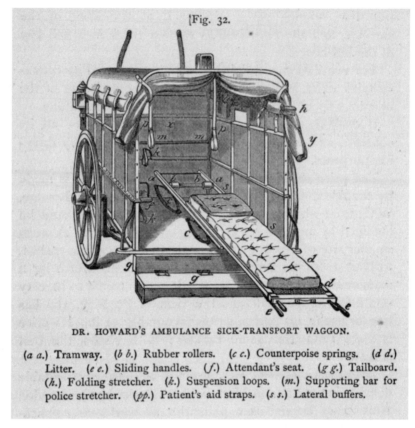

[Fig. 32.

DR. HOWARD'S AMBULANCE SICK-TRANSPORT WAGGON.

(*a a.*) **Tramway.** (*b b.*) **Rubber rollers.** (*c c.*) **Counterpoise springs.** (*d d.*) **Litter.** (*e e.*) **Sliding handles.** (*f.*) **Attendant's seat.** (*g g.*) **Tailboard.** (*h.*) **Folding stretcher.** (*k.*) **Suspension loops.** (*m.*) **Supporting bar for police stretcher.** (*pp.*) **Patient's aid straps.** (*s s.*) **Lateral buffers.**

FIGURE 23. "Dr Howard's Ambulance Sick-Transport Waggon." One of a number of more specialist vehicles that emerged in the 1880s for civilian purposes and that were generally purchased by larger local authorities. Source: G. J. H. Evatt, *Ambulance Organization, Equipment and Transport* (London: William Clowes, 1884), 83. © The Bodleian Libraries, The University of Oxford.

South (Rotherhithe), and West (Fulham).[127] Direct telephone lines were established with the MAB's central office on the Strand, where on receipt of a notification from a MOH, calls were made to the relevant land station (see figure 24). In 1891, the MAB's chief clerk suggested that ambulances were dispatched within only five minutes once the office had been notified; and by making for speed and rapid response, there was less chance of the infected coming into contact with others prior to their removal.[128] As the MOH for St. Pancras enthused: "It enables hospitals to be placed at a distance, and yet to be in instant communication with the central board. To a large extent the risks of visits to the infectious sick may be avoided

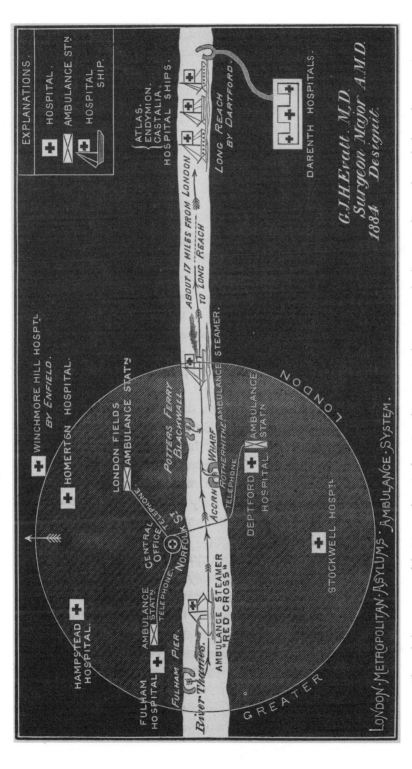

FIGURE 24. The ambulance system of the Metropolitan Asylums Board in 1884. At this point, as the diagram indicates, three telephones lines were in use. Source: G.J.H. Evatt, *Ambulance Organization, Equipment and Transport* (London: William Clowes and Sons, 1884), 29. © The Bodleian Libraries, The University of Oxford.

with such a ready means of inquiry at hand."[129] The traffic was immense: in 1898 alone, the land service made some thirty-five thousand removals, and by this point, so the MAB claimed, it was the largest integrated civilian ambulance system in the world.[130]

Isolating Persons

Ambulances were not always required. In those cases permitted to remain at home by a MOH the provision of a separate room and bed was judged sufficient accommodation, albeit preferably a room on the top floor: it made for better ventilation and was less likely to see familial traffic across the doorway. Above all, the room had to be stripped bare of any needless bedding, upholstery, and fabrics such as carpets that might harbor germs. Such practices were promoted in domestic manuals and by visiting MOsH and inspectors; but wealth determined quite how and to what extent they might be observed. Middle- and upper-class households had more and bigger rooms, and could rely on a servant to act as a nurse.[131]

Hospitals for infectious diseases afforded a greater degree of control, as indeed they had to, for besides the risk of cross-infection they were also porous institutions, as Graham Mooney has emphasized.[132] The human traffic included nursing and ambulance staff; contractors supplying items such as food, bedding, and disinfectants; as well as visitors. Little wonder that some suggested they should be called "aggregation hospitals."[133] Crucial, then, was regulating access and spatial contact. The most extreme expression of this was the "cubicle" or "barrier system," where the patient was provided with his or her own "box," completely cut off from others via glass partitions and served by its own door. First promoted by Plymouth's MOH in 1871, the city's council subsequently sought approval for a modified variant in 1890 but was refused by the LGB. The system enjoyed a revival in the Edwardian period, however, owing to the example of two Parisian hospitals, the Pasteur Hospital and the city's Hospital for Sick Children. In 1906, Walthamstow district council built a small hospital in Chingford composed of twelve cubicles situated in a single ward. A handful of councils followed suit, including Norwich, Enfield, and Croydon, while the LGB provided a model (a new plan D) of how a cubicle system might be built.[134]

The majority of hospitals relied on French-style pavilion wards combined with a set of regulations encouraged by the LGB and overseen by MOsH and hospital managers. A degree of discretion was urged in the case of visitors, especially when it came to mothers, who might need to suckle their young. Rules were relaxed when a patient was suffering from typhoid or near death. Otherwise visiting was strongly discouraged: as one survey of hospital hygiene put it in 1892, visiting introduced "a very considerable element of risk into the sanitation of the ward."[135] Thorne Thorne's 1882 survey had earlier expressed surprise at how strict some of the practices were. It was common to permit visiting only at set times and in limited numbers. In places it was restricted to looking through the window of a nurse's duty room that adjoined a ward.[136] Rules formulated by the MAB in 1877 allowed just one visitor at a time for up to fifteen minutes; specified that only vaccinated persons could visit smallpox patients; and advised that no contact should be made with the patient.[137]

In spatial terms, the key units were the ward and the bed. It seems in all new hospitals patients were afforded at least two thousand cubic feet of air, as specified by the LGB. Further common features included the establishment of a "neutral zone" of land between a hospital and a surrounding neighborhood (the LGB recommended at least forty feet); different entrances for staff and patients; easily cleansed surfaces (e.g., iron bedsteads and wax-polished wooden floorboards); and plentiful access to fresh air in keeping with the pavilion system (e.g., large windows, and verandas and airing courts). Mortuaries also featured, which were managed with just the same risk-averse attention to detail: viewing windows were installed, for instance, so that friends and family were "able to have a look at the dead without danger."[138] The key point of difference was the degree of ward-based classification. Rural hospitals of only two wards, each containing as few as two or three beds, were able to separate male and female patients, or two infections when required. By contrast, city-based institutions, which normally contained upward of forty beds, were able to provide separate wards for different infections, as well as special pavilions for cases that were of "uncertain diagnosis": a case of classifying the unclassified, if only for a while, as their symptoms did or did not develop. In some hospitals, such as Salford's Ladywell Sanatorium, opened in 1891, separate wards were also provided for convalescent patients.[139] The variations were many, but the general principle was to segregate as much as possible, in keeping with the overall size of an establishment.

Managing risk, then, was partly about managing space and bodies—access to space; the space between bodies; and the movement of bodies—and all of this had to be synchronized as quickly as possible, which meant it was also a matter of *speed*. The final element of stamping out was disinfection. Here too statute was more than generous, empowering sanitary authorities to enforce the disinfection of property and to build specialist disinfection facilities; and these powers were readily drawn upon, reflecting a desire to act in *all* circumstances and to target *all* means of transmission, regardless of whether or not an outbreak had developed—in other words, safety first. It was about closing down epidemiological possibilities, however slight, and even in the absence of any certainty as to what the "seed" was from a microbiological perspective. In the case of smallpox, for instance, the 1882 royal commission highlighted no fewer than seven specific "elements of danger" in relation to hospitals, extending from the arrival of ambulances and the letters dispatched by staff to the sewerage arrangements.[140] In practice, it made for a twofold kind of rigor: the mobilization of new and improved material substances and technologies, together with their utilization at each (temporal) stage and at every (spatial) point in the movement and management of an infected or suspect person.

Sanitary inspectors were charged with initiating actions in the home. Fumigating rooms where an infected person had resided was one tactic. Rooms were sealed up with tape, fumigated, and left for twenty-four hours; surfaces were then wiped with a disinfectant solution; wallpaper was replaced. Burning sulphur remained popular, but alternatives included the use of formaldehyde gas, a German innovation introduced in the 1890s.[141] In cases of typhoid especially, soiled linen and foodstuffs were destroyed and the drains disinfected using substances such as copperas. In pail-closet towns, inhabitants were supplied with colored vessels to mark them for special treatment at the dust depot. Meanwhile, clothing, bedding, and mattresses were dispatched to disinfecting machines, whether situated in an isolation hospital or in a special municipal station. Birmingham and Ipswich councils were among the first to build the latter, building specialized disinfecting stations in 1876.[142] By the 1890s, they had become standard in large cities: a survey for the LCC in 1893 revealed that the capital was home to sixteen municipal steam machines, plus fourteen that relied on dry heat.[143]

In cases of home isolation, members of the public played their part, drawing on the advice of sanitary officials and a medley of other agents, including voluntary societies and the authors of home-nursing manuals. "Burn everything that can be burnt; boil anything that can be so treated; wash and scrub well and expose to fresh air and sunlight; and send woolen articles, mattresses, etc., to be disinfected by steam by professional disinfectors," was the general advice given by the National Health Society in a penny pamphlet published in 1895.[144] Other tactics included hanging a sheet saturated with a solution of carbolic acid over the door of the sickroom; disinfecting all cups, glasses, spoons, bedpans, and spittoons used by the infected person; limiting all visiting; keeping the nurse or the person in attendance as separate as possible from other householders; and then fumigating the sickroom once the patient had recovered.

It was in hospitals where something like a total hygiene developed, amplifying the stricter practices that had begun to emerge as part of the diffusion of pavilion-style wards and growing resort to antiseptic and aseptic surgical practices.[145] The "rituals" were many, as they were sometimes styled. One set focused on managing the possibilities for transmission between the inside and outside of a hospital. Ambulances and bedding vans, for instance, were disinfected using a variety of phenol-based sprays. Particular attention was paid to the passage of new and convalescing patients. On arrival they had to give up their clothes, which were disinfected and stored in a locker; a bath followed. From the 1890s, new hospitals incorporated special discharge rooms containing slipper baths and dressing boxes. The "Bathing-out Rules" put in place in 1896 in Birmingham's Fever Hospital indicate something of the risk-averse intensity that developed. Patients were washed in bathwater mixed with Izal. The heads of children were rubbed with carbolic oil; noses and ears were syringed with a weak solution of formalin. A hot drink and food were provided, before the patient was examined by the medical superintendent and signed out.[146] Nothing so exacting was applied in the case of visitors, but all had to partake of a modicum of risk-averse ritual. Visitors might be required to don surgical-style, rubberized mackintoshes, or at least some kind of washable overall. Hands had to be washed in carbolic soap on entrance and exit. As early the 1880s, visitors to Huddersfield's hospital even had to take a bath on leaving and have their clothes disinfected—which, unsurprisingly, did much to deter visiting.[147]

The other principal set of practices focused on closing down the risk of cross-infection within hospitals, and especially wards. Separate laundry and disinfection blocks formed a crucial point of passage for all bedding, clothing, and towels, where they were subject to steaming and boil-washing. Destructors, of the kind found in municipal dust yards, were used for burning bed linen, sponges, and paper tissues; disinfectants were immediately applied to patients' excreta. Nurses wore cotton rather than woolen dresses, which were less liable to harbor germs; sleeves were rolled up. Hands were washed with carbolic soap or methylated spirits following any contact with a patient.[148] General regimen of this sort was encouraged from the 1870s and it was joined in the 1890s by more bespoke practices for cases of diphtheria and scarlet fever. Patients' fauces, for instance, were douched with Izal or Lysol; nasal and aural discharges were similarly treated. At Manchester's Monsall Hospital nurses applied mild disinfectant to the throats of scarlet fever patients using sterilized nozzles and rubber gloves, all part of what the medical superintendent described as "surgical cleanliness."[149]

THE "ENGLISH SYSTEM"

What, finally, of ports? The product of multiple initiatives inland, stamping out continued to travel, pursuing a twofold translocal journey in the context of England's coastal gateways to the world. On the one hand, stamping out was reworked in a domestic portside setting; on the other, it moved through the ISCs that first emerged in the 1850s, eventually becoming the international model. It traveled in this fashion underpinned by a sense of its humanitarian and liberal qualities, despite having been criticized by some as quite the opposite in the context of towns and cities. The contrast here, however, was not with the absence of compulsion, but with quarantine, a contrast that built on the midcentury arguments of the GBH and the NAPSS. The difference was that a discernible system had now emerged, one that paralleled measures inland. In 1887, speaking on the subject of cholera at a BMA conference, Thorne Thorne of the LGB drew a stark contrast between "European measures of restriction" and "British measures of prevention": "The one is the quarantine system; the other is our system of medical inspection and isolation."[150] Ten years later, addressing the Royal College of Physicians, the MOH for the Port of London, William Collingridge, outlined the history of what he called the "English system," a term first used in this context in 1875.[151] "This is a system which, while in no way interfering with trade, affords the utmost protection which is possible or even desirable," he stated, reminding his audience that the port of departure was of no concern, only what officials were presented with after inspection. The "isolation of the sick and the disinfection of the vessel follow exactly the same lines as those employed on shore," he added, before claiming that the wealth of the British Empire depended on it.[152]

In each direction the LGB was at the heart of the making of the system. In 1873, as British ports were threatened by another pandemic of cholera, the LGB took responsibility for prescribing measures, making for the first official appearance of the English system at home. A year later, beginning with the fourth ISC in Vienna, the combination of inspection, disinfection, and isolation became the signal system urged by British delegations; and in particular, from the sixth conference (Rome, 1885), by the LGB's Thorne Thorne, who in 1892 became the board's chief medical officer.[153] The conflicts that flourished at this level have been brilliantly reconstructed by Peter Baldwin and Krista Maglen in what made for a complex mix of contested science (including Robert Koch's bacteriological findings), and considerations of commerce, geopolitics, and administrative capacity.[154] And Britain's responsibilities were many, given its multiple possessions and protectorates abroad, including India and Hong Kong, and Egypt and the Suez Canal.

In the end, practices converged around the English model, culminating in the 1903 International Sanitary Convention, which was designed to standardize four earlier conventions formulated in the 1890s that applied to cholera and plague. It prescribed the key elements of the English system; compulsory notification *between* nation-states; as well as the foundation of a permanent bureaucracy, which in 1907 took the form of the Office international d'hygiène publique, based in Paris. The 1903 convention was presented as a triumph for British efforts, though there were compromises.[155] The 1903 agreement, for instance, allowed for a five-day period of "observation" in the case of all those that had been on board an infected vessel, healthy, suspect, or stricken; whereas in England the healthy were required only to provide information as to their destination inland, or what was styled as a system of "surveillance" as opposed to one of "observation." Ultimately, the "uniformity of system" sought by the British since the 1840s remained frustrated. Yet, compared to the variations that had been detailed by the NAPSS in the early 1860s, the 1903 convention made for relative uniformity. The twenty signatories included Germany, Austria-Hungary, Brazil, the United States, France, and Russia.

The English system, then, if it helped to secure freedom of commerce and movement, did so, it could be argued, on the basis of *more* and not less interference. Either way, it was about institutionalizing the same kind of risk-based readiness and attention to individual bodies and spaces characteristic of stamping out inland. The crucial development was the formation of port sanitary authorities (PSAs) to constitute what was termed "a first line of defence" against "foreign attacks." The LGB began putting together PSAs from its inception. Forty-six were established by LGB orders between 1872 and 1880; by 1904, there were fifty-nine permanent authorities, which between them encompassed all the major and minor ports in England and Wales.[156] Each was charged with applying the resources of existing urban and rural districts in order to fulfil two principal duties: securing the sanitary state of ships; and preventing the introduction of sea-borne cases of infectious disease, including familiar zymotic diseases such as smallpox and typhoid.

In this way, the LGB began to home in on the coastline and reforming practices specific to ports. All could agree that ports were first and foremost economic spaces, and this meant clarifying the role of customs officials, their principal gatekeepers in this respect. Relations between customs and sanitary officials seem to have been good from the start, with the former obliged to report any actual or suspected cases of infectious disease to the latter. Yet, as the LGB and PSAs complained, this was not so in all cases given that the 1825 Quarantine Act remained in force. Centrally, it meant the Privy Council remained an administrative agent and it did occasionally make orders on this front post-1872, despite the country's ailing infrastructure: a single functioning quarantine station on the Solent by the 1880s. More importantly, it meant customs officials could order quarantine in cases of yellow fever and plague, bypassing PSAs entirely.[157] The situation was not resolved until the 1896 Public Health Act, when quarantine was abolished, making the LGB the sole central authority and enabling PSA officials to inspect all vessels in all cases, regardless of the opinions of customs officers.

The more pressing problem was ensuring that PSAs were as best equipped as they might be. The administrative variations were many and were detailed in two major surveys by the LGB in 1884–85 and 1893–94. Each was prompted by further "cholera scares" in 1884 and 1892–93, and each doubled as opportunities for the central inspectors to urge more systematic administration on the part of PSAs.[158] Certainly there was resistance. Curiously, one of the attractions of quarantine was that it was paid for centrally through "imperial taxation," rather than locally from the rates. In 1892, Grimsby town council led a deputation to the LGB on behalf of twenty-six other PSAs urging the reinstatement of quarantine for cholera on these grounds.[159] In 1898, when a national association of PSAs was formed, questions of cost topped its list of lobbying priorities, even if quarantine was now off the agenda (though to no avail, for the actions of PSAs would remain a local charge).[160] Still, a basic pattern gradually emerged: the busier, the better equipped. London was rare in having its own MOH; other PSAs, such as Hull, Bristol, and Tyne, pos-

sessed their own teams of inspectors; most co-opted existing local officials. By the mid-1890s, isolation hospitals ranged from bespoke floating
hospitals (e.g., the Tees PSA) and portside establishments (London) to
converted railway carriages (New Shoreham) and ad hoc tents (Lancaster) in very minor ports (see figure 25). The majority resorted to inland
facilities run by sanitary authorities.

PSAs were thus probed and prodded by the LGB in the same fashion
as their mainland counterparts, and they drew on a similar repertoire of
measures, including the 1889 Notification Act. The major ports readily
took advantage of these powers. Sanitary inspections took place on
much the same lines, resulting in notices for whitewashing and altera-
tions to onboard plumbing and ventilation. In 1890, Collingridge
detailed that in the first six months of the year some 7,500 vessels had
been inspected in the Port of London, of which 347 were subject to
whitewashing. It brought the cumulative total of inspections since 1873
up to almost 309,000.[161] In Hull, tens of thousands of emigrants were
inspected each summer during the late 1880s and early 1890s, and
indeed inspected again at the railway station, where they boarded trains
for Liverpool or Glasgow.[162] When a case was reported onboard a ship,
a medley of practices was set in motion that recalled those used inland.
In 1888, Tyne PSA's MOH—also that of Newcastle—detailed the following "routine" once intelligence had been received from a customs
officer. It began with the chief inspector boarding the vessel and verifying
or not the initial assessment, or admission from a captain. In the event of
infection, the inspector certified the removal of the individual to the
floating hospital; ensured that the vessel was cleansed and fumigated;
and telephoned the MOH, who alerted the inland hospital. The captain
and the customs officer were then given certificates granting clearance to
proceed to harbor, where the ship was placed under supervision.[163]

These were indeed routine duties as applied to "indigenous" diseases
such as smallpox and typhus. Of a different order again were the measures put in place when cholera and then plague threatened at the turn of
the century, for this is when governing epidemiological risks reached its
acme. On the one hand, there was plentiful early warning. The LGB,
GRO, newspapers, and sanitary and maritime publications maintained
a keen eye on their progress abroad detailing their devastation and next
steps. There was no shortage of information, as well as public alarm at
times, not least when cholera was wreaking deadly havoc in Hamburg
in 1892.[164] On the other hand, as "exotic" diseases, the stakes were
raised and there was still much that could *not* be known, in particular

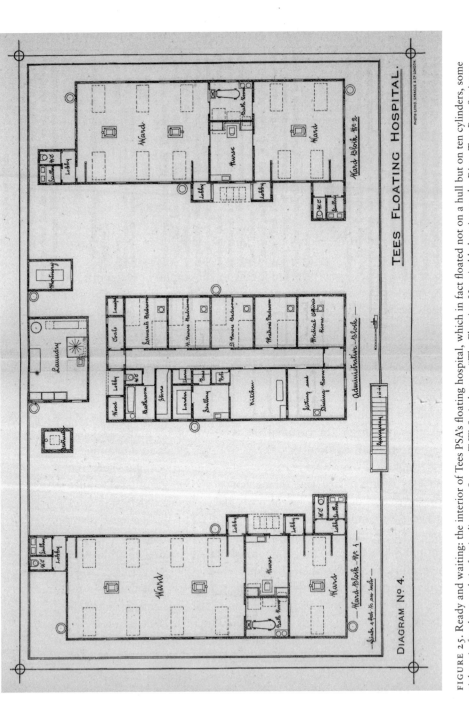

FIGURE 25. Ready and waiting: the interior of Tees PSA's floating hospital, which in fact floated not on a hull but on ten cylinders, some eighty-six feet long and six feet in diameter. Source: T. W. Stainthorpe, "The Floating Hospital belonging to the River Tees Port Sanitary Authority," *Proceedings of the Incorporated Association of Municipal and County Engineers*, vol. 21, 1894–95 (London: E. and F.N. Spon,

the condition of any given ship and its cargo, crew, and passengers, even if it had sailed from an infected or suspect port. Ultimately, one could not be sure that portside measures would prove successful. The result was that cholera and plague were subject to special measures, and not only to provide for their portside "exclusion," but also to allow for their "control" should the former fail: a strategy of safety first, and on a national scale. The measures were subsequently judged a success: the biggest crisis came in 1893, when cholera claimed only 135 lives.

In terms of their control and limitation, it was partly about the LGB performing the same regulatory function as the GBH and MDPC had before it. Orders and official memoranda were issued to all urban and rural authorities, reminding them of the symptoms to look out for, and urging the speedy isolation of suspect cases and measures of disinfection. By the 1890s the LGB could build on the stamping-out culture that had emerged. A general memorandum issued in 1892 discussed cholera—already subject to official notification—alongside "diphtheria, fever and any other epidemic disease." It was simply that "greater vigilance" should be exercised with respect to matters of sanitation and inspecting the poor.[165] In 1900, the LGB made plague a notifiable disease, urging that it be treated in the same way as indigenous ones.[166] The most responsive authorities were those most at risk. In 1892, Newcastle's sanitary committee readied itself following the death of a cholera patient on the Tyne PSA's floating hospital. A "second line of defence" was thus put into place, which included stockpiling disinfectants and co-opting the police station's telephone system for notification purposes.[167] Similarly, Liverpool's sanitary committee contracted eight additional inspectors during the 1900–1901 plague scare. When a handful of suspected plague cases were found on shore, the same measures were deployed that applied in cases of smallpox and typhus: hospital isolation for the afflicted; the disinfection of their clothing and bedding; and return visits to the houses in question and to friends and neighbors.[168]

At the same time, these efforts were fused with those of PSAs as agents of exclusion, making for dense compounds of localized-centralized agency and international flows of information. During the mid-1880s, the LGB imposed a set of temporary bans relating to imported rags in keeping with the spread of cholera abroad, first from Spain (in June 1885 and February 1886), then from Italy (July 1886), and then from Austria-Hungary (October).[169] Placed on alert, PSAs stepped up their efforts. During the same period, Tyne PSA employed an extra inspector to target vessels from infected and suspect ports according to information gleaned from newspapers, the medical press, and the *Shipping Gazette*.[170] Later, in 1893, it again intensified its efforts, recruiting two extra inspectors to work days and nights, and providing a special disinfection launch comprising cylinders of pressurized chlorine, a receptacle for bales of rags, and a steam machine.

The most notable development was the attention given to rats in the case of plague, which first arrived in Europe (at Oporto, Portugal) in July 1899. In 1900 and 1901, the LGB issued memoranda which besides encouraging standard stamping-out measures urged special attention "to the risk of importing plague into the country by means of plague-infected rats"; a recommendation that built on growing international consensus regarding its epidemiology.[171] The memoranda galvanized what would become a long-standing war on rats. In 1903 alone, some seventy-six thousand were destroyed by hired rat catchers on vessels moored in London's docks.[172] Destruction, however, was only the end point of a long chain of precautionary measures. In 1902, Bristol's MOH detailed some of the extra practices employed there and at other leading ports. They included consulting the weekly updates issued by the U.S. Marine Hospital regarding infected ports; ensuring that infected ports were kept on the in-house list for three months even after their official clearance abroad; and placing all ships sailing from suspect or infected ports under the immediate twenty-four-hour supervision of watchmen to guard against the escape of rats along gangways and mooring cables.[173] Nothing was left to chance, not even the ingenuity of rodents, in this particular plague-based variant of portside risk-aversion.

CONCLUSION

It had been long in the making and was of truly zigzagging and contingent gestation; but by roughly 1900 something like a common stamping-out system was in place, in both ports and inland areas, for governing the danger and spread of infectious diseases. Further innovations would follow. In 1912, an ISC convention applied its own model fully to yellow fever. In 1913, tuberculosis was made a compulsory notifiable disease at home, following experiments in Brighton, Manchester, Liverpool, and Sheffield. It is tempting to interpret this as part of the rise of a modern and more muscular state that acted on the basis of the growing precision and ambitions of sanitary science; but this reading obscures just as much as it illuminates.

Two concluding points might be made in this respect. The first is that the modernity of stamping out resides less in the incursions or agency of a growing and more powerful state, and more in the antagonisms and tensions in which it was assembled and legitimized as a system. Contemporaries certainly thought of stamping out in terms of the state and the power to interfere with personal liberty. Quite rightly in some respects: it was indeed about interfering, and doing so, ultimately, on the basis of legal compulsion. Yet, there was no guiding supra-agent such as a state at work in terms of how stamping out emerged. Rather, its various threads and facets were figured out and put together as part of a modern system of central-local relations and a field of governance that extended much beyond public health professionals. Equally, the very meaning of "liberty" was up for grabs. Ultimately, the English, who so prided themselves on their historical attachments to liberty, opted for security; or rather, since it could be argued either way, liberty *as* security, and in particular freedom from the danger of infected others. It was a moot point perhaps, a matter of perspective; but it was certainly part of how the problem of governing infectious diseases was posed and practiced.

The second point is that stamping out was a logistical art, and of a piece with an emerging culture of modern governance that combined time and space in ever-more dense and compressed ways. It is certainly possible to discern its key elements—surveillance, isolation, and disinfection—amid the emergency responses to cholera. But these measures were only of a temporary character, and it is this dimension that partly distinguishes stamping out as it began to coalesce during the 1860s: its application, that is, to a range of zymotic diseases and on a permanent basis, so that local authorities were in a constant state of alert, ready to react as quickly as possible across time and space. And this is bound up with the risk-oriented nature of stamping out. It was not only a matter of applying the insights of sanitary science, as in the differential, disease-specific application of disinfectants and tactics of hospital isolation. It was also about a risk-averse precision of practice which, paradoxically perhaps, meant a certain kind of prophylactic indiscrimination in the attention given to individual bodies and spaces—precision, that is, as practical rigor in the way one eliminated possibilities (possible further infections) stemming from known dangers (notified, infected persons). It is no coincidence that the last decades of the century also witnessed the professionalization of local fire services; the advent of civic ambulance groups providing military-style first-aid relief; and the further tightening of practices introduced in the 1840s regarding the compulsory notification of accidents in factories.[174]

Such were the measures that evolved when a private body was a public danger and a risk to other bodies; but as we shall now see, the public health system also required these same bodies to engage in preventive practices that, by contrast, were much more routine, daily, and habitual.

CHAPTER 7

Personal Hygiene

Cleanliness, Class, and the Habitual Self

Public health reformers did not shy from stating the obvious: that improving collective health, for all that it required the mobilization of taxes and laws, technologies and expertise, also required the cooperation of the public. This is partly what defines the modernity of England's public health system as it developed during the Victorian period: namely, the problem of working with the public as both an object and a subject of governance. This was not the only ethos of governing. Compulsion was required in places, or at least the threat of legal action in the event of noncompliance, as in smallpox vaccination and nuisance administration. Still, a broad strategy of public cooperation and co-option formed a touchstone throughout, evident in the very architecture of center-local relations, and extending to the provision of GRO statistics, and the work and doorstep encounters of officials such as sanitary inspectors. As has been argued, one of the drawbacks of thinking in terms of a modern state is that it obscures the way governing public health worked through an intensification of the agency of multiple actors, whether local or central, or of a political, nonprofessional sort, such as MPs and councillors. This is where the modernity of the system resides.

Another instance is the home, which was objectified, distanced, and gendered as a discrete domain of governance; *and* mobilized, formalized, and positioned as a crucial agent and ally of reform.[1] Indeed, the home was sometimes figured as part of a series of interlocking local "centers" of action. In 1858, the Earl of Shaftesbury, a former member of Chadwick's GBH, sought to dismiss claims of "centralization" before the NAPSS's health section. In fact, he suggested, the aim of bodies like the GBH and NAPSS was to make every locality and every family "the fountain, the centre, the alpha and omega" of all sanitary "operations." He added: "so far from seeking centralization, we seek only to make it [sanitary reform] central in so far as it shall be confined to localities, and in so far as it shall be found the dominant, prevalent and active principle in every household and domestic assemblage."[2] Sentiments of this sort were widespread. "It is in those millions of centres we call the home that sanitary science must have its true birth," declared Benjamin Ward Richardson in the course of addressing the SIGB in 1880 on "woman as sanitary reformer": "It is from those centres that the river of health must rise."[3]

This chapter examines the intensification of a still more intimate center of modern governance: namely, a *personal* sphere of governance, and in particular practices of personal cleanliness. There was a definite inheritance in this respect, notably the practices based on the regimen of the "nonnaturals," which stretched back to the ancient Greeks and that enjoyed a revival in Europe between the sixteenth and eighteenth centuries.[4] There were six canonical categories in all: exposure to air; food and drink; sleeping and waking; movement and rest; retentions and evacuations, including sexual activities; and the emotions and passions. All of these areas of individual attention remained crucial during the Victorian period, when they were joined by washing the body. One might speak, then, of a linear, centuries-long process of hygienic individualization, much as modernity more generally is sometimes equated with the inexorable rise of "the individual."

Yet, it was only during the Victorian period when these practices were consistently positioned and promoted as "personal" and "private," as opposed to "public." Crucially, this was not only in a spatial and bodily sense; it was also in terms of their governance, and thinking about what did and did not lie within the sphere of the state and legal regulation.[5] The nature of the problem was not dissimilar to that which gave birth to a local level of governance, which blended considerations of logistics with those of liberty. On the one hand, it was moral and political; or in this case, of not interfering with the liberty of the subject, yet mobilizing this liberty all the same. On the other hand, it was organizational and epistemological, in the sense that it was impossible to know and regulate the individual peculiarities of an expanding mass of human bodies. And in the case of personal cleanliness, what mattered was the administration of that most intimate of surfaces, the skin, not to mention other embodied particulars, such as the hair and the feet.

The term *hygiene* played a role here, a word inherited from the Greeks via Latin and then French, and used with increasing frequency from the early nineteenth century to refer to all of those "arts" essential to preserving health.[6] One of the first texts to distinguish with any rigor between public and private hygiene was authored by the Scottish physician Alexander Kilgour, entitled *Lectures on the Ordinary Agents of Life as Applicable to Therapeutics and Hygiène* (1834). There were two subjects for consideration, he suggested: "the means which will be taken by Communities—or by the Government—for the public health; and the means which each individual will pursue for the preservation of his own health—or PUBLIC and PRIVATE hygiène."[7] The distinction had become commonplace by midcentury, featuring in and structuring the contents of a growing number of manuals and handbooks pitched at the public. "The sanitary legislation of our time is a work of the greatest value," stated the celebrated military physician E. A. Parkes in his popular guidebook *On Personal Care of Health,* first published in 1876:

> but it would be a fatal error to suppose it can do everything. It deals with many conditions which the individual man is powerless to control, but it cannot deal with others which belong only to the individual. From within this proceed many diseases, which no public hygiene can remove. There is, so to speak, an individual or private hygiene which must also be brought into action and without which half the work must remain undone, and the burden of sickness and suffering be but half removed.[8]

In the same year, a *Dictionary of Hygiène and Public Health* divided the subject into two spheres, public and private. Of the latter, it noted some general rules of conduct—regular exercise and fresh air; sensible clothing; personal cleanliness; and moderate intake of food and drink—while acknowledging that the precise management of these elements was something for the subject to determine, in keeping with his or her constitution. "Know thyself," the *Dictionary* urged, recalling the ancient Greek maxim.[9]

A repertoire of activities was thus devolved to the personal sphere of the self, of which cleanliness was a key part. These were the activities which, as John Simon tellingly put it in 1874, "the law does not, and generally could not, take within its scope."[10] From where, then, at this especially vulnerable point, the private or personal sphere, did the public health system draw its energy? The answer was *habit*, another term subject to innovation. Previously it had connoted inherited customs, clothes, and the condition of any given thing. These associations diminished as the term became synonymous with another earlier application: the repetitive actions of an individual's body and mind. "Custom supposes an act of the will; habit implies an involuntary movement," clarified one dictionary in 1846: "a custom is followed; a habit is acquired . . . Custom is applicable to bodies of men; habit is confined to the individual."[11] "Habit" was thus individualized and used principally to refer to a subjective tendency, acquired through practice, and rooted in the mind and body rather than in collective laws. Samuel Smiles's *Self-Help* (1859) was among the more popular texts to insist that the real source of social progress lay not in government legislation but in habits. "But no laws, however stringent, can make the idle industrious, the thriftless provident or the drunken sober," he wrote in the opening pages. "Such reforms can only be effected by means of individual action, economy, and self-denial; by better habits, rather than by greater rights."[12]

Just this aspiration is evident in the case of personal cleanliness: not only that it might be a matter of personal self-governance, but also that it might be habitual, and therefore relied upon in the absence of any state interference and legal regulation. Habits, after all, were thought of as a "second nature," a naturally occurring and predictable disposition of body and mind. Yet, as we shall see, these habits still had to be *made,* for the Victorians—who were incredibly conflicted on the question of free will, much as we still are today—were just as emphatic that (a) habit *formation* was a complex process, requiring environmental and educational stimulus as much as any interior moral will power; and (b) that these habits then had to be *maintained* over time.[13] Habits of cleanliness are a case in point. They were certainly private in the sense that they were a question of the self-governance of bodily details. But they were also a matter of governance much beyond the self, relying on novel technologies and the ongoing promotion of a medley of moral and physical norms of conduct; and the promoters of the latter were truly multiple.

The contingencies were thus immense, and making these habits was further complicated by the persistence and reclamation of older bathing practices. We shall turn to the revival of Roman-Turkish bathing in the final section. More importantly, making these habits entailed confronting one of the key axes of English society, class, and working with a public fractured by differential wealth and status. It is no coincidence that the variable realization of these habits gave birth to one of the more notorious mass nouns of the nineteenth century: "the Great Unwashed."

"Indeed, want of ordinary personal cleanliness has come to be regarded as a distinguishing characteristic of that section of the community included under the term 'lower orders,'" noted Birkenhead's MOH in 1876. "A Frenchman contemptuously refers to this class among his people as *sanculottes* (the breechless), a German playfully dubs this class among his people *grobiane* (clumsy Jacks); while in this country one of the most familiar expressions used to designate the masses is 'the great unwashed.'"[14] The phrase, it seems, was coined in 1830 to refer to journalists; but it only became a derogatory term for the lower classes once a washed society had become established as a work in progress.[15]

In all these respects, making personal habits constitutes the least systematic of all the areas of modern public health reform examined in this book; by the same token, it also constitutes the most *systemic,* in the sense of requiring the articulation and combination of multiple norms, technologies, and agents. This chapter attempts to reconstruct this diffuse and complex systemic mix, beginning with the provision of technologies for washing the body.

PUBLIC AND PRIVATE TECHNOLOGIES

There were two basic assumptions that underpinned the encouragement of personal cleanliness. One is that it required some kind of technological accompaniment and stimulus. As Chadwick pithily put it in an address called "Skin Cleanliness," delivered to the Society of Arts in 1877: "Provision of mechanical conveniences and appliances must precede and facilitate the formation of habits."[16] The second sustained and framed the more general gestation of public health as a modern system of governance: simply that it was a matter of historical progress and civilizational development. Indeed, much like debating the merits of centralization, reforming bathing habits entailed engaging with an inheritance that now stretched back over centuries; but in this case there was much more consensus regarding the past, and the narratives were often crude. Briefly, apparently "filth-loving" primitive peoples represented the absence of hygiene; Jewish practices and Mosaic laws, a good start; Roman society, the zenith of past achievements; early Christendom, a step back; and reformed, early-modern Christianity, a tentative step forward. "When the civilisation of the Egyptians, the Jews, the Greeks and the Romans faded, the world passed through dark ages of mental and physical barbarism," declared Lyon Playfair in 1874, addressing the NAPSS's health section. "For a thousand years there was not a man or woman in Europe that ever took a bath," he suggested, before applauding the revival of hygiene in the nineteenth century.[17]

One lockable door; one slipper-style bathtub in which the whole body could be immersed; and one set of taps, providing hot and cold water: it was this particular combination of technologies that was upheld as the best means of securing ablutionary habits and civilizational progress. The pioneers of fixed installations were public baths establishments, which began to emerge in the 1840s. Their number underwent a gradual expansion up to the 1880s, before taking off in the 1890s. In 1877, one survey put the number in England at forty-nine; by 1914 it had grown to more than three hundred.[18] Domestic bathrooms of a similar kind—plumbed and fixed—developed during the latter third of the century. A variety of portable baths were a common feature in the homes of the wealthy by midcentury, where they might be prepared by servants and used in bedrooms. During the 1830s and 1840s, advice literature dwelled on the subject: Thomas Webster's *Encyclopaedia of Domestic Economy* (1844), for instance, detailed portable shower, leg and hip, and slipper baths.[19] By the 1880s, it seems that fixed slipper baths situated in a plumbed bathroom had come to be regarded as a necessity among the wealthy and they soon became standard. "All the houses built nowadays for the accommodation of the middle and upper classes are provided with bathrooms," noted one review of the latest literature on bathing in 1892.[20]

Public baths represent the boldest intervention in terms of encouraging habits of cleanliness among the public at large, and they also included swimming baths and, in some cases, attached laundries. They were initially provided using both municipal and philanthropic sources of funding. In terms of the latter, the key development came in London in 1844, when a meeting held at Mansion House led to the establishment of the Committee for Promoting the Establishment of Baths and Washhouses for the Labouring Classes. The committee financed three establishments and donors included Queen Victoria and the Archbishop of Canterbury.[21] Philanthropic sentiments continued to inspire the input of finance until the end of the century. As late as 1896, a small establishment opened in Market Harborough that had been partly funded by the railway contractor and local MP J. W. Logan.[22] The dominant course was to raise the finance on the security of the rates through an agreement with the Public Works Loan Commissioners, in which case it required vetting by the Treasury and then, from the 1870s, the LGB. Municipal input featured from the start. The first establishment to provide plumbed baths for "the lower orders" was built by Liverpool's corporation in

1842 on a site in Frederick Street, which housed ten slipper baths. Two more were built by the council in the following decade, one at Paul Street in 1846, containing forty-five warm baths, and one at Cornwallis Street in 1851, containing sixty-three.

Public baths certainly proved popular. Precise statistics were generated regarding the number of bathers, a product of the routine bookkeeping systems that all baths were expected to maintain in the interests of public accountability. In 1857, the deputy chairman of the London Committee, William Hawes, spoke before the NAPSS, where he detailed that between 1847 and 1854 the total number of private baths taken within the capital's twelve establishments was over five million.[23] Similar levels of consumption were later reported in the provinces. In 1876, a committee of Manchester's council presented a report advocating municipal ownership and investment. There was much demand, it suggested, noting that in 1875 the number of baths taken in Birmingham, Bristol, and Liverpool was roughly 286,000, 88,000, and 430,000 respectively.[24] And numbers continued to expand into the Edwardian period. In 1915, an LCC manual entitled *Comparative Municipal Statistics* detailed that over three million private baths had been taken in 1911 in London's fifty establishments; 430,000 in Manchester's sixteen; and 360,000 in Birmingham's fourteen.[25]

Quite how regularly they were visited and by whom is another matter. It was never part of the bureaucracy of public baths to gather information on the occupational identity of their users, though contemporaries suggested they were frequented by all classes with the exclusion of those at either end of the social scale.[26] What is clear is that they were part of an evolving hierarchy of technologies that was shaped by just this: class, and what the public could afford in terms of its hugely stratified levels of income. This was crucial in terms of the provision of facilities in the homes of the wealthy, where it was a question of catering to shifting tastes amid an expanding marketplace of products offered by commercial agents, such as Doulton and Shanks. But it was also a consideration that defined public baths, which, somehow, were supposed to be financially self-supporting—much indeed like the subjects they hoped to create and cater for—and publicly accessible in terms of their admission costs.

Decisive here was the provision of different classes of facilities, charged at different prices. It was taken for granted that different facilities should be provided for men and women, and that more should be furnished for the former; it was the class dimension that was subject to regulation. Another contribution of the London Committee came in the form of political lobbying and eventually legislation, which was steered through parliament by the Tory peer and committee member Sir Henry Dukinfield: the 1846 Baths and Washhouses Act, supplemented by an amending act in the next year. Besides empowering local authorities to borrow money on the security of the rates, the 1846–47 legislation prescribed the pricing and provision of facilities. Warm baths for "the labouring classes" were fixed at a maximum of two pence, and those of a "higher class" at no more than six pence; lower class baths were to be no fewer than twice the number of the better class. As contemporaries explained, it was about reconciling the need to maximize revenue, whereby first-class facilities would help to pay for the second, while providing for those sections of the community most in want. The same provisions were reaffirmed later in the 1875 Public Health Act.

The result was that all baths provided at least two classes of facilities—some provided three, such as Liverpool's Cornwallis Street establishment, and London's Paddington Baths built in 1874—and that the most numerous were second-class facilities for men. St. Giles and Bloomsbury Baths for example, built in 1853, provided seventy-three slipper baths in all: women were furnished with seven first-class and sixteen second-class baths; men with sixteen first-class and thirty-four second-class (see figure 26). Similarly, the establishment opened in 1895 on Tibberton Square, Islington, housed almost one hundred slipper baths: ten first-class female; twenty-three second-class female; eighteen first-class male; and forty-six second-class male.[27] The problem was that, for all the meticulous statutory specifications, public baths rarely proved self-supporting.[28] It meant that popular access to state-of-the-art technologies was reliant, ultimately, on the willingness of local authorities to bear a financial burden. A case in point is Manchester, where in 1854 the Manchester and Salford Baths and Laundry Company was founded, "consisting of about fifty of the city's leading men," and promising a 5 percent annual return for each investor. The company built baths in Greengate, Salford (1856), Ardwick (1857), and Hulme (1860); but none proved financially feasible, still less profitable, and in 1877 the latter two were taken over by the city council.[29]

This is also why they proved politically problematic, attracting, as was only legitimate, public scrutiny on the part of ratepayers and councillors. This was evident throughout. In 1853, a vestry meeting of St. Mary's parish, Southwark, was called to discuss plans for an establishment costing fourteen thousand pounds and comprising eighty slipper baths. The local

BLOOMSBURY BATHS AND WASHHOUSES.

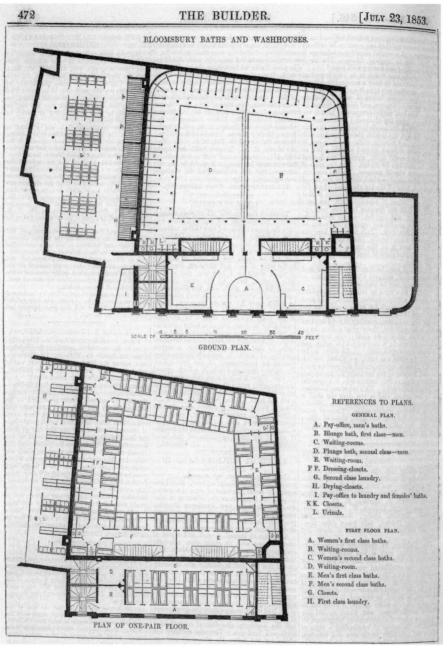

SCALE OF 10 5 0 10 20 30 40 FEET

GROUND PLAN.

PLAN OF ONE-PAIR FLOOR.

REFERENCES TO PLANS.

GENERAL PLAN.

A. Pay-office, men's baths.
B. Blunge bath, first class—men.
C. Waiting-rooms.
D. Plunge bath, second class—men.
E. Waiting-room.
F F. Dressing-closets.
G. Second class laundry.
H. Drying-closets.
I. Pay-office to laundry and females' baths.
K K. Closets.
L. Urinals.

FIRST FLOOR PLAN.

A. Women's first class baths.
B. Waiting-rooms.
C. Women's second class baths.
D. Waiting-room.
E. Men's first class baths.
F. Men's second class baths.
G. Closets.
H. First class laundry.

FIGURE 26. Bloomsbury baths and washhouses. The establishment also contained "plunge baths" (B and D), which were designed for both washing and swimming. Swimming pools proper only became standard from the 1870s. Source: "St Giles and Bloomsbury Public Baths and Washhouses," *Builder*, July 23, 1853, 472. © The Bodleian Libraries, The University of Oxford.

poor law surgeon moved the motion in support of the project, but it met with little favor among the ratepayers. According to the *Morning Post,* following "a scene of confusion scarcely equalled in the annals of the most disorderly parish," the meeting was hastily adjourned.[30] Still in the 1870s the parish was without an establishment. Councillors remained wary. In Birkenhead, plans were first put before the council in 1863; it was not until 1883 when the first establishment was opened.[31] In 1876, the town's MOH bemoaned the intransigence of his local authority employers: "Excellent reasons for not proceeding with the works have been plentiful; the most frequently urged being that the state of the finances of the town do not warrant it."[32] Even amid the expansion at the turn of the century, public skepticism remained pronounced. In 1901, during an LGB hearing, a solicitor for the Manchester and Salford Property Owners' Association opposed—to no avail, as it happened—a council proposal for a set of baths in Chorlton-upon-Medlock. Similar opposition was encountered—which here proved successful—in 1908 in Preston, where an LGB inquiry heard representations from ratepayers complaining "that the rates were already excessive and the baths would be a loss to the town."[33]

The flipside was that public baths were promoted by the same agents that at other times and in other places opposed them. They could hardly have expanded without this. Candidates spoke up for them in election addresses; councillors defended their merits in meetings; and ratepayers petitioned for their installation. Above all, it was civic sentiments that overrode any misgivings about their financial feasibility, even if this remained a critical consideration. Just such sentiments were expressed in the midcentury, when they mixed with a sense of elite civic stewardship; and they became still more pronounced during the 1880s and 1890s, when these same sentiments assumed a more social and democratic form. "It would be difficult in small houses of only five shillings rent per week to have all the perfect arrangements of a bath," declared the Liberal MP, William Mather, during a speech to mark the opening of Gorton baths in Manchester in 1890: "what the individual could not do for himself the community could carry out collectively."[34] The Liverpudlian magistrate and Tory alderman Thomas Hughes was quite explicit about the matter when he appeared before a select committee on municipal trading in 1900. "We have established a number of baths and washhouses, not with the idea of making money, or rather, not with the idea of losing money, although that has been the result," he explained. "The desire of Liverpool has so far been to improve the health of the poor and to give them facilities . . . which they would not have at home."[35]

The goal, then, was to strike some kind of balance, reaching out to the public while not engaging in anything too financially ruinous—a goal that was not easy to achieve under the watchful eyes of empowered ratepayers and councillors. Indeed, the public reach of public baths was limited precisely because of this concern and the charges imposed on customers. Competing among the multiple demands placed on the budgets of working-class families in particular was difficult. "The ordinary warm bath and public swimming bath are usually within the scope of the artisan, the youth and the unmarried men of the labouring classes," noted one delegate before the SIGB in 1888. The same was not true of "married labourers and their families" who could only afford to use public baths occasionally, "the reason being that the price charged, though so low, is still too much for their means."[36] It was just this conundrum that prompted interest in continental innovations, notably the People's Bath (*Volksbad*) pioneered by the German dermatologist Oscar Lassar, which was first displayed at the 1883 Berlin Hygiene Exhibition. Designed for use by the poorest classes and costing only a penny, the facilities consisted of a small, corrugated-iron shelter partitioned into shower cubicles. (It was in fact a development of some recent practices introduced in the French and German armies.) In the 1880s and 1890s, People's Baths were championed by councillors and architects in the interests of placing still cheaper facilities at the heart of working-class districts.[37] But although there was growing resort to showers within old and new establishments (as well as within middle-class homes), the impact of Lassar's model was modest. Among the larger authorities, only Liverpool and Bristol opted to provide these especially austere institutions.[38]

The result was that the plumbed baths on offer in public establishments came to occupy a technological middle ground between the more luxurious facilities to be had in upper- and middle-class homes, and those that might be had in working-class dwellings. In the 1890s, bathrooms began to feature in philanthropic and municipal housing schemes, as well as in the bylaw terraces pitched at the upper end of the working-class market; but this was a late and restricted development, and the majority of working-class households had to do without, supplementing whatever visits were made to public baths with the use of improvised arrangements.[39] These were of two principal sorts. One option was to wash next to a kitchen sink or in a curtained-off corner of a bedroom with the aid of a basin of water and a washstand. A series of "Lectures for the People" delivered in the 1880s by the MSSA recommended just this combination.[40] The other option was to buy a cheap variant of the portable baths that had been popular among the middle and upper classes during the first half of the century. In 1879, as part of an "Address to the Wage Classes," Benjamin Ward Richardson dismissed claims that bathing at home was too inconvenient or costly: "A shallow tub, or a shallow metal bath . . . a good sponge; a piece of soap; two gallons of water; and a good large towel, are quite sufficient for every purpose of health."[41] Both options were indeed sufficient and not ideal; and yet it was impossible not to be pragmatic. As in the case of public baths, it was about working with what was affordable and feasible.

Between them these technologies constituted the basic repertoire of technologies for washing the body that developed during the Victorian period. It made for a stratified mix of technological sophistication and degrees of privacy: a private space within a private space (the domestic bathroom); a private space within a public, segregated space (the public baths cubicle); and an improvised, semiprivate space (the tub or washbasin in a kitchen or bedroom). And not everyone was able to partake of these technologies. Limited access to bathing technologies among the poor was the principal inspiration for the establishment of public baths during the midcentury; and these limits, if no longer quite so extensive, were still painfully apparent later on. Public health officials, domestic visitors, and social investigators continued to publicize the existence of an "outcast" population accustomed to bodily and domestic dirt; or what for some signified a lack of "personal civilization." In 1895, one MOH dwelled on the neglect of personal cleanliness among "the submerged tenth," a term he borrowed from William Booth's social investigation, *In Darkest England* (1890), where it referred to a residual stratum of the poor who lived in slums and survived on itinerant labor and begging. Given their intense poverty and irregular lives, it was no surprise, the MOH noted, "that they get out of the habit of washing, until in the end they get positively afraid of a bath, lest it should kill them."[42]

Quite when and where the very poorest washed is difficult to know, for we know most about their dirt rather than their cleanliness. We do know that workhouses, poor law infirmaries, and pauper schools provided baths, making for a final spatial-technological variation at the bottom of the social scale: the institutional bath, undertaken whether one liked it or not. By the 1870s, children in metropolitan pauper schools were being washed at least once a week in plumbed baths, and

in some places nightly under the supervision of a teacher.[43] Adult paupers were bathed less regularly but with no less institutional insistence.
A circular issued by the LGB in 1886 to its poor law inspectors urged
the encouragement of the following in workhouses: a bath on entrance
for every inmate and then one every month; or perhaps every two weeks,
should it be sought by a pauper.[44] In these instances, habits of cleanliness, such as they were, were largely a matter of institutional discipline
in contrast to the more subjective, self-formed habits beyond.

ENGINEERING HABITS

Either way, the technological dependencies did not end here, for these
habits required plumbing, which in turn required a range of further technological innovations that extended much beyond a tub and a tap, a
home or a public baths establishment. The most complex was the building of water-supply systems, the scale of which rivaled that of the sewerage systems considered in chapter 5. The infrastructural technologies
that required integrating and maintaining were at once manifold and
immense, among others street mains, pumping engines, and filtering
beds, as well as aqueducts and reservoirs. Ultimately, the intimate habits
performed in and around baths, washstands, and showers depended on
material systems that stretched out toward rivers and the countryside
and then back again, where they ran beneath streets and pavements
before emerging in the form of a domestic tap or standpipe. The lathered
hands of a cleanly subject would have been impossible without a great
chain of technological being that began with the distant capture of spring
and rainwater.

There were multiple other considerations besides washing. Questions
of cost and ownership were the subject of dispute among MPs, councillors, and ratepayers; and water was also used for drinking and cooking,
washing clothes, flushing toilets, and extinguishing fires.[45] But washing
the body was part of the mix, and it was during the 1840s when the
variable quality of water supplies was first linked to the question of
encouraging hygienic habits en masse. Chadwick's *Sanitary Report* discussed the matter in this fashion, and it was posed in these terms during
the Royal Commission on the Health of Towns (1843–45), which
included gathering information on Liverpool's pioneering Frederick
Street establishment.[46] It was returned to again by the GBH during its
inquiry into metropolitan water supplies in 1850, when evidence was
gathered on domestic baths and bathing habits, and how much water

might be required were popular demand to outstrip the seven public baths then operating in London.[47] It became an established preoccupation. Later royal commission and select committee inquiries received evidence on the matter as part of a broader interest in levels of water consumption, industrial, municipal, and domestic.

In terms of domestic practices, the key development was the introduction of constant systems of supply, which took place principally from the 1870s, and where water was available when required at the turn of a tap. It led to the eclipse of two earlier and more inconvenient methods: intermittent systems of supply, where water was provided only at particular times, and so had to be stored; and resort to local wells and rivers, and even murky canals. Constant systems, however, developed in the same uneven fashion as sewerage systems, and for similar reasons of variable geography and local-political willingness to engage in reform. Meanwhile, within towns and cities, variations of access were shaped by levels of income, and what householders and landlords could afford or were prepared to install. The principal problem here emerged as part of the same specifications that sought to encourage constant supplies: the meticulous plumbing regulations against wastage that had to be met in order to obtain a connection from either a private company or, increasingly, a municipal provider. Beginning with the 1847 Waterworks Clauses Act, the burden was thrown on consumers in terms of getting the details right. Regulations issued in Sheffield in 1870, for instance, specified the size and position of pipes, the design of ballcocks, and the placement of cisterns. The plumbing of water closets was minutely specified, as was that of baths. All baths had to feature "perfectly watertight plugs," while overflow pipes were banned.[48] Only once company approval had been granted following an inspection was a constant supply turned on.

Getting connected was thus a costly and intricate business, so it is no surprise that the poorest were among the last to enjoy the convenience of a free flowing tap. In all towns and cities there remained pockets of the population that relied on intermittent systems and communal standpipes. Still in 1900 some 5 percent of houses in London were without a constant service.[49] Nonetheless, slowly but surely, constant water was democratized, allowing an increase in domestic consumption and a corresponding change in habits. In 1884, Newcastle's borough engineer reported on the improvements that had taken place in the town's supply over the preceding twenty or so years, including the recent addition of another large-scale reservoir at Colt Crag—capable in fact of holding more than 1,000 million gallons of water—bringing the total that served the city and neighboring Gateshead to four. One fact was especially gratifying, he suggested: a rise in daily per capita water consumption from roughly twenty-eight gallons to thirty-eight, something he attributed to "improved habits of cleanliness among the people," and growing resort to water closets and baths among the wealthy.[50]

Public baths, by contrast, were a priority and the 1846–47 statute provided for a free water supply, which most seemed to have enjoyed thereafter. Swimming pools might require as much as one hundred thousand gallons when full; and though fifty was thought sufficient for a slipper bath, each might be used by as many as twenty customers per day. The problem in the case of public baths was ensuring overall efficiency as part of their quest to be self-supporting. Statute dealt with the provision and pricing of different classes of facilities, but there was still the question of quite how an establishment should be designed and managed. Efforts were especially intense during the 1840s and 1850s, and included the promotion of standard-setting buildings. In 1851, the London Committee opened a "model" establishment in Whitechapel, further publishing advice regarding how to build and manage baths according to the "utmost economy."[51] The work of the committee in fact traveled much beyond England, attracting interest from sanitary reformers in France and the United States (in particular New York's People's Bathing and Washing Association), and even inspiring, so it was claimed, the establishment of public baths in Hamburg, Berlin, and Brussels; but on the domestic front at least, the London Committee was not the only initial source of good practice.[52] In 1851, a London-based duo, Arthur Ashpitel and John Whichcord, published *Observations on Bath and Wash-houses*. Designed to provide an accessible introduction for architects, engineers, and councillors—it also contained a brief history of bathing, and an abstract of the 1846–47 legislation—it quickly went through three editions.[53]

During the 1870s the management of public baths was codified by the LGB in its first set of model bylaws (1877), which further specified the roles and imperatives outlined in the initial wave of promotional activity. No agent escaped regulatory attention, from the masters and matrons in charge to their many subordinates, including money-takers, baths attendants, and on-site engineers. The clocked paperwork that had to be generated was immense, extending from daily accounts of ticket receipts and weekly statements of fuel consumption to annual reports regarding the work of an entire establishment for the scrutiny of local councillors.[54] The act of washing may have been obscure and situated behind a locked door; but everything that made it possible—the coal and soap consumed; the tickets exchanged; the hire and cost of staff—was subject to meticulous accounting.

This particular amalgam of centralized-localized agency was peculiar to public baths. Domestic baths were more discrete technologies, administratively and spatially, even if surveyors might have to sign off the plans for new houses and water inspectors check the plumbing. Either way, when it came to the material construction of baths and systems for supplying hot water, both domestic and public installations relied on the same set of agents responsible for making the infrastructural connections in the first place: engineers, architects, and plumbers. As detailed in the pages of an expanding professional press, notably the *Builder* (established in 1842) and the *Building News* (1855), the choices were many and much discussed, not least with an eye to catering to the different demands of customers, municipal or private. As early as 1847, a correspondent of the *Builder* summed up what would remain the key considerations when it came to the private baths of public baths: "There are two most important requisites for baths: 1. Durability. 2. Cleanliness. There is a third, though of less importance: 3. Beauty."[55] Copper, cast iron, and zinc baths were all tried before the 1880s, when preferences began to settle on the use of glazed fireclay baths. They were not without defects: as the architect Robert Owen Allsop noted in his handbook, *Public Baths and Washhouses* (1894), compared to other kinds, heavy porcelain baths were not quite so efficient when it came to conserving the heat of water.[56] But unlike metallic baths, which required considerable scrubbing, they were easily cleansed by a mop and had rounded, dirt-resisting angles.

This was one of many cost-saving design features. Baths were arranged in pairs between slate partitions to economize on plumbing; decorative embellishments were ruled out; and in order to discourage water waste, nonconcussive taps were installed that, once activated, automatically began shutting off. In upper- and middle-class homes the details still mattered: according to S. Stevens Hellyer's *Plumber and Sanitary Houses,* in the interests of efficiently flushing out an interior bath trap, plug holes had to be of such dimensions as to allow for the discharge of thirty gallons per minute—one among a multitude of technical-systemic minutiae that were obsessively refined and reflected upon.[57] Otherwise the room for maneuver was considerable. Baths might be housed in decorative wooden paneling or furnished with enameled designs around the sides: Shanks's Fin de Siècle bath of 1899, for instance, was available in no fewer than sixteen different exterior patterns.[58] A range of tiling and furnishing options allowed for further expressions of domestic taste. Fashions came and went, however. Among the middle and the lower-middle classes at least, the general trend was toward more serviceable sanitary arrangements that dispensed with any extras that might harbor dirt and were not easily cleansed.[59] It was a step in the direction of the kind of functional materiality that characterized public baths cubicles.

The options were just as varied in the case of hot water systems. Portable baths with their own source of heat first emerged during the 1830s, principally in the form of a tub attached to a coal-fired stove and miniature boiler. Later variants included the gas-powered "geyser."[60] The key Victorian innovation was the provision of circulating systems, combining cisterns and pipes, tanks and boilers. The first public baths relied on one or two coal-fired single-flue Cornish boilers. They were still in use at the end of the century in smaller establishments; but larger establishments came to rely on double-flue Lancashire boilers, normally twenty-five feet in length and seven feet in diameter, which had earlier been pioneered in the 1840s by the Scottish engineer William Fairbairn. Cold water was supplied via a feed pump before leaving via networks of circulating copper pipes running under the floors of slipper baths. Lancashire boilers were capable of heating up to fifteen hundred gallons of water per hour and were complex systems in themselves, comprising "economizers" to recycle heat, and water gauges and thermometers. Set side by side in a row of three or four, boilers were usually situated in a basement-level engineering room, home also to a coal store and the opening of the establishment chimney shaft.[61]

In homes the first arrangements were based on the so-called tank system pioneered in Britain during the 1850s, which consisted of a kitchen-range boiler together with a cold water cistern and hot water tank, both situated in the loft or on the top floor. Once the boiler was fired, convection currents rose up the pipes while the heavier cold water flowed down, creating a rudimentary feed and return circuit. The problems were many, however—for one thing it allowed the mixing of cold and hot water at any given tap—and the principal alternative was the cylinder system, an export from the United States which was first marketed in Britain in 1868 by a company based in Camden, London.[62] Refined thereafter by British manufacturers, its distinguishing features were a cylinder instead of a box-shaped hot water tank; shorter and more heat-efficient pipe networks by virtue of placing the cylinder near the boiler; and ready access to hot water, which could be drawn directly from the cylinder without mixing with cold water (see figure 27). Crucially, it was also safer and more reliable. As one sanitary engineer explained in 1885, compared to "what our Trans-Atlantic brethren call the English system," the "American [cylinder] system" was much less vulnerable to frost-induced blockages and explosions; and this was principally because the distance between a boiler and a cylinder was much less than between a boiler and a loft-based tank.[63]

Class remained crucial: before the interwar period, systems of this sort were largely confined to the homes of the upper and middle classes. The majority of homes relied on kettles and pots for hot water, prepared on wood-, coal- or gas-powered stoves. Nonetheless, however patchy and class-variable, the formation and performance of habits of cleanliness were gradually folded into remarkably dense and expansive technological systems: even the single domestic tap dispensing only cold water relied on networks that stretched for miles beyond. Yet, if (human) hygienic habits were gradually technologized, it also worked the other way, to the extent that technological complexity made for fragility and the need for (human) maintenance. Plumbers were the key agents in homes and their work was gradually subject to regulation: in 1885 the Worshipful Company of Plumbers instituted a system of registration based on the completion of a training certificate; in 1906, a national Institute of Plumbers was formed.[64] In public baths, in-house engineers were provided with workshops to undertake the repair of pipes, tap heads and plug holes. Outside agents might be enlisted: during the early 1880s, the Manchester Steam Users' Association began undertaking monthly inspections of the boilers located in the city's public baths, a type of service it also provided to homes.[65]

This particular kind of maintenance paid off. Domestic boiler explosions were rare, though they were sufficiently frequent—and fatal—for plumbers to obsess about the matter. Equally, as Vanessa Taylor and Frank Trentmann have argued, there were two further sources of public sensitivity, both of which developed as sites of political mobilization during the latter decades of the century.[66] One of these was money; or rather, water rates, and the bewildering means of rate assessment employed by companies and elected municipal authorities, which included charging extra for baths and water closets. Disputes flared up in all major towns and cities, as ratepayers and self-styled consumers argued for lower charges and more uniform means of determining prices. Such was the angst in Sheffield that a short-lived Bath Defence Association was set up in 1880 to protest against the surcharges imposed on the two thousand and more homes with fixed provisions.[67]

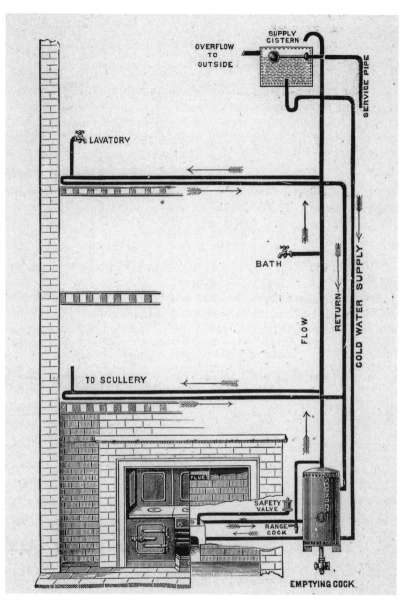

FIGURE 27. Domestic baths apparatus and plumbing according to the cylinder system. Source: Walter Jones, *Heating by Hot Water, Ventilation and Hot Water Supply*, 3rd ed. (London: Crosby Lockwood, 1903), 258. © The Bodleian Libraries, The University of Oxford.

The other source of political mobilization was more basic, if also more revealing, of the systemic and infrastructural dependencies of water-based habits: quite simply, water itself, and the fact that a free-flowing tap ultimately relied on the weather, and in particular rainfall. The threat of "water famines" during summer and autumn was a recurrent source of anxiety, feeding into local debates about the adequacy of costly water-supply systems, as in Bradford in 1884, Liverpool in 1885, and Leicester in 1894.[68] When droughts did strike, the normal course was to revert to intermittent supplies, along with pleas to the public to prevent wastage and limit usage; but this was not without considerable public anguish, which only increased as constant systems became the norm. In 1898, for instance, when shortages returned to the capital for the fourth summer running, public meetings were held that brought together MPs, LCC representatives, and the East London Water Consumer Defence League, culminating in deputations to the LGB and rallies in Victoria Park and Trafalgar Square.[69]

For most of the time and for most people, perhaps, things worked as they were supposed to. Even so, habits of cleanliness were only as habitual as technological systems would allow, and they might be rudely interrupted or curtailed, even after more convenient constant connections had been made. We shall turn to the act of washing in a moment. First, a more basic question: why were these habits encouraged at all, and by whom?

THE "GOSPEL OF CLEANLINESS"

In some instances people had little choice in the matter, such as the paupers noted above; to which we might add prisoners, soldiers, and hospital patients. Public baths in fact partook of something of the culture of disciplinary institutions, where subjects were posed as objects of regulated upkeep and supervision. Besides their architecture with its strict class- and gender-based distributions of space, they also relied on turnstiles, tickets, and wall-mounted clocks to help manage the flow of people. In the case of slipper baths, most establishments insisted on a maximum of thirty minutes per session; anything beyond this, an attendant would come knocking on the cubicle door.[70] They were also promoted in disciplinary terms. "Professionally speaking," stated one poor law doctor in 1853, "I would declare that no one remedy could be devised to counteract the evils of our overcrowded dwellings, so much as the establishment of Public Baths"; and these evils were many, including poor law dependency and an aversion toward hard work.[71] Drunkenness was another: "as truly and naturally as drink leads to dirt, so equally and obviously does dirt lead to drink," noted one temperance reformer and public baths advocate in 1884.[72] Others still suggested personal cleanliness made working-class minds more receptive to the ministrations of domestic missionaries.[73] Such sentiments were widespread, especially at midcentury, when one enthusiast suggested that public baths might be thought of as "schools for the moral training of the people."[74]

The problem, however—the very modern problem that meant that public baths were institutions at once civic, class-based, and commercial—was that they were a matter of choice: of a multitude of possible bathers, who as active subjects could choose whether or not to avail themselves of a bath, and at the cost of at least a penny. They were a standing invitation, perhaps, but no more than that. Henry Rumsey put the matter succinctly in 1868 before the NAPSS: "You may erect baths and washhouses, but no act of Parliament can compel their use."[75] Others did the same: "It is no good setting up baths or washhouses if people don't care to use them," stated the Tory MP Lord Derby in 1872, in a speech on "sanitary duties."[76] And the problem extended much beyond public baths and washing the body: it was *the* problem when it came to all those practices positioned as part of a personal sphere of governance, such as drinking, smoking, and exercising.

Yet, if it was a limit internalized and reflected on at the time—and indeed few subjects were forced into washing, with the exception of those in disciplinary settings—there was no shortage of agents beyond the government or the state encouraging habits of cleanliness. Health was the principal rationale. Cleanliness, it was suggested, made for good health in general, the absence of skin complaints, and rendered one less likely to contract infectious diseases. Equally, however, health was rarely elevated into a goal in and of itself. Instead, it was folded into ethical schemas that transcended the self and the body in one way or another, meaning that subjects were exposed to a medley of maxims and injunctions that mixed the sanitary and the moral. In practice, what was dubbed the "gospel of cleanliness" comprised multiple agents and rationales, which between them operated in all manner of settings.

One premise was Christian, as captured in the phrase "Cleanliness is next to Godliness." Coined by John Wesley in the 1780s with reference only to cleanliness of dress, it was developed by the Victorians to include cleanliness in all of its manifestations, especially of the body and home. This no doubt struck the strongest chord among the faithful, and it was issued most forcefully via pulpits and the immense industry of domestic visiting societies. As early as 1836, a pamphlet encouraging the formation of district visiting societies urged that "habits of personal cleanliness ought to be insisted upon."[77] Even here there were variations, among them fiery, finger-wagging evangelical ones. In 1858, the renowned Liverpudlian Baptist minister Hugh Stowell Brown delivered a sermon on the subject—then published as a pamphlet—warning his audience that "dirt and drink are the devil's foremen." He went on: "I believe that the devil the hates the gospel and dreads the gospel; I believe he also dreads soap and water. He is no great admirer of churches; as little does he admire public baths and washhouses."[78] Like others of an evangelical ilk, Brown conflated literal and metaphorical forms of filth. Cleanliness of speech and dress, soul and body: all were part of the same spiritual-hygienic whole.

Meanwhile, more moderate clergymen and more sanitary-oriented domestic visitors—such as members of the ladies' sanitary associations discussed in chapter 4—might invoke "Nature" or a "Supreme Author," whose laws of health had to be adhered to simply because they were of divine origin. Personal cleanliness was part of what made the universe tick over in a benign, uniform fashion. References could also be entirely fleeting. In 1887, the sanitary engineer Major Lamorock Flower addressed an audience of workingmen in Bolton on the subject of cleanliness. "Order is Heaven's first law," he stated, adding: "the cleanly person is a creature of order. We never find a disorderly person smart and cleanly"; and that was it.[79] More broadly, the phrase "Cleanliness is next to Godliness" spilled casually into the daily press, where it featured in items reporting sermons, election addresses, and the work of local authorities; but often with nothing in the way of elaboration.

Moving in a more secular direction, cleanliness was also understood in social terms, as one of the many ingredients that made up a diligent and conscientious member of society. As noted above, it was hoped that public baths would fulfil a school-like function, whereby they enabled and encouraged the subjective self-discipline associated with cleanliness. This particular rationale was most pronounced in schools proper, notably—for they contained by far the most children—in grant-maintained elementary schools, governed as they were by an evolving set of national inspection standards. Despite much lobbying, hygiene never achieved the privileged status of other subjects in the national education codes that emerged from the 1860s, most famously reading, writing, and arithmetic, or the so-called three R's. Instead, cleanliness was bound up with a series of attributes that fell under the category of "discipline." The first mention of this was made in the 1875 code, and it was formally incorporated into the criteria of a new merit grant in 1882, which detailed that heads and teachers were expected "to satisfy the inspector that all reasonable care is taken . . . to bring up the children in habits of punctuality, cleanliness and neatness." Further habits included "cheerful obedience to duty, of consideration and respect for others, and of honour and truthfulness in word and act."[80]

This was official recognition of what was already being encouraged by teachers, at least on the evidence of the school manuals published between the 1850s and 1870s.[81] Indeed, rules might be issued requiring—if to little effect in poorer areas—that parents send their children to school clean and neatly dressed. Encouraging habits of cleanliness remained crucial, and from the 1880s it formed part of a broader national educational endeavor that was increasingly understood in terms of promoting "citizenship," and even maintaining the "health of the race," physical and moral.[82] At the same time, concessions were made by the central Board of Education that allowed for money to be spent on specific hygiene-related activities, including swimming lessons.[83] In Manchester, for instance, the number of visits by children to public baths increased from 133,000 in 1897, when classes were first introduced, to over 570,000 in 1907.[84] Much less fun, no doubt, were in-class lessons on how to wash the hands and face, and on the rudiments of human biology.

Perhaps the emphasis on citizenship increased toward the end of the century; but even in schools it is difficult to dissociate the social from the religious, for the vast majority of children were daily exposed to some kind of Christian teaching by way of fostering a sense of social duty and self-discipline. In any case, neither the social nor the religious premise is easy to disentangle from a final and more intimate one: manners, and the obligation not to offend oneself, or one's immediate company, with unpleasant sights and smells. This was of long descent, having informed codes of aristocratic sociability in the seventeenth and eighteenth centuries, when great store was placed on the cleanliness of hands and faces, cuffs and collars.[85] The Victorians retained the emphasis on exterior stylization, but pitched the message at all classes while urging more bodily thoroughness. A key medium was the genre of etiquette and domestic advice manuals, which proliferated from the 1830s and 1840s, and in various forms, popular and elite, male and female.[86] Meanwhile, schools provided a space for the diffusion of this particular premise among children, where personal cleanliness mixed with considerations of speech, dress, and table conduct.

For those higher up the social scale in particular, etiquette opened up a whole world of carefully regulated nuances: of gestures and words, bodily postures and sartorial trimmings, all of which had to be modulated according to occasion and audience (birthdays, weddings, and so on). The rituals were many, and one of them was securing cleanliness. Combined, they made for a repertoire of habits that were commonly described in terms of "civility," "refinement," "gentility," and "breeding." In the case of cleanliness, it seems the keyword was *decency*. During the 1870s, the metropolitan MOH for Paddington, William Hardwicke, outlined the utility of public baths, writing that cleanliness should be encouraged on two grounds besides that of health: "decency and morality." "Upon the first point, decency, but little need be said," he wrote, urging his readers "that each one of them owes a respect to himself as well as to the society in which he moves." "It is from the latter motive that he is, as he ought to be, rigidly scrupulous in preserving those parts of the body which are exposed to view from the disfigurement of dirt of every kind."[87] Crudely put, cleanliness was also a matter of appearances and self-esteem.

It would not be wholly wrong to differentiate the gospel of cleanliness into three facets, the religious, the social, and the individual, if only because the Victorians did so themselves. In 1855, one pamphleteer suggested that there "are many considerations which ought to induce all to attend to the duty of cleanliness": "It is a *personal* duty, that is, a duty we owe to ourselves individually; it is a *social* duty, that is, a duty which we owe to society; and it is a *religious* duty, that is, a duty which we owe to God." For this particular author the most important rationale was the religious one, and he reminded his readers that "God is to be worshipped with outward reverence, as well as with inward reverence, with clean bodies as well as clean hearts."[88] But there was no necessary antagonism between the three. On the contrary, they reinforced one another, and this form of ethical-sanitary eclecticism was commonplace. It even extended to attempts to prove that hygiene had always been a personal obligation, at least within civilized societies. In 1884, the MOH Alfred Carpenter addressed the SIGB on the subject of "education by proverb in sanitary work," where he cherry-picked maxims and anecdotes from across different ages and cultures—Greek, Roman, and Jewish in particular—by way of demonstrating the universal wisdom of caring for one's health.[89]

At the same time, it is difficult to dissociate moral imperatives from considerations of social stigma, and the dynamics of searching for status both between and within classes. The phrase "the Great Unwashed" merely encapsulated what was a matter of routine comment and exposure among middle- and upper-class readers of social investigations and journalistic reportage: simply that more and more dirt could be found the further one penetrated the depths of society. The reality was more nuanced, of course, just as were the depictions themselves, where fear and pathos, disgust and fascination, propelled a new eye for the moral and physical details of working-class life. Yet, the currency and crudity of the phrase are suggestive of the class-based prejudice—and pride—that evidently informed the use of soap and water, just as it did other habits relating to language and dress. It is significant that when it came to *forming* these habits the utility of shame was acknowledged. "You will never induce men to habits of cleanliness simply by dangling before them the fear of getting a skin eruption, or a dirty complexion, or harbouring vermin," noted the dermatologist H. G. Brooke in 1884, as he delivered a popular lecture in Manchester on washing the body. He was thinking in particular of those who ended up in prisons and workhouses. "They will never be clean," he went on, "until either their pride is touched and they are shamed into cleanliness, or until they learn to appreciate the feeling of self-respect which cleanliness brings with it."[90]

In this way, general norms of personal hygiene perhaps operated quietly and subtly, indeed habitually, to the extent that they became part of an unreflective—if still class-inflected—performance of body, mind, and morals: a matter of comment among social equals and family only when infringed. Equally, this particular dimension hardly operated in a subterranean fashion, and this was largely thanks to a final agent that might be noted: a flourishing soap industry.[91] The industry expanded markedly during the second half of the century, following the abolition of soap duty—otherwise styled as a "tax on cleanliness"—by William Gladstone as chancellor of the exchequer in 1853. In 1850, it was estimated that the annual production of soap in Britain was roughly 80,000 tons a year; in 1893, a book on soap manufacturing put the figure at over 330,000.[92] In terms of marketing and production, the key shift was from unbranded blocks that were cut and sold in shops to pre-prepared tablets wrapped in packaging. The result was a sprawling marketplace of products, extending from soaps for washing clothes and household surfaces to the "toilet soap" used for washing bodies. The brands were many, among others Pears', Hudson's, Lever's, and Brooke's.

Crucially, competition entailed advertising and the use of billboards, shop displays, and, above all, the clocked pages of magazines and newspapers. Adverts composed of a handful of pithy, eye-catching sentences were crammed into pages alongside other adverts, which was the dominant mode midcentury. The broad shift from the 1870s was toward larger, more elaborate adverts. The variations were many: some were almost entirely pictorial; others were composed only of text. But in whatever form they appeared, soap adverts were rarely subtle when it came to promoting the virtues of cleanliness, disclosing as they did so some of the prejudices they appealed to—and encouraged—including of a racial sort (see figure 28).[93] Boasts of commercial popularity and endorsements from experts and celebrities also featured, as well as claims that a particular brand combined all manner of wholesome qualities. "Pears' Soap means health; Pears' Soap means purity; Pears' Soap means honesty," noted a full-page advert published in the London-based *Penny Illustrated Paper* in 1896.[94] "Prior to soap was barbarism," it baldly stated. Others proclaimed that soap was a vital ingredient in the generation of healthy habits and happy homes (see figure 29). Quite how these adverts were read and received is difficult to recover, of course, but they were certainly hard to avoid: the magazine and newspaper press teems with these crude, commercially driven inducements to personal cleanliness.

Beyond the commitment to forming habits, it is incredibly difficult to identify any kind of coherent or singular modern subject in relation to cleanliness. The moral elements that went into the making of these habits were not so different from the technological ones, in the sense that they were multiple, interconnected, and widely diffused; not to mention infused with a sense of class-based hierarchy and civilizational development. To the extent that any kind of *popular* subjectivity was associated with cleanliness, then it is the one Brooke invoked when he spoke of a "feeling of self-respect"; or rather, the respectable subject, and a basic core of values that included hard work, sobriety, and the thrifty management of household resources. Bathrooms came to be regarded as something "no self-respecting householder can do without," and cleanliness and a healthy body were consistently talked of in these and associated terms.[95] "Cleanliness is more than wholesomeness. It furnishes an atmosphere of self-respect," wrote Samuel Smiles in his best-selling *Thrift* (1875). "People are cleanly in proportion as they are decent, industrious, and self-respecting."[96]

Of course, devolved to a personal sphere of governance, free of any legal prescription or official supervision, the complexities of performance

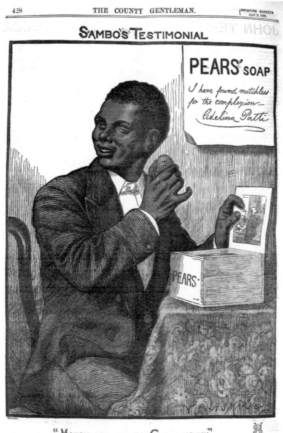

FIGURE 28. In the top corner is an endorsement from the famous (white) opera singer, Adelina Patti, who finds Pears' soap "matchless for the complexion"—as does Sambo, in his own misspelled way. Source: *County Gentleman: A Sporting Gazette and Agricultural Journal*, April 3, 1886, 428. © The British Library Board.

and realization are immense. As we might imagine—and contrary to the reformist rhetoric—a clean body did not necessarily make for a pure mind or further respectable habits. The "journeyman engineer" Thomas Wright, in *Some Habits and Customs of the Working Classes* (1867), noted the practice among working men of visiting public baths on a Saturday afternoon, putting on their best suits afterward, and then venturing

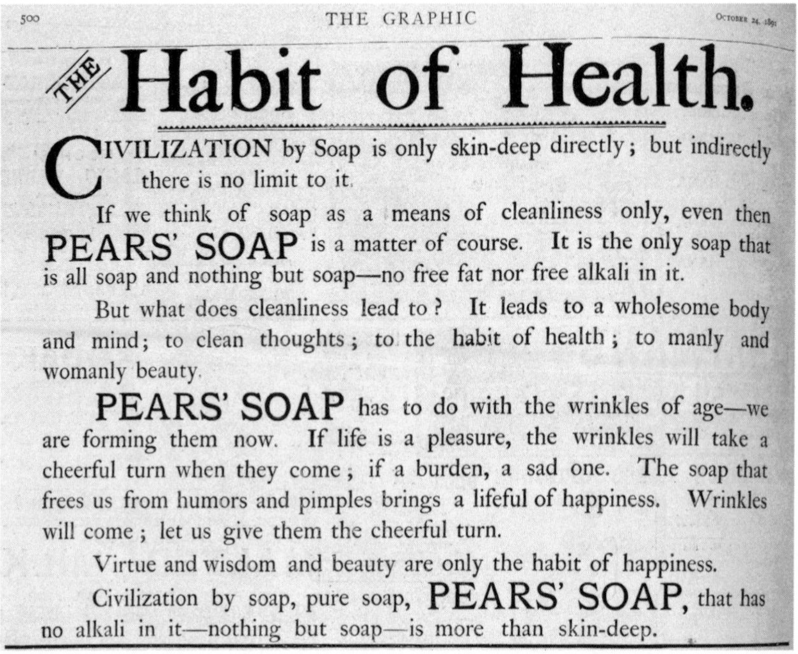

500   THE GRAPHIC   October 24, 1891

THE Habit of Health.

CIVILIZATION by Soap is only skin-deep directly; but indirectly there is no limit to it.

If we think of soap as a means of cleanliness only, even then PEARS' SOAP is a matter of course. It is the only soap that is all soap and nothing but soap—no free fat nor free alkali in it.

But what does cleanliness lead to ? It leads to a wholesome body and mind; to clean thoughts; to the habit of health; to manly and womanly beauty.

PEARS' SOAP has to do with the wrinkles of age—we are forming them now. If life is a pleasure, the wrinkles will take a cheerful turn when they come; if a burden, a sad one. The soap that frees us from humors and pimples brings a lifeful of happiness. Wrinkles will come; let us give them the cheerful turn.

Virtue and wisdom and beauty are only the habit of happiness.

Civilization by soap, pure soap, PEARS' SOAP, that has no alkali in it—nothing but soap—is more than skin-deep.

FIGURE 29. A text-only advert for Pears' soap proclaiming, in typical fashion, that cleanliness is "more than skin-deep" and essential to "the habit of happiness." Source: "The Habit of Health," *Graphic*, October 24, 1891, 500. © The Bodleian Libraries, The University of Oxford.

into town in the evening in search of drink and amusement.[97] Nonetheless, in the case of working-class families, it seems that personal cleanliness, when and where it was practiced regularly, was born of the same culture of self-improvement and modest aspiration that informed the reading of respectable literature and membership of churches and friendly societies. It is no coincidence that from the 1880s public baths were sometimes situated alongside municipal libraries.

WASHING THE BODY

Whatever the precise mix of motivations and moral prods that applied in individual cases, the body itself intensified as a site of hygienic self-management. The same applies to the home, which, as noted above, was also posited as a discrete sphere of governance. Victoria Kelley has detailed the rituals that emerged over the course of the second half of the century, as performed by a housewife or one or more female servants.[98]

Clothes, linen, plates, pans, rugs, and even the front doorstep: all of these items and more became part of weekly cleansing schedules. Thresholds of tolerance were raised as the most minuscule manifestations of dirt were hunted down. "Make war on dust!" was one rallying cry. The body underwent a similar hygienic reformation. Previously, as Georges Vigarello and Keith Thomas have described, washing had largely been restricted to the face, hands, and neck, extending to the torso and legs only occasionally.[99] Now regular, all-over washing became the ideal. It constitutes a key moment in the history of the bath, which was increasingly considered a means of securing cleanliness. It was a relative reappraisal, for its earlier status as a therapeutic technology enjoyed a new lease of life, as we shall see below. But within the broader scheme of practices, there was a gradual shift toward the predominance of bathing-as-washing. And it was here, in and around the tub or washstand, where a final set of elements was brought into play that realized "the personal" as a matter of embodied self-governance: the skin and hands; soap and warm water; and an assortment of utensils and accessories.

The shift was underway by the 1840s, when public baths first began to appear. "This bath [the tepid bath] is rather a means of *preserving* health than a very powerful curative agent," noted one metropolitan physician in 1842. "As a means of securing personal cleanliness it is unequalled; and it is chiefly as subservient to this end that tepid bathing is becoming so prevalent."[100] One might attribute this to the promotion of cleanliness in all its forms and it was to some extent; but it also turned on a quite specific reappraisal of the skin and the uses of water.[101] In terms of the latter, water was reconceived as a sanitary agent. Prior to the nineteenth century, it had largely been prized for its ability to rebalance the body's liquids and solids, whether bathed in or ingested, hot or cold. Neither hot nor cold water went out of fashion: that cold baths constituted a useful and refreshing "tonic" was still being endorsed in mainstream hygiene manuals in the early twentieth century. Even so, water was now privileged as a means of external purification and for this tepid or warm water of between twenty-five and thirty-five degrees Celsius was generally judged the best. "Hot baths are relaxing and unnecessary for cleansing purposes," noted Brooke, "but a warm bath melts up the fat on the skin and dissolves other impurities which do not dissolve easily in cold water, and thus renders the cleansing action of the soap much more thorough."[102]

At the same time, the skin was grasped as organ in and of itself, rather than as a fleshly medium via which certain qualities, such as hardness or softness, might be imparted to the subject's constitution as he or she bathed. The structural and functional intricacies of the skin would soon become the preserve of the science of dermatology: the first specialist journals emerged in the 1860s and by the end of the century dermatology was the subject of international conferences, the first of which took place in Paris in 1889.[103] For popular purposes much less detail was required, and from the 1840s most texts or lectures of this sort pointed to three layers: the epidermis or scarf skin, the layer that was easily shed; the mucous coat or protective layer, which contained the skin's pigment; and the true skin or corium, the layer responsible for touch and situated just above the sweat glands (figure 30). The same texts also set out the role of the skin within the broader economy of the body, foregrounding the excretory and respiratory work it performed. "To reduce the functional activity of the skin is to throw more work on the lungs," stated Richardson in a popular lecture entitled "The Next to Godliness," which he first delivered at Newcastle town hall in 1882. This, he went on, interfered with "the airing of the blood" and made "sluggish the action of the stomach, the liver and other secreting organs," finally "dulling the brain."[104] One frequently cited fact plucked from what became the leading treatise on the subject, Erasmus Wilson's *Healthy Skin,* first published in 1845, was the number of pores that drained a single square inch of flesh: roughly three thousand; or for an average-sized man, about seven million over the entire body. Another was the total length of sweat glands in an adult body, which Wilson reckoned was about twenty-eight miles.[105]

Corporeal thoroughness was thus one norm that began to take root in the 1840s, thereby encouraging a tactile intimacy between subjects and their bodies. "First of all, then, keep yourselves scrupulously clean," urged one *Pocket Manual of Etiquette, and Guide to Correct Personal Habits* (1865), noting that "Cleanliness is next to Godliness" and was no less close to "gentility." It added: "[and] not your hands and face merely, but your whole person from the crown of your head to the sole of your foot."[106] What kind of self-governance was this, physically speaking? On the rare occasions when it was described, it was suggested that it was about enacting a kind of instinctive, bodily intelligence. The "hand is a sentient rubber," "a rubber endowed with mind," declared Wilson in his *Healthy Skin,* as he set out the proper procedure for washing the face: "it knows when and where to rub hard, where softly, where to bend here and there, into the little hollows and crevices where dust is apt to congregate; or where to find little ugly clusters of black-nosed grubs, which are

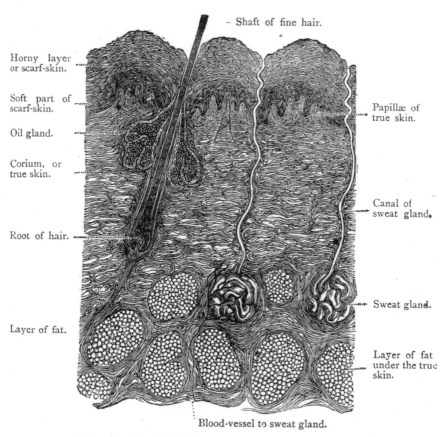

- Shaft of fine hair.

Horny layer or scarf-skin.

Soft part of scarf-skin.

Oil gland.

Corium, or true skin.

Root of hair.

Layer of fat.

Papillæ of true skin.

Canal of sweat gland.

Sweat gland.

Layer of fat under the true skin.

Blood-vessel to sweat gland.

FIG. 2.—MAGNIFIED PORTION OF THE SKIN.*

FIGURE 30. There was remarkable consistency of popular, diagrammatic exposition between the 1840s and the late Victorian period. Wilson's *Healthy Skin* seems to have been responsible. Source: Arthur Ransome, "Water: Its Work of Purification," *Health Lectures for the People Delivered in Manchester, 1879–80*, vol. 3 (Manchester: John Heywood, 1880), 67. © The Bodleian Libraries, The University of Oxford.

rubbed out and off and dissolved by soap and water. In a word, the hand enables you to combine efficient friction of the skin with complete ablution."[107] It was not unlike the embodied knowledge that sanitary inspectors relied on as they sought to determine problems: a matter, that is, of mobilizing the senses in conjunction with particular microtechnologies. The other norm was chronological regularity, the very essence of habits. As early as the 1840s, the Health of Towns Association and its offshoots recommended that "the whole surface of the body, from head to foot" should be washed daily.[108] The rationale was simple. It was a matter of keeping up with the skin and the multiple operations it undertook on an ongoing basis: processes of waste removal and sweating, for instance, and the fleshly renewal of scales. Some areas required more attention than others, in particular the face and armpits. There was also the danger of overwashing and robbing the skin of its natural oils and moisture; but the general consensus was that a bath should feature "among the regular occupations of life," and preferably daily.[109]

Ideally at least, washing was a matter of timetabled maintenance and chronological repetition. The term *maintenance* in fact was often used in this context, and mechanical analogies were common. In 1846, one Mancunian physician and public-baths enthusiast compared the skin to the "governor" of a steam engine, for in much the same way the skin either released or conserved the heat of the body, depending on the needs of its inner components, the kidneys and lungs especially: "maintaining a healthy action of the surface of the body" thus required "regular washing, bathing and friction."[110] Perhaps for some, then, washing was a routine chore on this account; and yet, however vexatious it might have been, there was also the stimulus of the modest pleasures to be had. Most of all, there was the sensory pleasure of feeling clean. Hardwicke, quoted above, suggested that "the capacity for gratification resides not in the eye, the ear or the palate, but in that wondrous fabric, the skin." Cleanliness was one of nature's "tranquil pleasures," providing a vibrant, sensory clarity.[111] The act, too, was pleasurable. If cold baths refreshed, then warm baths relieved. The warm bath "has a soothing effect on the nervous system," noted one manual, "and is exceedingly gratifying after a day's fatigue and worry."[112]

The pleasure of feeling clean was open to all classes, but this is not true of the pleasure of combining hands and soap with a plumbed bath and warm water, which remained beyond the reach of great swaths of the population. By the Edwardian period, it seems all but the very poorest engaged in daily washing, but this could be restricted to the hands and face. All-over washing was a weekly affair, and even then it might take place in a copper tub, or around a washstand or a domestic sink.[113] Class remained the master determinant, here governing the details of bodily indulgence. The act itself went under different names: as Thomas Wright noted, "cleaning-up" was the term of choice among the lower classes; higher up, it was "performing your toilet."[114] The differences were immense, even when it came to basic technologies. An 1877 primer on domestic economy quoted Hippolyte Taine's *Notes on England* (1871), where the Frenchman described what he regarded as an unusually luxurious abundance of instruments that accompanied two dressing tables in a London mansion. One had a mirror; the other doubled as a washstand: the "second is furnished with one large jug, one small one, a medium one for hot water, two porcelain basins, a dish for tooth-brushes, two soap dishes, a water-bottle with its tumbler, a finger-glass with its glass." A shallow zinc bath was contained underneath, while an adjacent cupboard contained four towels. Taine was amused by the array of utensils, joking that an Englishman probably spent "a fifth of his life in his tub." The author that quoted Taine was not so amused, recommending a more modest array of "necessaries": soap, sponge, towel, and toothbrush.[115]

The range of possibilities was just as pronounced in the case of plumbed arrangements. Upper-class bathrooms constituted one extreme. By the 1890s they contained lavatories (plumbed sinks), framed mirrors, heated towel rails, bidets, curtained showers, and bathtubs; and as with all domestic bathrooms, there were no time limits governing use.[116] The handful of People's Baths, of the sort pioneered by Lassar in Germany, occupied the other end of the spectrum. In 1888, the industrialist Charles Clement Walker built what seems to have been the first Lassar-style unit in England at his factory in Donnington, Shropshire. Partitioned with corrugated iron, each of the six cubicle chambers contained a shower and a shallow cast-iron, circular bath, eight inches deep. Micromechanisms sought to ensure compliant behavior: each door was numbered; a place in the corner was marked "Boots"; and directions for use were posted on the walls. According to Walker, the establishment could wash eighteen men per hour, affording each twenty minutes. Standardized, functional, efficient—it was entirely in keeping with the industrial setting.[117]

Public baths did at least furnish the same kind of space for all classes: the slipper bath cubicle, of roughly six feet by seven. Privacy was granted to all. Model LGB regulations specified that it was something that was not to be "interfered with" or "intruded upon." The differences began once the door was closed. All public baths provided different classes of facilities, commonly two, which furnished a different set of technologies for tub-based self-fashioning. The journalist Hugh Shimmin, writing for the *Liverpool Mercury* in 1856, detailed the facilities at the city's Cornwallis Street establishment, where there were three classes:

> In the first we find a carpet, two chairs, a bootjack, boothooks, shoehorn, fleshbrush, hairbrush, and comb, a large looking-glass, hand ewer and soap, and three towels. We notice further the fleshbrush has a long handle. There

is also a tap by which the bather can regulate the temperature. In the second class we find a carpet, a chair, a small looking-glass, a fleshbrush without a handle, a tap, and two towels. In the third class we see no carpet, no flesh-brush, no tap, one towel, and no looking-glass.

Degrees of wealth thus translated as degrees of comfort and the possibilities for hygienic precision: a mirror (looking-glass) for the face; a bristled fleshbrush for the skin; a comb for the hair—or not, of course. At Cornwallis Street, third-class customers were even denied the opportunity of gazing at themselves in a mirror and running their own water. Shimmin quoted a "gruff-looking mechanic—probably a Chartist," who drew the following implication: "That a poor fellow who can only pay twopence is not worth looking at, and it would do him no good to be allowed to see himself."[118]

Shimmin's mechanic had a point, and it would remain valid for the rest of the century and beyond. Simply put, the higher one's class, the more one could explore the nooks and crannies of the body, and the utility of technologies such as fleshbrushes and looking-glasses. "It is curious to note how much of a man's individuality lies simply in the skin," noted the dermatologist, Malcolm Morris, before an audience at the 1884 International Health Exhibition. He was in the midst of celebrating its remarkable anatomy: the "vitalising tubes called blood vessels, others called lymphatics; the wondrous telegraphic system of nerves . . . the sacs in which the hair grows and little bags or receptacles for fat."[119] All shared this same intricate skin, but not all could govern it with the same care and habitual regularity. Some bodies were more personal than others.

TURKISH BATHING

It would be wrong to speak of anything like a homogenization of washing practices, even if by the end of the century the English as a whole were thought to be relatively clean. "Compared with many of the Continental nations—we might make bold to say with any," noted an editorial in the *Sanitary Record* in 1893, "the English will certainly hold their own in the matter of cleanliness, and perhaps they might be found standing at the top of the list."[120] Only the Japanese were considered competitors in this respect, as were the Germans by the Edwardian period. Equally, bathing per se remained a varied practice, as inherited methods premised on the bath as a therapeutic technology were reworked and refreshed. "Local baths," for instance, which were designed to relieve pain in a specific part of the body, were still being recommended at the end of the century, including the portable feet and hip baths that had earlier been popular in middle-class dressing rooms.[121] The hydropathic work of the Silesian peasant, Vincent Priessnitz, who had set up an establishment during the 1820s at Gräfenberg, was promoted in England from the 1840s, affording a variety of water cures that recalled those of the eighteenth century.[122] Meanwhile, spa and sea bathing towns were transformed into tourist centers, building on the mobility made possible within and beyond England by the advent of railway systems.[123]

These practices might be considered alternative, given the eventual popularity of washing using slipper baths, showers, and washstands. They had their place and purpose, however, commercially as much as therapeutically. They were also of a piece with a modern culture of governance that looked backward as much as forward when it came to posing problems and solutions, and situating the relative advance or backwardness of present endeavors. The best instance of this is Turkish bathing, which was based on the reclamation of the classical practices that otherwise formed such an important point of reference when it came to judging—and historicizing—the sanitary progress of the Victorians. Moving forward and securing "progress" did not preclude insisting on the vitality and relevance of past practices, in this case from the relatively deep past of antiquity.

One individual in particular was credited with having inspired the introduction of Turkish bathing to the British Isles: the one-time diplomat, Tory-radical MP, arch-anti-centralizer, and leading Turcophile, David Urquhart. The key text was his travel memoir *The Pillars of Hercules* (1850), which contained a lengthy evocation of what Urquhart regarded as the only kind of bath: the Greek *balineum* or Roman *thermae,* but especially the Turkish variant, the *hammam,* where a ritualized "drama" was performed consisting of sweating, soaping, massaging, and recuperating. To find the real "standard of cleanliness," "we must look for one tested by long experience and fixed from ancient days," insisted Urquhart, mocking European pretensions to hygienic civilization.[124] But if the past was much ahead of the present in this respect, it was to the public baths and washhouses of contemporary London that Urquhart looked in order to substantiate his claim that Turkish baths might become truly popular institutions in Britain, quoting figures relating to their prices, usage, and running costs.[125] The first establishment inspired by Urquhart was built in 1856 by the Irish hydropathist, Richard Barter, at his bathing complex in Blarney, County Cork. They spread from here into Britain, and by the late 1870s there were thought to be over one hundred private Turkish baths in the United Kingdom, including in industrial centers such as Manchester and Birmingham.[126] In fact, Turkish baths enjoyed a surge of interest in the 1860s and 1870s that rivaled that of public baths in the 1840s and 1850s—which is one reason, perhaps, why the expansion of public baths slowed around the same time, before picking up once more in the 1880s.

It proved a contested, not to say confused, historical resurrection, and quickly gave birth to what in 1860 was dubbed the "Turkish bath question."[127] For one thing, enthusiasts disagreed about the precise temperatures that should be secured and whether or not it was desirable to supply only hot dry air (which was more Roman) or to furnish a degree of air-borne moisture (more Turkish). A related issue was quite what constituted a "Turkish bath" in the first place. Accounts differed, just as did the names employed: Roman-Turkish bath; Improved Turkish bath; Eastern bath; Oriental bath; Anglo-Roman bath; and *hammam* (in honor of Barter, it was known as the Roman-Irish bath when this style of bathing later traveled to Germany). A final set of considerations concerned the curative utility of the Turkish bath. Converts suggested it could help to cure all kinds of afflictions, among others scrofula, rheumatism, consumption, and sciatica. Hot air was invested with the same kind of polyvalent powers that had surrounded the use of cold water in the eighteenth century, and that remained current in some forms of hydropathy. The only difference was that Turkish baths also possessed a sanitary function: a deep cleansing action that purified all layers of the skin. An emerging medical profession was more skeptical. In 1861, the *BMJ* critiqued "Turkish bath mania," urging a more nuanced and considered appraisal of its benefits.[128] Evidently professional opinions remained mixed: still in the late Victorian period, advocates saw fit to note what for them was the ill-founded hostility of much of the medical community.[129]

Ironically, the term *Turkish bath* came to predominate in the 1880s, just as practices settled around the (originally Roman) use of hot dry air and a standard set of processes: immersion in a moderately hot room (the *tepidarium* room), followed by one or more hotter rooms (*calidarium* and *laconicum*); then a full body massage and shampooing (in the *lavatorium*), followed by a cold plunge or shower; and then a final period of relaxation (*frigidarium*). All in, it could take up to two and a half hours.[130] At the same time, the desire to remain faithful to Roman-Turkish practices combined with resort to state-of-the-art technologies. Early baths, especially those in Ireland, simulated ancient hypocaust arrangements, perhaps in conjunction with side flues allowing heat to flow directly into the bathing room.[131] By contrast, later baths relied on industrial apparatus, in particular coke-fired stoves with an iron or brick radiating surface situated beneath the floors. Patents began to emerge in the 1860s and the preferred model became the Convoluted Stove, pioneered in 1866 by two Manchester-based Turkish bath owners, Joseph Constantine and Thomas Whitaker.[132] A dash of contemporary morality was added in some establishments in the shape of bathing and changing cubicles, offering a more secure alternative to a suitably placed towel around the waist. Liverpool's Mulberry Street Oriental Baths, which opened in 1861, comprised a ladies' and a gentlemen's section, plus a private wing containing a *tepidarium, calidarium,* and *frigidarium.*[133]

There were variations of the bathing process, in keeping with the baths themselves, which were of varying size and location. Some were attached to residential houses, allowing for only one hot room. The capital was home to the most luxurious, including the celebrated Jermyn Street Hammam, built in 1862 by the London and Provincial Turkish Bath Company under the supervision of Urquhart. The *frigidarium* featured a fountain and Moorish, iron-wrought hanging lanterns, while the domed, Greek-style, cross-shaped *calidarium* contained a large marble slab on which bathers could recline (see figure 31). Turkish facilities also featured in public baths. The Leaf Street Baths in Hulme, built by the Manchester and Salford Baths and Laundry Company in 1860, seems to have been the first to incorporate a Turkish bath, followed by public baths in Bradford, Hanley, and Stalybridge during the 1860s and 1870s.[134] By the end of the century, Turkish baths were an established part of the facilities offered by large city-center complexes, even if they had failed to become the truly popular, cross-class institutions that Urquhart and others had envisaged in the 1850s and 1860s. Indeed, their prices meant that they catered to a restricted and largely middle-class market. At the turn of the century, the Turkish facilities at Manchester's Leaf Street and Whitworth baths cost one shilling, more than ten times the price of the cheapest slipper bath at just a penny. The costs were higher still in London, where the Jermyn Street Hammam, for instance, charged no less than four shillings for the full ritual.[135]

Hospitals, asylums, and hydropathic establishments also featured Turkish baths and clearly they were used by some with curative intent. But skeptical or otherwise, all medical professionals could agree that Turkish baths were good for cleansing the skin, and even better as a

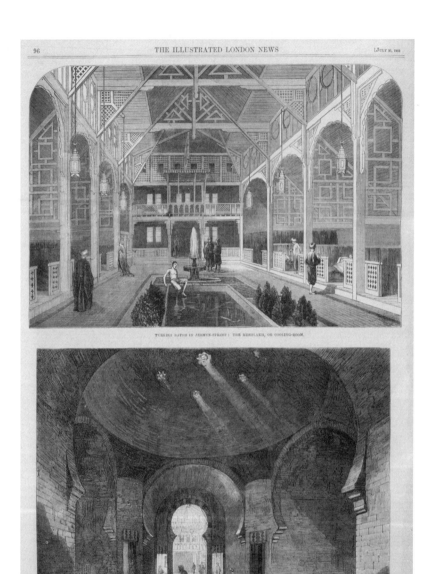

TURKISH BATHS IN JERMYN-STREET : THE MESHLAKH, OR COOLING-ROOM.

TURKISH BATHS IN JERMYN-STREET : THE HARARAH, OR HOT-CHAMBER.—SEE SUPPLEMENT, PAGE 111.

FIGURE 31. The "*meshlakh,* or cooling-room" (top) and the "*hararah,* or hot-chamber" (bottom) of London's Jermyn Street Hammam. Source: *Illustrated London News,* July 26, 1862, 96. It is a rare instance of a truly large-scale Turkish bathing establishment. Most were small and required nothing like the investment for municipal public baths. © The Bodleian Libraries, The University of Oxford.

means of refreshing the mind and body. None other than Erasmus Wilson praised the sweet sensation of shampooing by an attendant— "the pressing and kneading of the muscles, the traction of the sinews"— while celebrating the experience of the *calidarium:* "All care, all anxiety, all trouble, all memory of the external world and its miserable littleness is chased from the mind." The body enjoyed a similar kind of liberation: "PAIN ENTERS NOT HERE."[136] As early as the 1860s, Turkish baths were being recommended for all those "who are chained to the desk," and exposed to the strains and stresses of commerce.[137] Ultimately, the end product was much the same as that sought by public baths: a subject refreshed, healthy, clear-headed, and clean. What Turkish baths offered was a sensory journey en route, where the self was dissolved a little prior to the consolidating experience of the cooling room. In 1898, one West Country doctor conjured the image of a businessman "reclining in the tropical atmosphere and soothing semi-obscurity of a Turkish bath": "There, lulled to rest by the faint sound of trickling water . . . undisturbed by any noise louder than the soft tread of a bare-footed ministrant, the weary body, disembarrassed of all its habitual sumptuary restraints, passes into a blissful condition of absolute repose and the overwrought brain—its tension mercifully relaxed for the nonce—is refreshed by brief intervals of dreamless oblivion."[138] Such were the delights of Roman bathing remade in a modern, Victorian fashion. Or rather, "revived" as "Turkish bathing"; placed on a new technological footing with the aid of industrial heating systems; and sold as an antidote to the pressures of civilization and bureaucracy.

CONCLUSION

The broad point argued for above is as follows: namely, that public health reform in Victorian and Edwardian England did not entail the eclipse or erasure of a personal sphere (or indeed "center") of governing. Quite the contrary: it turned upon the intensification, reanimation, and indeed formalization of a personal or private sphere of hygiene. This is not to deny the advent of more impersonal, centralized, and bureaucratic forms of governing, instances of which have been discussed at length in previous chapters. Rather, it is to suggest that these forms of governing developed in tandem, moving together as part of a complex and modern articulation of multiple levels and agents of governance.

In the process, a domain of individual habits emerged as both a problem and a solution. Good habits were a good thing, enabling the public health system to function in a zone that was difficult to know and regulate, and beyond recourse to any kind of state compulsion or bureaucratic supervision. Conversely, however, there was the possibility of forming bad habits, besides the struggle to maintain good ones. This kind of habitual co-option and cooperation was certainly required in the case of washing the body, for it was an intrinsically intimate practice, and one that all could agree was best performed behind a locked door; but it extended to *all* health-related habits. In 1875, for instance, the physician Daniel Noble delivered the first of a new series of popular lectures for the MSSA (some of which have been quoted above), entitled "Causes Reducing the Effects of Sanitary Reform." Why, he asked, given all the efforts and exertions of local authorities and ministers since Chadwick's 1842 *Sanitary Report,* had there been no significant reduction in the GRO's death rates? He attributed this "to the thoughtless action and perverted conduct of the people." For "it is clear that whatever be the good you would render to individuals or to the masses, it can only be made fully available by suitable cooperation on the part of those for whom it is intended."[139] His list of bad habits included overwork, excess alcohol consumption, smoking, and a lack of recreation. There was, evidently, only so much that could be done.

Nonetheless, efforts were made, as we have seen. However good or bad, useful or obstructive, habits were *governed,* and governed intensely, even in the absence of what the Victorians referred to as "State" or "Government interference." Habits of cleanliness had to be made and unmade, formed and sustained, and they were hardly the discrete or detached phenomena implied by the terms *personal cleanliness* and *private hygiene.* MPs and councillors; clergymen and schoolteachers; public baths and residential houses; sanitaryware companies, soap manufactures, and water-supply systems, among others: the formation and performance of hygienic habits brought into play all of these agents, as part of a diffuse field of human-technological governance. In this respect, perhaps an analogy might be made with the statistical "facts" examined in chapter 3, for habits also had to be made and composed, even if they too were thought to have a kind of natural and objective status that existed independently of conscious human efforts and systems of governing.

A final point: personal cleanliness was profoundly *social.* Besides being promoted in these terms—as a "social duty," say—it also functioned as an index of class. Slowly but surely habits of cleanliness became embedded among the public at large. Cruelly perhaps, just as they did so, not only were standards raised but the possibilities for their performance became more elaborate and nuanced; and these possibilities were principally determined by a subject's wealth and status. Accordingly, for all the progress that was made, the function of cleanliness as a source of class-based prejudice only increased rather than diminished. "For the cults of religion and pedigree we have substituted the cult of soap and water," wrote the social commentator Stephen Reynolds in 1909. "Cleanliness is our greatest class-symbol," he went on, "for nothing else rouses so instantaneously and violently the latent snobbery that one would fain be rid of. . . . The bathroom is the inmost, the strongest fortress, of our English snobbery."[140] Reynolds may have been exaggerating; but in terms of everyday practices of social acknowledgment and interaction it was here where the variable, class-specific functioning of the public health system assumed its most potent, visceral form.

CHAPTER 8

Conclusion

Systems, Variations, Politics

This book has sought to avoid constructing any straw men. Throughout, it has aimed to work with rather than against the grain of the "antiheroic" historiography discussed in chapter 1. Contingency and choice, variation and conflict, and the multiple interrelations of expertise, politics, and administrative practice: all this has formed the analytical point of departure—the very stuff we might make better sense of, even as we luxuriate in it. Of course, no period has a monopoly on this kind of complexity, and it extended much beyond 1910. Something of the new shape of public health can be glimpsed in George Newman's *Outline of the Practice of Preventive Medicine,* which he authored in his capacity as chief medical officer to the newly formed Ministry of Health in 1919. He detailed ten "elements of a national policy," recalling some of the priorities of the Victorian period, such as the "influence of the environment," the "prevention and treatment of infectious disease," and "public education in hygiene."[1] But it also singled out "heredity and race," "infant welfare," and the "school child": all preoccupations that might be discerned in the mid- to late Victorian period, and still more in the early twentieth century, but which become more pronounced and institutionalized during the interwar years. Finally, the *Outline* urged attention to more chronic conditions, including heart disease, which Newman discussed under the heading "Prevention and Treatment of Non-Infectious Disease."

This was a reflection of the shifting epidemiological profile of the English population—indeed, it was partly a reflection of the achievements of the Victorians examined here, as the deadliness of the so-called zymotic class of infectious diseases gradually withered and faded.[2] Certainly, in this sense, England's public health system required updating. Yet, as a voluminous literature has detailed, quite how these novel points and priorities of reform were administered was, as before, subject to considerable contestation and local variation.[3] And so it would continue. The National Health Service, for instance, the most iconic and brave of all the postwar developments in what some now dubbed "social medicine"—another twist in the institutional meanings of public health—is now seen as a fragile achievement amid the emergence of an only patchy social-democratic "consensus."[4] The examples might be multiplied up to the present. Indeed, understood as an institutional assemblage, perhaps we might all agree that "public health" has neither an essence nor a telos, and that it is impossible to point to any reform that was not mangled in practice and subject to partial and variable realization. The argument of this book, however, is that none of this unbridled contingency and administrative complexity should preclude seeking to identify modern transformations, and the work of structural factors and dynamics.

So when and how did public health become modern in England? This transformation took place during the early to mid-Victorian period, when the *problem* of public health first assumed a modern form and structural dynamism. To be clear: it is not that the origins of what would follow can be found here. Rather, it was at this point when a modern sense of historical progress and administrative—even utopian—possibility began to inform public health reform, which henceforth became a matter of building bureaucratic and technological systems of unprecedented size and intricacy. It was also at this point when a series of modern dynamics concerning different levels, agents, and temporalities of governance began to combine, thereby structuring how England's public health system was conceived and practiced, reformed and frustrated. In some respects, the guiding interpretive thread has been quite simple: namely, that it is a matter of historical processes that are dialectical in nature, whereby more of one does not preclude more of the other. Among other examples: centralization *and* localization; bureaucratization *and* democratization; growing systemic scale *and* growing attention to systemic detail; or again, greater chronological compression *and* greater temporal depth and historicity.

Such has been the general design of the argument presented here. There are three aspects in particular that might be highlighted in conclusion.

SYSTEMS

One of these is the question of where we should locate the quality of modernity. This book has argued that modernity is best located in the making and remaking of systems, rather than in the making and remaking of a state. It has done so in the context of England, but the limitations of thinking in terms of a state are especially apparent in a comparative context. Take France, which began establishing local health councils in 1802, and set up a permanent central public health office much earlier than in England, doing so in 1822 in the form of a Conseil supérieur de santé, before establishing a Comité consultatif d'hygiène publique in 1848.[5] Yet, comparative assessments suggest that the French state remained relatively weak, if also centralized, a quality otherwise seen as a sign of the "strength" and "size" of a state. "Fearing both revolution and despotism," writes Dorothy Porter, "the French state remained centralized but noninterventionist, delegating its responsibilities for achieving national reforms to the individual operations of local and regional authorities."[6] And so it did, and these "operations" made for local public health systems that were just as complex, innovative, and fraught as those in England. Another useful example here is the United States, where a permanent, central-federal bureaucracy developed much later in the form of the U.S. Public Health Service, established in 1912. This was as much a product of long-standing, state-based antipathy toward federal regulation and broader struggles regarding nation-building, as it was logistical factors and the sheer geographical size of the United States (which expanded considerably during the nineteenth century, of course). Yet the absence of a centralized (federal) state in the United States hardly made for the absence of public health systems. This is most of all the case in cities, east and west, but it is also evident at the level of individual states, a level that began to coalesce in the late 1860s and 1870s, when the first state boards of health were established.[7]

Small wonder, then, that it is no longer original or provocative to suggest that states are not monolithic or one-dimensional entities, but in fact are complex, contradictory, and multidimensional. These kinds of arguments are especially pronounced in the historiography of public health in the British Empire, where historians have identified a diversity of imperial and colonial state formations, each determined by the size of the territory in question, and the precise interplay of commercial, military, professional, and subaltern forms of agency.[8] But these arguments can be found elsewhere, forming something like the new orthodoxy in relation to how we understand the state. As Peter Baldwin has argued, in an essay where he seeks to move beyond thinking in terms of "weak" and "strong" states: "Should we expect states to be uniformly one thing or the other? States are lumpy. They may focus their energies and attention on certain matters while ignoring others. They may not be consistently laissez-faire or interventionist."[9] Baldwin is quite right, as are all those who argue for a more nuanced understanding of the state.

Thinking in terms of systems helps us to move beyond the now tired and overburdened paradigm of the state. Simply put, this is what governing *is*—designing, operating, and critiquing systems—and it is here where we can accurately locate contingency and choice, and variations of development. To be sure, the term *system* is a slippery one. It means a combination of parts that form a whole, as well as a combination of parts that function as a whole in a way that is methodical, orderly, and efficient, which is to say, systematic. The term is useful, however, precisely because of this slippage, which became more pronounced and endemic in the wake of the new sense of historical-administrative possibility that emerged during the Victorian period. No system was systematic: this much is obvious. And yet, the *desire* for greater system, even for total system, was an important driver of reform and critique. It was evident, for instance, in the grandiose and agenda-setting—if also alternate—visions of system offered by the likes of Chadwick (more sanitary and infrastructural) and Rumsey (more state-medical and person-centered). But it was also evident in the routine grumbling about the need for more efficiency and coordination. Monotonous moaning that systems are not quite working as they should is just as much a defining feature of modernity as the generation of imposing visions promising a new order of things.

Thinking in terms of systems also helps us to grasp the interrelations that emerged between different levels of governance—levels indeed that extended at once below and beyond a central state. This book has argued that the modernity of England's public health system as it emerged from the 1830s resides not in the ascendancy of one level over another. Rather, it lies in an intensification of multiple levels, which once formalized as such—as "local," "central," "personal," and "international" in particular—then entered into new and complex systemic combinations. Historiographically speaking, the biggest loser has perhaps been the local, which is often seen as the preeminent site of premodern forms of governance. The argument here, however, is that the local should be understood as a fully modern site of power, and more especially as a product of a new form of multi-tiered governance that involved logistical-political processes of mutual elaboration. It is no coincidence that the local flourished as a site of popular consciousness and civic identity during the second half of the nineteenth century, just as London's Whitehall district and Downing Street became the symbolic centers of national governance.[10] It is also an argument in keeping with recent reappraisals of "the local." As historians have argued, for all the growing transnationalism of urban policy formation from midcentury onward, the agency of cities and towns remained crucial. It was here where novel policies and systems were generated and tried out; and it was here where those from elsewhere were either directly borrowed, reworked, or rejected entirely. The local is not a premodern residue or survivor: it is a constitutive and dynamic part of the administrative landscape of modernity.[11]

The same applies to the two levels that seem the most distant, namely the personal and the international. One might argue, for instance, that the international level remained relatively undeveloped in the nineteenth century compared to the personal, which, as chapter 7 detailed, emerged as a novel site of governance during the same stretch of time. Certainly one of the most striking developments of the twentieth century was the further internationalization of public health. This included the emergence of the Health Organization of the League of Nations in 1922, and the establishment of the World Health Organization in 1948.[12] Yet scholars have also identified a shift toward "the personal" during the twentieth century, with the rise of "individual responsibility" for chronic conditions such as heart disease and obesity, and associated bad habits such as smoking and a lack of exercise.[13] But to repeat: the argument of this book is that we need not choose between the personal and the international, however far apart they might seem. Instead, they should be historicized together, as part of the elaboration of a modern field of governance that emerged, in England at least, in the early and mid-Victorian periods. Smoking, obesity, excess drinking, and venereal disease: all of these public health problems located in personal habits of conduct have become the subject of international campaigns that seek to advance the work of national governments and local authorities.

VARIATIONS

The argument advanced here also has implications for how we think about the question of variation. As chapter 1 noted, in the absence of any modernizing trajectory, of which England might be seen as either an exemplary or an imperfect instance, variations of institutional development have been to the fore in the "antiheroic" historiography. This is with good empirical reason, for public health was indeed subject to variable realization, at all levels, at all times, and in all places. No two cities were the same, let alone any two countries. We should surely speak, as Porter and others have done, of multiple and nationally specific "models" of public health, rather than a single exemplar.[14] Yet, the recovery and consciousness of variation should also be seen as an integral feature of modernity. Put another way, while we might affirm the fact of variation in retrospect, this should not obscure the way variation formed a crucial and obsessive preoccupation in the past. Modernity is partly defined by the continual processing of administrative successes and failures, and differential rates of progress and development.

What is at stake here is less a set of individual ideas about time and space (histories of which abound), and more a general culture of interrogation regarding what has been done and what might be done, and whether we are regressing or progressing. On the one hand, different spaces and all that they contain—particular people, practices, and systems—are thought to inhabit the same ticking clock and chronological calendar; on the other, these spaces are also thought to embody differential rates of progress, and thus relative "advance" or "backwardness." It is no coincidence that the spatial dynamics of governing began to change in the 1830s and 1840s, just as public health was conceived as a historical endeavor comprising immense future possibilities as well as a weighty past; and no coincidence, either, that England's public health system was henceforth subject to ongoing, statisticalized time serialization. Where are we now in the present year, month, or week? How much progress has been made, and what might be achieved in the future? How do we stand in relation to elsewhere, ahead or behind; and if behind, what might be learned from there, borrowed, emulated, or adapted? Such questions were often posed explicitly; but they were also institutionalized, as evident, for instance, in the routine reflexive reporting of central bureaucracies such as the GRO, GBH, and LGB, and the deliberations of professional associations.

To be sure, this consciousness of variation was perhaps most pronounced in the imperial sphere, where British efforts to enhance the health of indigenous populations were thought of in terms of reforming "habits" and "customs" that reflected "arrested civilizations," and backward and barbaric societies.[15] It would also flourish in the twentieth century, amid an international discourse of "developed" and "developing countries." This even included looking to the Soviet Union during the interwar period; Scandinavian systems would prove popular in the post-war decades.[16] The examples are many, but clearly this same modern consciousness was already at work in the nineteenth-century metropole, shaping both perceptions and practices of reform.

This is one reason why historians have emphasized the porosity of the modern state, and the need for comparative and "connected" accounts.[17] Two points might be made here. The first is that this consciousness of variation was made possible by the work of novel administrative and technological systems. The best example of this perhaps is the GRO, which developed an elaborate system for the publication of spatial-temporal variations of death rates, among other measures in a remarkable step-change in the volume of vital statistics that was produced. But whatever the type of variation in question, whether it concerned the means of public health or the success of these means, its recovery and articulation relied on systems of writing and classification, as well as systems for the speedy transmission of information, such as railway, postal, and telegraphic networks.

The second point is that variations of progress and systemic successes were grasped both within and across national boundaries, making for complex, multilayered circuits of emulation and borrowing. Localities looked to other localities, domestic, foreign, and imperial; nations looked to other nations; and international organizations provided forums where both kinds of governmental gaze might be exercised. As we have seen, within England, local authorities routinely sought guidance in the work of other local authorities; but England was also home to some crucial exports that crossed national borders, most of all "the sanitary idea" and large-scale sewerage systems. The work of English engineers was a crucial point of reference in the United States, France, and Germany, and the multiple parts of the British Empire, where it seems there was still more intense dispute about the merits of combined and separate waterborne systems, as well as conservancy systems.[18] Another crucial export, of course, was the "English system," which was promoted via the ISCs of the late nineteenth century, and that offered an alternative to crude practices of quarantine dating back to the late medieval period.

It was not all one-way traffic, however. Examples not considered in this book include burial reform, which was informed by French and German practices; or again, the reform of milk supplies and the establishment of municipal milk depots at the turn of the century, which built on French innovations.[19] Even where particular systems were *not* modeled on those abroad, this did not preclude constant reference to continental and imperial practices. A striking instance is furnished by the CDAs of the 1860s. The British CDAs were explicitly fashioned and defended as an alternative to "continental systems" of policing venereal disease, which were based on the regulation of brothels, as in France and a number of German cities, but also across the British Empire. Continental forms of governance were first introduced in Hong Kong in 1857, before spreading in the 1860s to places as diverse as India, Malta, the Cape Colony, Barbados, and Queensland, Australia. Strictly speaking, the British system—which was also limited to military towns—was indeed different. But systemic subtleties of administration did nothing to quell domestic opposition; and as Philippa Levine has detailed, once the British laws had been scrapped in 1886, the repeal lobby was able to focus its attention on quashing imperial practices.[20]

Crucially, the porous nature of the modern English state is also evident in terms of bigger considerations about the priorities and scope of "public health" as a national enterprise. Chadwick's sanitary approach was partly informed by the work of French hygienists, even if Chadwick developed their insights in an altogether partial fashion.[21] Equally, more expansive, non-Chadwickian visions of public health drew their inspiration from beyond England. A notable example is Rumsey's attempt to "anglicize," as he put it, German and French practices of medical police in the form of state medicine, a much more palatable reformist idiom in England.[22] It may have failed by its own self-consciously high standards, but it also stirred ambitions and framed new possibilities, ultimately setting an agenda that would inform the formation of the LGB in 1871. More might be said in this vein; but evidently "policy tourism" and transnational processes of "policy transfer" are not recent phenomena.[23] Rather, they are a defining feature of modernity, and should be understood as part and parcel of a novel consciousness of spatial-temporal variations of "progress" that first flourished in the nineteenth century.

POLITICS

Finally, the argument advanced here can also help us to rethink the politics of modern public health. This, too, is another key feature of the "antiheroic" historiography. It is not uncommon to find arguments which suggest that public health is inescapably a matter of politics.

"Public health is inherently political," writes one recent comparative history of the United States, Canada, Britain, and France, and their efforts to combat infant mortality, tuberculosis, lung cancer, and HIV/AIDS.[24] So it is; but what is this politics a product of, precisely? The answers are various, of course, ranging from the articulation of class-based and professional interests to the need for social discipline and the assertion of shared cultural values. Clearly these are all important, and can help to explain the peculiar national trajectories of modern public health, as well as the peculiar institutional formations that have surrounded—and continue to surround—particular afflictions. The politics of modern public health, however, can also be grasped as the structural product of the dual status of the public as both an object and a subject of governance: the public, that is, as the object of laws, regulations, and disciplinary forms of expert knowledge and prescription; *and* the public as the recognized subject of rights, opinions, liberties, interests, and a capacity for self-government.

To be sure, in Victorian and Edwardian England there were many "publics," a plurality that was partly determined by considerations of class, race, and gender. The advent of a more egalitarian and social-democratic culture of political subjectivities would have to wait until the mid-twentieth century, as part of the emergence of a welfare state. But this need not preclude insisting on an underlying dynamic that can be seen in the *joint* emergence—and fractious entanglement—of both a modern state and a modern democracy and civil society. We have seen this dynamic at work in various places in this book, from the emergence and contestation of center-local relations (chapter 2) and national systems of statistical scrutiny (chapter 3), to the everyday work of officials (chapter 4) and the encouragement of personal habits of conduct (chapter 7). Much like spatial-temporal variations of progress, this too emerged as an articulate problem during the Victorian period. It is evident, for instance, in the popularization of terms such as *centralization* and *bureaucracy*, as well as in the use of distinctions between official "facts" and public "opinions," and "professional" and "nonprofessional" agents.

The term *liberal* best captures the politics of Victorian and Edwardian public health reform, and it has been used in places here, deploying the more diffuse and cultural understanding evident in recent scholarship.[25] In particular, it captures a broad culture of governance that was at once mindful of the need for central regulation and the authority of officials and elites, *and* respectful of the public's right to property, privacy, local self-government, and representative (if not yet fully democratic) institutions. But the account here also suggests that we should be wary of invoking an overarching and diffuse political quality, liberal or otherwise. The principal reason for this is because it risks obscuring the way the very distinction between the "political" and the "nonpolitical" was itself up for grabs, and was constantly being affirmed and dissolved, drawn and erased. This is not a marginal point: it was crucial to how public health was assembled and contested as a modern system of governance. The administrative independence claimed by and accorded to professionals and officials was constantly being revoked and withdrawn; or at the very least, judged with suspicion by a public and its representatives conscious that expert and official actions cost time and money, constituted a possible threat to private interests and liberties, and even rested on shaky evidence. This is not to deny that public health is political, even inherently so; but it is to insist that notions of "political action" and of what constitutes "politics" should not be taken for granted. Rather, they should be treated as historical and organizational variables in and of themselves.

Doing so can help us to better understand the production of political struggle. All historians of public health recognize the novelty of the forms of expertise, science, and professional association that developed in the Victorian period; but just as novel and important was the development of more formalized forms of political agency, such as a more expansive and partisan press, and higher levels of party-based organization both within and outside parliament. Both were crucial, and the consequence was variable relations of conflict and cooperation between professionals and officials on the one hand, and members of the public and its representatives on the other. To be sure, the dominant ethos on the part of professionals was to seek cooperative relations with those who were distinguished from the official core of public health. But it is testament to the modernity of this struggle that some professionals and bureaucrats argued that solutions lay in *transcending* a realm of politics and public opinion. A technocratic itch was always at work.

Historians tend to associate this with Chadwick, who has been upheld (much as he was at the time) as the archetypal Benthamite bureaucrat; but it extended much beyond, as the professionalization of public health deepened during the latter half of the century. "Is it not time for politicians to shake hands over measures which are called for by sanitarians because they influence the health of the people?" asked one MOH, Alfred Carpenter, before the SIGB in 1884, assuming that his audience of fellow professionals felt the same. "Why should not measures be taken out of the range of politics and put before the House and our town councils as non-political measures, to be judged upon their own merits?"[26] Carpenter, it seems, was objecting to the undue *party*-politicization of public health reform. And yet, his sentiments are no less political for that, for they point in the direction of unencumbered bureaucratic empowerment and unaccountable governance. Put another way, in order to understand fully the politics of modern public health we also need to recognize the historical novelty of boundary disputes about the limits and nature of "politics" and "the political."

Ultimately, the deeper issue at stake in these struggles was liberty and what it meant. It is once again symptomatic of the underlying structural dynamics of modernity that the meaning of liberty was much disputed. The right to be spared regulation was certainly one measure of liberty, as in the debates over sanitary centralization and the stamping out of infectious diseases. Yet regulation, of one sort or another, could also secure and enhance liberty, at least when public health was understood as a constituent ingredient of freedom. According to some, central regulation made for enhanced powers of local self-government; equally, notifying and isolating cases of infectious disease secured freedom for both the individual concerned and the community at large. The same point was made in relation to the provision of sewerage systems. How, after all, could one be free if sick or even dead—and what of freedom from insanitary environments, and those known to be infected? Certainly the conundrum did not go unnoticed at the time, finding its way into even the most humdrum fields of administration. "Sanitary inspection, however coercive or restraining it might superficially appear, was really contributory to personal liberty and made for a wider freedom," stated the president of the 1907 annual conference of inspectors. "Its mission was to emancipate. There was no tyranny as cruel and oppressive as that of disease."[27] Perhaps this is what is meant by "the rule of freedom," as Patrick Joyce has memorably put it.[28] But only, we might add, if we allow that freedom was a protean and slippery ideal, open to both "negative" and more "positive" meanings—indeed, only if we allow that *freedom* functioned as a kind of empty signifier, around which all manner of administrative signifieds gathered and competed.

A final word: the aim of this book has been to offer an understanding of modernity that makes better sense of the contested and contingent formation of public health in Victorian and Edwardian England. Quite whether the argument can do the same interpretive work elsewhere and on into the twentieth century must remain a moot point for the moment. The brief and patchy comparative comments made above only gesture in this direction, and do not pretend to do anything more. The book, however, has also sought to make a historiographical argument, for the underlying conviction has been that affirming complexity, contingency, and spatial-temporal variations of practice need not preclude affirming a "bigger picture," in this case the bigger picture of modernity. Too often, peculiar details and exceptions—the nitty-gritty richness of the historical record—are wielded as a warning against the search for structural factors and dynamics in explaining the past. But this is to indulge in our empirical instincts as historians, rather than to take conceptual risks: to retreat to a comfort zone of detail and variation. In truth, the two might go together, with one illuminating the other. And however much we might shrink from the category, "the modern" remains crucial to making sense of who and what we are now, in the present.

Notes

CHAPTER I. IN SEARCH OF HYGEIA

1. Benjamin Ward Richardson, *Vita Medica: Chapters of Medical Life and Work* (London: Longmans, Green, 1897), 238.

2. Benjamin Ward Richardson, "Address on Health," *TNAPSS: 1875* (London: Longmans, Green, 1876), 119.

3. Ibid., 105, 120.

4. There is still debate about the precise causes and contours of this transition, which continues to unfold today. For an excellent summation on the period under question here see Simon Szreter and Anne Hardy, "Urban Fertility and Mortality Patterns," in *The Cambridge Urban History of Britain*, vol. 3, 1840–1950, ed. Martin Daunton (Cambridge: Cambridge University Press, 2000), 629–72.

5. *Times*, October 13, 1875, 9.

6. *The New Oxford Dictionary of English* (Oxford: Clarendon, 1998), 1883.

7. Samuel Johnson, *A Dictionary of the English Language,* facsimile ed. (London: Times Books, 1979), s.v. "Sys"; and Hyde Clarke, *A New and Comprehensive Dictionary of the English Language* (London: John Weale, 1855), 392.

8. Johnson, *Dictionary of the English Language,* s.v. "Sys."

9. James Henry Murray, ed., *Johnson's Dictionary* (London: George Routledge, 1874), 177; *The Concise Oxford Dictionary of Current English* (Oxford: Clarendon, 1914), 895.

10. See, most recently, Christopher Hamlin, "Public Health," in *The Oxford Handbook of the History of Medicine,* ed. Mark Jackson (Oxford: Oxford University Press, 2011), 411–28.

11. Dorothy Porter, introduction to *The History of Public Health and the Modern State,* ed. Dorothy Porter (Amsterdam: Rodopi, 1994), 1–3.

12. See esp. S. E. Finer, *The Life and Times of Sir Edwin Chadwick* (London: Methuen, 1952); R. A. Lewis, *Edwin Chadwick and the Public Health Movement* (London: Longmans and Green, 1952); and Royston Lambert, *Sir John Simon, 1816–1904, and English Sanitary Administration* (London: Macgibbon and Kee, 1963).

13. George Rosen, *A History of Public Health,* expanded ed. (Baltimore: Johns Hopkins University Press, 1993). See esp. chaps. 5–6.

14. Richard Price, *British Society, 1680–1880: Dynamism, Containment and Change* (Cambridge: Cambridge University Press, 1999), 4. The "history of social policy," he suggests, is a "notorious example."

15. See, for instance, David Roberts, *Victorian Origins of the British Welfare State* (New Haven, CT: Yale University Press, 1960); Ruth G. Hodgkinson, *The Origins of the National Health Service: The Medical Services of the New Poor Law, 1834–1871* (London: Wellcome Library, 1967); and J. N. Tarn, *Five Per Cent Philanthropy: An Account of Housing in Urban Areas between 1840 and 1914* (London: Cambridge University Press, 1973).

16. Oliver MacDonagh, "The Nineteenth-Century Revolution in Government: A Reappraisal," *Historical Journal* 1, no. 1 (1958): 52–67. Overviews of the historiography include Valerie Cromwell, ed., *Revolution or Evolution: British Government in the Nineteenth Century* (London: Longman, 1977); and Peter Mandler, "Introduction: State and Society in Victorian Britain," in *Liberty and Authority in Victorian Britain,* ed. Peter Mandler (Oxford: Oxford University Press, 2006), 1–21.

17. Peter Baldwin, *Contagion and the State in Europe, 1830–1930* (Cambridge: Cambridge University Press, 1999).

18. Erwin H. Ackerknecht, "Anticontagionism between 1821 and 1867," *Bulletin of the History of Medicine* 22, no. 5 (1948): 562–93.

19. Recent examples of local, British, European, and imperial studies include Nigel Richardson, *Typhoid in Uppingham: Analysis of a Victorian Town and School in Crisis, 1875–1877* (London: Pickering and Chatto, 2008); Deborah Brunton, *The Politics of Vaccination: Practice and Policy in England, Wales, Ireland, and Scotland, 1800–1874* (Rochester, NY: University of Rochester Press, 2008); Donnacha Seán Lucey and Virginia Crossman, eds., *Healthcare in Ireland and Britain from 1850: Voluntary, Regional and Comparative Perspectives* (London: Institute of Historical Research, 2014); E. P. Hennock, "The Urban Sanitary Movement in England and Germany, 1838–1914: A Comparison," *Continuity and Change* 15, no. 2 (2000): 269–96; Constance A. Nathanson, *Disease Prevention as Social Change: The State, Society, and Public Health in the United States, France, Great Britain, and Canada* (New York: Russell Sage Foundation, 2007); and Ryan Johnson and Amna Khalid, eds., *Public Health in the British Empire: Intermediaries, Subordinates, and the Practice of Public Health, 1850–1960* (New York: Routledge, 2012).

20. See, among multiple other accounts, Mark Harrison, *Public Health in British India: Anglo-Indian Preventive Medicine, 1859–1914* (Cambridge: Cambridge University Press, 1994); Martin V. Melosi, *The Sanitary City: Urban*

Infrastructure in America from Colonial Times to the Present (Baltimore: Johns Hopkins University Press, 2000); and Linda Bryder, "A New World? Two Hundred Years of Public Health in Australia and New Zealand," in Porter, ed., *History of Public Health and the Modern State*, 313–34.

21. See esp. Christopher Hamlin, *A Science of Impurity: Water Analysis in Nineteenth Century Britain* (Berkeley: University of California Press, 1990); Anne Hardy, "On the Cusp: Epidemiology and Bacteriology at the Local Government Board, 1890–1905," *Medical History* 42, no. 3 (1998): 328–46; Michael Worboys, *Spreading Germs: Disease Theories and Medical Practice in Britain, 1865–1900* (Cambridge: Cambridge University Press, 2000); Michael Worboys, "Was There a Bacteriological Revolution in Late Nineteenth-Century Medicine?" *Studies in History and Philosophy of Biological and Biomedical Sciences* 38, no. 1 (2007): 20–42; and James F. Stark, *The Making of Modern Anthrax, 1875–1920: Uniting Local, National and Global Histories of Disease* (London: Pickering and Chatto, 2013).

22. See esp. David Arnold, *Colonizing the Body: State Medicine and Epidemic Disease in Nineteenth-Century India* (Berkeley: University of California Press, 1993); Philippa Levine, *Prostitution, Race, and Politics: Policing Venereal Disease in the British Empire* (New York: Routledge, 2003); and Hibba Abugideiri, *Gender and the Making of Modern Medicine in Colonial Egypt* (Farnham: Ashgate, 2010).

23. See esp. Mary Poovey, *Making a Social Body: British Cultural Formation, 1830–1864* (Chicago: University of Chicago Press, 1995); Frank Mort, *Dangerous Sexualities: Medico-Moral Politics in England since 1830*, 2nd ed. (London: Routledge, 2000); Nadja Durbach, *Bodily Matters: The Anti-Vaccination Movement in England, 1853–1907* (Durham, NC: Duke University Press, 2005); Pamela K. Gilbert, *The Citizen's Body: Desire, Health, and the Social in Victorian England* (Athens: Ohio State University Press, 2007); Michelle Allen, *Cleansing the City: Sanitary Geographies in Victorian London* (Athens: Ohio State University Press, 2008); and Pamela K. Gilbert, *Cholera and Nation: Doctoring the Social Body in Victorian England* (Albany: State University of New York Press, 2008).

24. B. R. Mitchell, *British Historical Statistics* (Cambridge: Cambridge University Press, 1988), 8–9.

25. See esp. Ann F. La Berge, "Edwin Chadwick and the French Connection," *Bulletin of the History of Medicine* 62, no. 1 (1988): 23–41; John V. Pickstone, "Dearth, Dirt and Fever Epidemics: Rewriting the History of British 'Public Health,' 1780–1850," in *Epidemics and Ideas: Essays on the Historical Perception of Pestilence*, ed. Terence Ranger and Paul Slack (Cambridge: Cambridge University Press, 1992), 125–48; and Christopher Hamlin, *Public Health and Social Justice in the Age of Chadwick: Britain, 1800–1854* (Cambridge: Cambridge University Press, 1998).

26. Hamlin, "Public Health," 411–12.

27. Dorothy Porter, *Health, Civilization and the State: A History of Public Health from Ancient to Modern Times* (London: Routledge, 1999), 3–4.

28. See, most recently, Frank Trentmann, "Materiality in the Future of History: Things, Practices and Politics," *Journal of British Studies* 48, no. 2 (2009):

283–307; and Tony Bennett and Patrick Joyce, eds., *Material Powers: Cultural Studies, History and the Material Turn* (London: Routledge, 2010).

29. Joanna Innes, "Central Government 'Interference': Changing Conceptions, Practices, and Concerns, *c.* 1700–1850," in *Civil Society in British History: Ideas, Identities, Institutions,* ed. Jose Harris (Oxford: Oxford University Press, 2003), 42–43.

30. The work of Hobbes marks the crucial intervention here, even if it was not necessarily a common point of reference at the time. Quentin Skinner, "The State," in *Political Innovation and Conceptual Change,* ed. Terence Ball, James Farr, and Russell L. Hanson (Cambridge: Cambridge University Press, 1989), 90–126.

31. James Meadowcroft, *Conceptualizing the State: Innovation and Dispute in British Political Thought, 1880–1914* (Oxford: Clarendon, 1995), chap. 1.

32. See, for instance, George Steinmetz, *State/Culture: State-Formation after the Cultural Turn* (Ithaca, NY: Cornell University Press, 1999); and Bob Jessop, *State Power* (Cambridge: Polity, 2007).

33. Mark Bevir, *Governance: A Very Short Introduction* (Oxford: Oxford University Press, 2012), 1.

34. Robert J. Morris, "Governance: Two Centuries of Urban Growth," in *Urban Governance: Britain and Beyond since 1750,* ed. Robert J. Morris and Richard H. Trainor (Ashgate: Aldershot, 2000), 1.

35. Patrick Joyce, *The State of Freedom: A Social History of the British State since 1800* (Cambridge: Cambridge University Press, 2013); and Timothy Mitchell, *Rule of Experts: Egypt, Techno-Politics, Modernity* (Berkeley: University of California Press, 2002).

36. A useful overview is G. Geltner, "Public Health and the Pre-Modern City: A Research Agenda," *History Compass* 10, no. 3 (2012): 231–45.

37. Carole Rawcliffe, *Urban Bodies: Communal Health in Late Medieval English Towns and Cities* (Woodbridge: Boydell, 2013).

38. Peter Buck, "Seventeenth-Century Political Arithmetic: Civil Strife and Vital Statistics," *Isis* 68, no. 241 (1977): 67–84; William Blackstone, *Commentaries on the Laws of England, Book the Fourth* (Oxford: Clarendon, 1769), 161.

39. Paul Slack, *The Impact of Plague in Tudor and Stuart England* (Oxford: Clarendon, 1990).

40. Joanna Innes, "The Local Acts of a National Parliament: Parliament's Role in Sanctioning Local Action in Eighteenth-Century Britain," *Parliamentary History* 17, no. 1 (1998): 23–47.

41. Excellent surveys, both of which have informed the brief account here, include Paul Slack, *From Reformation to Improvement: Public Welfare in Early Modern England* (Oxford: Clarendon, 1999); and Michael J. Braddick, *State Formation in Early Modern England, c. 1550–1700* (Cambridge: Cambridge University Press, 2000).

42. Christopher Hamlin, "Public Sphere to Public Health: The Transformation of 'Nuisance,'" in *Medicine, Health and the Public Sphere in Britain, 1600–2000,* ed. Steve Sturdy (London: Routledge, 2002), 190–94.

43. On the office of the magistrate see Norma Landau, *The Justices of the Peace, 1679–1760* (Berkeley: University of California Press, 1984).

44. Useful summaries include Mary Lindemann, *Medicine and Society in Early Modern Europe,* 2nd ed. (Cambridge: Cambridge University Press, 2010), chap. 6; and James C. Riley, *The Eighteenth-Century Campaign to Avoid Disease* (Basingstoke: Macmillan, 1987).

45. Dolly Jørgensen, "'All Good Rule of the Citee': Sanitation and Civic Government in England, 1400–1600," *Journal of Urban History* 36, no. 3 (2010): 300–315.

46. *The Court Leet Records of the Manor of Manchester, from the Year 1552 to the Year 1686, and from the Year 1731 to the Year 1846,* vol. 7 (Manchester: Henry Blacklock, 1888).

47. David Eastwood, *Government and Community in the English Provinces, 1700–1870* (Basingstoke: Palgrave Macmillan, 1997), 66.

48. Valeska Huber, "The Unification of the Globe by Disease? The International Sanitary Conferences on Cholera, 1851–1894," *Historical Journal* 49, no. 2 (2006): 458.

49. Anthony Giddens, *The Consequences of Modernity* (Oxford: Polity, 2004), 21–29.

50. For reflections see Bernhard Struck, Kate Ferris, and Jacques Revel, "Introduction: Space and Scale in Transnational History," *International History Review* 33, no. 4 (2011): 573–84; and Michael Zürn, "Global Governance as Multi-Level Governance," in *The Oxford Handbook of Governance,* ed. David Levi-Faur (Oxford: Oxford University Press, 2012), 730–44.

51. David Vincent, *The Culture of Secrecy: Britain, 1832–1998* (Oxford: Oxford University Press, 1998), 45–46; Roy MacLeod, introduction to *Government and Expertise: Specialists, Administrators and Professionals, 1860–1919,* ed. Roy MacLeod (Cambridge: Cambridge University Press, 1988), 3 and 256 n. 11.

52. Anne Hardy, "The Public in Public Health," in *Beyond Habermas: Democracy, Knowledge, and the Public Sphere,* ed. Christian J. Emden and David Midgley (New York: Berghahn Books, 2013), 87–98. On the vitality of voluntary action more generally see Frank Prochaska, *Christianity and Social Service in Modern Britain: The Disinherited Spirit* (Oxford: Oxford University Press, 2006).

53. See esp. Martin Pugh, *The Making of Modern British Politics, 1867–1939,* 2nd ed. (Oxford: Basil Blackwell, 1996), chap. 1; and Matthew Roberts, *Political Movements in Urban England, 1832–1914* (Basingstoke: Palgrave Macmillan, 2009).

54. John Russell Vincent, *The Formation of the Liberal Party, 1857–1868* (London: Constable, 1966), 65. On public opinion see Jonathan Parry, *The Rise and Fall of Liberal Government in Victorian Britain* (New Haven, CT: Yale University Press, 1993), chap. 1.

55. Peter Wagner, *Modernity as Experience and Interpretation: A New Sociology of Modernity* (Cambridge: Polity, 2008); Pierre Manent, *A World beyond Politics? A Defense of the Nation-State,* trans. Marc LePain (Princeton, NJ: Princeton University Press, 2006), 1–9; and Marcel Gauchet, *The Disenchantment of the World: A Political History of Religion,* trans. Oscar Burge (Princeton, NJ: Princeton University Press, 1999), 180–85.

56. Michel Foucault, *"Society Must Be Defended": Lectures at the Collège de France, 1975–76*, ed. Mauro Bertani and Alessandro Fontana, trans. David Macey (London: Allen Lane, 2003), 37–38.

57. See esp. Reinhart Koselleck, *Futures Past: On the Semantics of Historical Time*, trans. Keith Tribe (New York: Columbia University Press, 2004); and Reinhart Koselleck, *The Practice of Conceptual History: Timing History, Spacing Concepts*, trans. Todd Samuel Presner (Stanford, CA: Stanford University Press, 2002).

58. Billie Melman, "The Pleasures of Victorian Horror: Popular Histories, Modernity, and Sensationalism in the Long Nineteenth Century," in *Tudorism: Historical Imagination and the Appropriation of the Sixteenth Century*, ed. Tatiana C. String and Marcus Bull (Oxford: Oxford University Press, 2011), 37–57.

59. Jerome Hamilton Buckley, *The Triumph of Time: A Study of the Victorian Concepts of Time, History, Progress, and Decadence* (Cambridge, MA: Belknap, 1967). Another useful overview is Robin Gilmour, *The Victorian Period: The Intellectual and Cultural Context of English Literature, 1830–1890* (Harlow: Pearson, 1993), chap. 1.

60. Reinhart Koselleck, "'Neuzeit': Remarks on the Semantics of Modern Concepts of Movement," in Koselleck, *Futures Past*, 248.

61. See esp. David Harvey, *The Condition of Postmodernity: An Enquiry into the Origin of Cultural Change* (Oxford: Basil Blackwell, 1989), chaps. 15–16; and Giddens, *Consequences of Modernity*, chap. 1.

62. Koselleck, "'Neuzeit': Remarks on the Semantics of Modern Concepts of Movement," 238. The classic account of this dialectic remains Johannes Fabian, *Time and the Other: How Anthropology Makes Its Object* (New York: Columbia University Press, 1983). See also Peter Osborne, *The Politics of Time: Modernity and Avant-Garde* (London: Verso, 1995), 16–17.

63. Most recently, see Sue Zemka, *Time and the Moment in Victorian Literature and Society* (Cambridge: Cambridge University Press, 2012).

64. Peter J. Hugill, "The Shrinking Victorian World," in *The Victorian World*, ed. Martin Hewitt (Abingdon: Routledge, 2012), 73–89.

65. James Vernon, *Distant Strangers: How Britain Became Modern* (Berkeley: University of California Press, 2014), 5–6. See also, and most recently, "AHR Roundtable: Historians and the Question of 'Modernity,'" *American Historical Review* 116, no. 3 (2011): 631–751.

66. See esp. Martin Hewitt, "Why the Notion of Victorian Britain *Does* Make Sense," *Victorian Studies* 48, no. 3 (2006): 395–438.

67. F. B. Smith, *The People's Health, 1830–1910* (London: Croom Helm, 1979); Anthony S. Wohl, *Endangered Lives: Public Health in Victorian Britain* (London: Methuen, 1984).

CHAPTER 2. A PERFECT CHAOS

1. Eric Hobsbawm, "Introduction: Inventing Traditions," in *The Invention of Tradition*, ed. Eric Hobsbawm and Terence Ranger (Cambridge: Cambridge University Press, 1984), 1–14; and J. C. D. Clark, *English Society, 1660–1832:*

Religion, Ideology and Politics during the Ancien Regime, 2nd ed. (Cambridge: Cambridge University Press, 2000), 12–13. Useful discussions on this theme also include Peter Fritzsche, *Stranded in the Present: Modern Time and the Melancholy of History* (Cambridge, MA: Harvard University Press, 2004).

2. Benjamin Disraeli, *The Chancellor of the Exchequer in Scotland, Being Two Speeches Delivered by Him in the City of Edinburgh on 29th and 30th October 1867* (Edinburgh: William Blackwood, 1867), 28.

3. Clark, *English Society*, 12.

4. J. W. Burrow, "'The Village Community' and the Uses of History in Late Nineteenth-Century England," in *Historical Perspectives: Studies in English Thought and Society in Honour of J. H. Plumb*, ed. Neil McKendrick (London: Europa, 1974), 255–84.

5. Edward Jenks, *An Outline of English Local Government* (London: Methuen, 1894), 1, 9.

6. Ibid., 9–10.

7. Joanna Innes, "Central Government 'Interference': Changing Conceptions, Practices, and Concerns, *c.* 1700–1850," in *Civil Society in British History: Ideas, Identities, Institutions*, ed. Jose Harris (Oxford: Oxford University Press, 2003), 42–43, 46.

8. Joanna Innes, "Forms of 'Government Growth,' 1780–1830," in *Structures and Transformations in Modern British History*, ed. David Feldman and Jon Lawrence (Cambridge: Cambridge University Press, 2011), 80.

9. M. D. Chalmers, *Local Government* (London: Macmillan, 1883), 10.

10. Edwin Chadwick, *Report on the Sanitary Condition of the Labouring Population of Great Britain*, ed. M. W. Flinn (Edinburgh: Edinburgh University Press, 1965), 425.

11. Herbert Page, "Our Sanitary System and Its Reorganisation," *Sanitary Record*, August 16, 1886, 52; and Herbert Page, "Our Sanitary System and Its Reorganisation," *Sanitary Record*, September 15, 1886, 101.

12. [Christopher Addison], *The Health of the People, and How It May be Improved, From a Speech Delivered by Dr Christopher Addison, MP, at the Whitehall Rooms, February, 6th, 1914* (London: University of London Press, 1914), 5–6.

13. The most thorough account of the early to mid-Victorian dominance of parliamentary liberalism remains Jonathan Parry, *The Rise and Fall of Liberal Government in Victorian Britain* (New Haven, CT: Yale University Press, 1993).

14. An excellent overview is John Davis, "Central Government and the Towns," in *The Cambridge Urban History of Britain*, vol. 3, 1840–1950, ed. Martin Daunton (Cambridge: Cambridge University Press, 2000), 261–86.

15. Among other accounts, see E. P. Hennock, *Fit and Proper Persons: Ideal and Reality in Nineteenth-Century Urban Government* (London: Edward Arnold, 1973); Derek Fraser, *Urban Politics in Victorian England: The Structure of Politics in Victorian Cities* (Leicester: Leicester University Press, 1976); Derek Fraser, *Power and Authority in the Victorian City* (Oxford: Basil Blackwell, 1979); Avner Offer, *Property and Politics, 1870–1914: Landownership, Law, Ideology, and Urban Development in England* (Cambridge: Cambridge University Press,

1981); and P. J. Waller, *Town, City and Nation: England, 1850–1914* (Oxford: Oxford University Press, 1983).

16. On civic pride see Philip Harling, "The Centrality of the Locality: The Local State, Local Democracy and Local Consciousness in Late-Victorian and Edwardian Britain," *Journal of Victorian Culture* 9, no. 2 (2004): 216–34.

17. David Eastwood, "'Amplifying the Province of the Legislature': The Flow of Information and the English State in the Early Nineteenth Century," *Historical Research* 62, no. 149 (1989): 291.

18. Christine Bellamy, *Administering Centre-Local Relations, 1871–1919: The Local Government Board in Its Fiscal and Cultural Context* (Manchester: Manchester University Press, 1988), chaps. 5–6.

19. Public health was not alone in this respect. The 1834 Poor Law Act had earlier established locally elected boards of guardians, while the 1870 Education Act established locally elected school boards. Other public health acts created elected nuisance boards, burial boards, and sewer authorities.

20. See, for instance, Mark Brayshay and Vivien F. T. Pointon, "Local Politics and Public Health in Mid-Nineteenth-Century Plymouth," *Medical History* 27, no. 2 (1983): 162–78; and John Prest, *Liberty and Locality: Parliament, Permissive Legislation and Ratepayers' Democracies in the Nineteenth Century* (Oxford: Clarendon, 1990).

21. An excellent overview is Barry M. Doyle, "The Changing Functions of Urban Governance: Councillors, Officials and Pressure Groups," in *The Cambridge Urban History of Britain*, vol. 3, 1840–1950, ed. Daunton, 287–313.

22. Hamish Fraser, "Municipal Socialism and Social Policy," in *The Victorian City: A Reader in British Urban History, 1820–1914*, ed. R. J. Morris and Richard Rodger (London: Longman, 1993), 258–80.

23. Sudhir Hazareesingh, *From Subject to Citizen: The Second Empire and the Emergence of Modern French Democracy* (Princeton, NJ: Princeton University Press, 1998), 13–14.

24. William C. Lubenow, *The Politics of Government Growth: Early Victorian Attitudes towards State Intervention, 1833–1848* (Newton Abbot: David and Charles, 1971), chap. 2.

25. Flinn, introduction to Chadwick, *Report on the Sanitary Condition of the Labouring Population of Great Britain*, 71.

26. *Second Report of the Commissioners for Inquiring into the State of Large Towns and Populous Districts*, No. 602 (1845), 6.

27. Ibid., 13, 19.

28. *Engineers and Officials: An Historical Sketch of the Progress of 'Health of Towns Works' in London and the Provinces* (London: Edward Stanford, 1856), 32.

29. Ibid., v, viii.

30. Ibid., iii.

31. [Edwin Chadwick], "Centralization: Public Charities in France," *London Review* 1, no. 2 (1829): 536–65. Innes notes that "I have not yet found references to 'centralization' or indeed to 'central government' in Britain before 1830." Chadwick's article is an exception, but it would seem, as Innes suggests,

that discussions were incredibly rare before the 1830s. Innes, "Central Government 'Interference,'" in Harris, ed., *Civil Society in British History*, 46.

32. [Chadwick], "Centralization," 542, 559.

33. Henry Lytton Bulwer, *The Monarchy of the Middle Classes: France, Social, Literary, Political*, 2 vols. (London: Richard Bentley, 1836), 2: 262–64.

34. Ibid., 142.

35. Bernard Porter, "'Bureau and Barrack': Early Victorian Attitudes towards the Continent," *Victorian Studies* 27, no. 4 (1984): 407–33. On attitudes to the continent see also Jonathan Parry, *The Politics of Patriotism: English Liberalism, National Identity and Europe, 1830–1886* (Cambridge: Cambridge University Press, 2006).

36. [John Austin], "Centralization," *Edinburgh Review* 85 (January 1847): 221–58.

37. Edwin Chadwick, *The Comparative Results of the Chief Principles of the Poor-Law Administration in England and Ireland, as Compared with That of Scotland* (London: E. Faithfull, 1864), 8.

38. See esp. Edwin Chadwick, *A Paper on the Chief Methods of Preparation for Legislation, Especially as Applicable to the Reform of Parliament* (London: Charles Knight, 1859).

39. On Chadwick's fall from office, see Anthony Brundage, *England's "Prussian Minister": Edwin Chadwick and the Politics of Government Growth, 1832–1854* (University Park: Pennsylvania State University Press, 1988), chap. 8.

40. Edwin Chadwick, *An Article on the Principles and Progress of the Poor Law Amendment Act; and Also on the Nature of the Central Control and Improved Local Administration Introduced by That Statute* (London: Charles Knight, 1837), 62–74.

41. Edwin Chadwick, *On the Evils of Disunity in Central and Local Administration, Especially with Reference to the Metropolis and Also on the New Centralisation for the People* (London: Longmans, Green, 1885), 77–79.

42. On the Scottish context see, most recently, Paul Laxton and Richard Rodger, *Insanitary City: Henry Littlejohn and the Condition of Edinburgh* (Lancaster: Carnegie, 2014), chap. 2.

43. J. Ingham Ikin, "On the Progress of Public Hygiène and Sanitary Legislation in England, and the Advantages to be Derived from Their Further Extension," *Provincial Medical and Surgical Journal*, September 17, 1851, 508–9.

44. "The Social Science Congress: Sir Stafford Northcote on State Medicine," *BMJ*, October 2, 1869, 383.

45. Patrick E. Carroll, "Medical Police and the History of Public Health," *Medical History* 46, no. 4 (2002): 461–94.

46. The work of John Simon is detailed in Royston Lambert, *Sir John Simon, 1816–1904, and English Sanitary Administration* (London: Macgibbon and Kee, 1963). See also Jeanne L. Brand, *Doctors and the State: The British Medical Profession and Government Action in Public Health, 1870–1912* (Baltimore: Johns Hopkins University Press, 1965).

47. On the Epidemiological Society—of which Simon was a member—see David E. Lilienfield, "'The Greening of Epidemiology': Sanitary Physicians and

the London Epidemiological Society (1830–1870)," *Bulletin of the History of Medicine* 52, no. 4 (1978): 503–28.

48. On the importance of professional interests, see Steven J. Novak, "Professionalism and Bureaucracy: English Doctors and the Victorian Public Health Administration," *Journal of Social History* 6, no. 4 (1973): 440–58.

49. On the formation of the committee, see Lawrence Goldman, *Science, Reform and Politics in Victorian Britain: The Social Science Association, 1857–1886* (Cambridge: Cambridge University Press, 2002), chap. 6.

50. Sir John Simon, *English Sanitary Institutions, Reviewed in Their Course of Development, and in Some of Their Political and Social Relations* (London: Cassell, 1890), 324; and Thomas Wrigley Grimshaw, "The Relations between Preventive Medicine and Vital Statistics," *Journal of State Medicine* 6, no. 9 (1898): 406–7. It was Rumsey's address to the BMA in Dublin in 1867 which first fired interest in the idea of a joint committee.

51. Henry Wyldbore Rumsey, *Essays on State Medicine* (London: John Churchill, 1856). Other key texts of his on state medicine include *On Sanitary Legislation and Administration in England: An Address* (London: John Churchill, 1857); and *On State Medicine in Great Britain and Ireland* (London: William Ridgway, 1867). Both were essentially condensed versions of his *Essays* of 1856.

52. Rumsey, *Essays on State Medicine*, 340–41; Rumsey, *On Sanitary Legislation and Administration*, 15.

53. Rumsey, *On Sanitary Legislation and Administration*, 44.

54. Ibid., 6.

55. Rumsey, *Essays on State Medicine*, 362. Rumsey was not the only doctor to take an interest in France and Germany. Continental developments routinely featured in the medical press, including, on occasions, comparative reviews. See "State Medicine in Prussia, France and England," *British and Foreign Medico-Chirurgical Review* 36 (October 1856): 366–87.

56. See Rumsey's testimony in House of Commons, "Report from the Select Committee on Medical Poor Relief," *Sessional Papers, 1854* (348), July 5, 1854, 139–42, where he also spoke of Italy, Austria, and France.

57. Rumsey, *Essays on State Medicine*, 5–6.

58. Ibid., ix.

59. Ibid., 120–21. On criticisms among the medical profession, see Margaret Pelling, *Cholera, Fever and English Medicine, 1825–1865* (Oxford: Oxford University Press, 1978), chap. 2.

60. Rumsey, *Essays on State Medicine*, 7–14, 101–21.

61. House of Commons, "Report from the Select Committee on Medical Poor Relief," *Sessional Papers, 1844* (531), July 29, 1844, 591–99; and [Henry W. Rumsey], "The Health and Sickness of Town Populations," *New Quarterly Review; or Home, Foreign and Colonial Journal* 13 (April 1846): 1–42.

62. Rumsey, *Essays on State Medicine*, vi, 56, 182, 218, 220, 234, 286, 399, 408.

63. Ibid., 46–49.

64. Ibid., 341–46.

65. Rumsey, *On Sanitary Legislation and Administration*, 53; Rumsey, *On State Medicine in Great Britain*, 33–34.

66. Rumsey, *Essays on State Medicine,* 50–54, 300–304.

67. Rumsey, *On State Medicine in Great Britain,* 35.

68. "State Medicine in Great Britain," *Journal of Public Health and Sanitary Review* 2 (July 1858): 111–12.

69. Rumsey, *On Sanitary Legislation and Administration,* 12–13.

70. Henry Wyldbore Rumsey, "The Memorial on State Medicine," *BMJ,* May 23, 1868, 520.

71. This is true of working-class opinions, which were just as complex as middle-class ones, and which were by no means ill-informed or oppositional. Michael Sigsworth and Michael Worboys, "The Public's View of Public Health in Mid-Victorian Britain," *Urban History* 21, no. 2 (1994): 237–50.

72. *The Times on Sanitary Misrule, Corporate and Parochial* (London: Effingham Wilson, 1851).

73. "Lord Morpeth's Sanitary Bill," *Liverpool Mercury,* April 4, 1848, 3.

74. A Citizen, *Centralization or Local Representation: Health of Towns' Bill: The Opinion of the Public Journals,* 3 vols. (London: Thomas Harreld, 1848), 1: 3.

75. Ibid., 3: 32.

76. Ibid., 1: 14.

77. Ibid., 1: 16.

78. *Hansard Parliamentary Debates,* 3rd ser., vol. 93 (1847), col. 1104.

79. *Hansard Parliamentary Debates,* 3rd ser., vol. 98 (1848), col. 772.

80. Ibid., cols. 713–14.

81. There is no space here to discuss the complexities of Smith's enormous body of work. The most extensive discussion is Ben Weinstein, "'Local Self-Government Is True Socialism': Joshua Toulmin Smith, the State and Character Formation," *English Historical Review* 123, no. 504 (2008): 1193–228.

82. On Smith's place in the politics of the City of London, see Ben Weinstein, *Liberalism and Local Government in Early Victorian London* (Woodbridge: Boydell and Brewer, 2011).

83. Fraser, *Power and Authority in the Victorian City,* 94, 117, 141–43.

84. Gregory Claeys, "Mazzini, Kossuth and British Radicalism, 1848–1854," *Journal of British Studies* 28, no. 3 (1989): 225–61. See also Miles Taylor, *The Decline of British Radicalism, 1847–1860* (Oxford: Clarendon, 1995), 87–92.

85. In terms of the latter, see J. Toulmin Smith, *The Metropolis and Its Municipal Management: Showing the Essentials of a Sound System of Municipal Self-Government as Applicable to All Town Populations* (London: Trelawny Saunders, 1852); Toulmin Smith, *The Metropolis Local Management Act, 1855* (London: Henry Sweet, 1855); and Toulmin Smith, *Practical Proceedings for the Removal of Nuisances and Execution of Drainage Works in Every Parish, Town and Place in England and Wales, under the Nuisances Removal Act, 1855* (London: Henry Sweet, 1855). In 1854, he began abbreviating his name to Toulmin Smith.

86. J. Toulmin Smith, *Local Self-Government and Centralization: The Characteristics of Each; and Its Practical Tendencies, as Affecting Social, Moral and Political Welfare and Progress* (London: John Chapman, 1851), 91–94.

87. J. Toulmin Smith, *The Laws of England Relating to Public Health* (London: S. Sweet, 1848), vii–viii, 11.

88. Smith, *Local Self-Government and Centralization*, 112.

89. On radical readings of the constitution more generally see Olive Anderson, *A Liberal State at War: English Politics and Economics during the Crimean War* (London: Macmillan, 1967), chap. 4; and James A. Epstein, *Radical Expression: Political Language, Ritual and Symbol in England, 1790–1840* (Oxford: Oxford University Press, 1994), chap. 1.

90. See esp. Smith, *Local Self-Government and Centralization*, chap. 14.

91. It was a label used by the *Times* in the early 1850s, for instance. *The Times on Sanitary Misrule, Corporate and Parochial,* 4.

92. Smith, *Practical Proceedings for the Removal of Nuisances,* 39.

93. Smith was opposed to all property qualifications, though he also thought criminals and those in receipt of alms should be excluded from the franchise. Smith, *Local Self-Government and Centralization,* 243–44. See also J. Toulmin Smith, *What Is the Corporation of London, and Who Are the Freemen?* (London: Effingham Wilson, 1850).

94. See, in particular, J. Toulmin Smith, *Government by Commissions Illegal and Pernicious: The Nature and Effects of All Commissions of Inquiry and Other Crown-Appointed Commissions* (London: S. Sweet, 1849), 106–20.

95. Toulmin Smith, *Local Self-Government Un-Mystified: A Vindication of Common Sense, Human Nature and Practical Improvement, against the Manifesto of Centralism Put Forth at the Social Science Association, 1857* (London: Edward Stanford, 1857), 4–5.

96. Toulmin Smith, *The Parish: Its Power and Obligations* (London: S. Sweet, 1854), 9–10.

97. Weinstein, "'Local Self-Government Is True Socialism,'" 1213–25.

98. J. W. Burrow, *A Liberal Descent: Victorian Historians and the English Past* (Cambridge: Cambridge University Press, 1981), chap. 7.

99. "How Is the Standard of Public Health to Be Raised?" *Lancet,* February 13, 1858, 170. The work it had in mind seems to have been Smith's *Local Self-Government Un-Mystified.*

100. Smith, *Local Self-Government Un-Mystified,* 53.

101. Peter Mandler, *Aristocratic Government in the Age of Reform: Whigs and Liberals, 1830–1852* (Oxford: Clarendon, 1990). Further complexities are discussed in Boyd Hilton, "Whiggery, Religion and Social Reform: The Case of Lord Morpeth," *Historical Journal* 37, no. 4 (1994): 829–59.

102. John Stuart Mill, *On Liberty and Other Essays,* ed. John Gray (Oxford: Oxford University Press, 1991), 291.

103. Ibid., 422.

104. Ibid., 423–24.

105. Ibid., 426.

106. Rumsey, *On Sanitary Legislation and Administration,* 39–44. The work he referred to was Mill's *Principles of Political Economy.*

107. According to Russell, the aim of the 1834 Act was "to establish self-government . . . acting centrally under general rules and principles . . . but with respect to details, acting according to the judgement of magistrates, county

gentlemen, and ratepayers connected with the district." Quoted in David East-wood, *Government and Community in the English Provinces, 1700–1870* (Basingstoke: Palgrave Macmillan, 1997), 164.

108. *Hansard Parliamentary Debates,* 3rd ser., vol. 96 (1848), cols. 388–89.

109. *Hansard Parliamentary Debates,* 3rd ser., vol. 93 (1847), cols. 1102–3.

110. Tom Taylor, "On Central and Local Action in Relation to Town Improvement," *TNAPSS: 1857* (London: John W. Parker, 1858), 476–77.

111. Ibid., 476.

112. Ibid., 479.

113. "Address by the Right Hon. W. Cowper, MP, on Public Health," *TNAPSS: 1859* (London: John W. Parker, 1860), 120.

114. On this particular constituency see Ben Weinstein, "Metropolitan Whiggery, 1832–1855," in *London Politics, 1760–1914,* ed. Matthew Cragoe and Antony Taylor (Basingstoke: Palgrave Macmillan, 2005), 57–74.

115. [William O'Brien], "Sanitary Reform," *Edinburgh Review* 91 (January 1850): 222.

116. On the use of organic analogies see, for example, [O'Brien], "Sanitary Reform," 220 and 226; and "Address by the Right Hon. W. Cowper, MP, on Public Health," 120–21.

117. We still know little about Ward save for an unflattering "sketch" which appeared in 1856 in *Engineers and Officials,* 56–58, 84–103, where Ward was presented as Chadwick's lackey and mouthpiece.

118. [F. O. Ward], "Sanitary Consolidation," *Quarterly Review* 88 (March 1851): 437–38.

119. Ibid., 438.

120. Ibid., 438–39.

121. Ibid., 440. Emphasis in original.

122. Ibid., 441.

123. Ibid., 436.

124. Ibid., 437.

125. Ibid., 448. Emphasis in original.

126. *Second Report of the Royal Sanitary Commission,* vol. 1, *The Report,* C. 281 (1871), 16, 35–36. Emphasis in original.

127. *Report of the Joint Committee on State Medicine of the British Medical and Social Science Associations on the Report of the Royal Sanitary Commission* (London: T. Richards, 1871).

128. Henry Wyldbore Rumsey, "Introductory Remarks Delivered in the Section of Public Medicine at the Annual Meeting of the British Medical Association, in Newcastle-upon-Tyne, August 1870," *BMJ,* August 27, 1870, 217.

129. *Second Report of the Royal Sanitary Commission,* vol. 1, *The Report,* 31–32. Emphasis in original.

130. On the fate of state medicine see esp. Brand, *Doctors and the State.*

131. Henry W. Acland, "An Address on Public Health," *BMJ,* September 28, 1872, 347.

132. Bellamy, *Administering Centre-Local Relations,* 115–41.

133. Recent revisionist works include Mark Bevir, *The Making of British Socialism* (Princeton, NJ: Princeton University Press, 2011).

134. J. A. Picton, "Self-Government in Towns," *Contemporary Review* 34 (March 1879): 696.

135. Burrow, "'The Village Community' and the Uses of History in Late Nineteenth-Century England."

136. Michael Bentley, "'Boundaries' in Theoretical Language about the British State," in *The Boundaries of the State in Modern Britain*, ed. S. J. D. Green and R. C. Whiting (Cambridge: Cambridge University Press, 1996), 29–56.

137. G. R. Searle, *Eugenics and Politics in Britain, 1900–1914* (Leyden: Noordhoff, 1976), chap. 6.

138. Frank M. Turner, *Contesting Cultural Authority: Essays in Victorian Intellectual Life* (Cambridge: Cambridge University Press, 1993), 208–28; and G. R. Searle, "Critics of Edwardian Society: The Case of the Radical Right," in *The Edwardian Age: Conflict and Stability, 1900–1914*, ed. Alan O'Day (London: Macmillan, 1979), 79–96. For a broader discussion see G. R. Searle, *The Quest for National Efficiency: A Study in British Politics and Political Thought, 1899–1914* (London: Ashfield, 1990).

139. J. R. Kellet, "Municipal Socialism, Enterprise and Trading in the Victorian City," *Urban History Yearbook* 5 (1978): 36–45.

140. H. M. Hyndman, *A Commune for London* (London: Justice Printery, 1887), 14–15.

141. Malcolm Falkus, "The Development of Municipal Trading in the Nineteenth Century," *Business History Review* 19 (1977): 134–61.

142. A useful overview is Offer, *Property and Politics*, chaps. 15 and 18.

143. W. C. Crofts, *Municipal Socialism* (London: Liberty and Property Defence League, 1892), 13–14.

144. Sidney Webb, *The Reform of London* (London: Eighty Club, 1894), 3, 30.

145. Bellamy, *Administering Centre-Local Relations*, 238–41.

146. Ernest Hart, "The Reform of Local Government," *Sanitary Record*, October 15, 1885, 142.

147. J. P. D. Dunbabin, "The Politics of the Establishment of County Councils," *Historical Journal* 6, no. 2 (1963): 226–52.

148. Alfred Carpenter, "Remarks on the General Working of the Public Health Administration in Great Britain," *BMJ*, October 16, 1880, 615.

149. H. Malet, "Some Philosophical Aspects of Public Health Work," *Public Health* 11, no. 4 (1898–99): 246–47.

150. Rumsey, *Essays on State Medicine*, 46–49; Rumsey, *On Sanitary Legislation and Administration*, 54–56.

151. Bellamy, *Administering Centre-Local Relations*, 112–15.

152. Waller, *Town, City and Nation*, 274–78.

153. Bellamy, *Administering Centre-Local Relations*, chap. 4.

154. Quoted in Waller, *Town, City and Nation*, 274.

155. Edwin Chadwick, *On the Requisite Attributions of a Minister of Health; and on the Principles of Central and Local Administrative Organisation and Action according to British Experiences* (London: n.p., 1878), 33.

156. Benjamin Ward Richardson, "A Ministry of Health," in *A Ministry of Health and Other Essays* (London: Chatto and Windus, 1879), 8.

157. Ibid., 25–27.

158. John Highet, "The Need of a State Department of Public Health," *Public Health* 12, no. 12 (1899–1900): 854–55.

159. Richardson, "A Ministry of Health," 14–25; A. Campbell Munro, "Public Health Administration in England and Scotland," *Public Health* 11, no. 1 (1898–99): 12.

160. Frank G. Bushnell, "The Appointment of a Minister of Health," *BMJ*, August 15, 1903, 354.

161. *Report of the Inter-Departmental Committee on Physical Deterioration*, vol. 1, *Report and Appendix*, Cd. 2175 (1904), 84–85.

162. The genesis and conduct of the commission has been reconstructed in meticulous detail. See A.M. McBriar, *An Edwardian Mixed Doubles: The Bosanquets versus the Webbs; A Study in British Social Policy, 1890–1929* (Oxford: Clarendon, 1987).

163. See esp. Bevir, *Making of British Socialism*, 188–93, where it contests the idea that there was a defining bureaucratic-elitist dimension to Sidney Webb's socialism. On the Webbs and their mixing with public health officials see John M. Eyler, *Sir Arthur Newsholme and State Medicine, 1885–1935* (Cambridge: Cambridge University Press, 1997), 207–19.

164. Mrs [Beatrice] Sidney Webb, "The Relation of Poor-Law Medical Relief to the Public Health Authorities," *Public Health* 19, no. 3 (1906–7): 129–44.

165. Eyler, *Sir Arthur Newsholme and State Medicine*, 211.

166. Arthur Newsholme, "A Discussion on the Coordination of the Public Medical Services," *BMJ*, September 14, 1907, 659–60.

167. A useful summary is Mrs Sidney [Beatrice] Webb, "The Minority Report in Its Relation to Public Health and the Medical Profession," *Public Health* 23, no. 5 (1909–10): 153–64.

168. Searle, *Quest for National Efficiency*, 243.

169. "The Report of the Poor Law Commission," *Public Health* 22, no. 6 (1908–9): 197–98.

170. McBriar, *Edwardian Mixed Doubles*, 295–302; Searle, *Quest for National Efficiency*, 237.

171. Bellamy, *Administering Centre-Local Relations*, 251–52.

172. Sidney Webb, *Grants In Aid: A Criticism and a Proposal* (London: Longmans, Green, 1911), 76–77.

173. Frank Honigsbaum, *The Struggle for the Ministry of Health* (London: G. Bell, 1970).

CHAPTER 3. NUMBERS, NORMS, AND OPINIONS

1. Ian Hacking, *The Taming of Chance* (Cambridge: Cambridge University Press, 1990), viii, 3.

2. House of Commons, "Copy of Second and Third Reports of the Official Statistics Committee; with the Minutes of Evidence and Appendix," *Sessional Papers, 1881* (39), January 27, 1881, iii.

3. Recent accounts include Andrea A. Rusnock, *Vital Accounts: Quantifying Health and Population in Eighteenth-Century England and France* (Cambridge:

Cambridge University Press, 2002); and Joanna Innes, *Inferior Politics: Social Problems and Social Policies in Eighteenth-Century Britain* (Oxford: Oxford University Press, 2009), chap. 4.

4. As Rusnock concludes: "The ability of the state and other bureaucratic institutions to provide continuity, centralization, and authenticity in record keeping increased significantly after 1800. In sharp contrast, the activities of eighteenth-century arithmeticians were voluntary, sporadic and highly contingent on particular controversies." Rusnock, *Vital Accounts,* 212.

5. *Prospectus of the Objects and Plan of the Operation of the Statistical Society of London* (London: n.p., 1834), 2–3.

6. "Sixth Annual Report of the Council of the Statistical Society of London," *JSSL* 3, no. 1 (1840): 2–5.

7. See esp. Nico Randeraad, *States and Statistics in the Nineteenth Century: Europe by Numbers,* trans. Debra Molnar (Manchester: Manchester University Press, 2010).

8. *Address of His Royal Highness the Prince Consort on the Opening of the International Statistical Congress, Held in London on the 16th of July, 1860* (London: William Clowes, 1860), 5.

9. François Ewald, "Norms, Discipline and the Law," *Representations* 30, no. 1 (1990): 150.

10. See esp. Theodore M. Porter, *Trust in Numbers: The Pursuit of Objectivity in Science and Public Life* (Princeton, NJ: Princeton University Press, 1996); and Peter Howlett and Mary S. Morgan, eds., *How Well Do Facts Travel? The Dissemination of Reliable Knowledge* (Cambridge: Cambridge University Press, 2011).

11. James C. Scott, *Seeing Like a State: How Certain Schemes to Improve the Human Condition Have Failed* (New Haven, CT: Yale University Press, 1998).

12. Mary Poovey, *A History of the Modern Fact: Problems of Knowledge in the Sciences of Wealth and Society* (Chicago: University of Chicago Press, 1998), chap. 7.

13. See in particular the definition given in the introduction to *JSSL* 1, no. 1 (1838): 1–5.

14. "Sixth Annual Report of the Council of the Statistical Society of London," 1–2, 6. Emphasis in original.

15. Theodore M. Porter, *The Rise of Statistical Thinking, 1820–1900* (Princeton, NJ: Princeton University Press, 1986), chaps. 8–9. An excellent summary of the differences between (nineteenth-century) "vital statistics" and (twentieth-century) "mathematical statistics" can be found in Eileen Magnello, "The Introduction of Mathematical Statistics into Medical Research: The Roles of Karl Pearson, Major Greenwood, and Austin Bradford Hill," in *The Road to Medical Statistics,* ed. Eileen Magnello and Anne Hardy (Amsterdam: Rodopi, 2002), 95–123.

16. It was not until the third edition of Notter and Firth's *The Theory and Practice of Hygiene,* published in 1908, that the work of Pearson and others was subject to elaboration. *The Theory and Practice of Hygiene, Revised and Largely Re-Written by R. H. Firth,* 3rd ed. (London: J. and A. Churchill, 1908), 810–30.

17. Edward Higgs, *Life, Death and Statistics: Civil Registration, Censuses and the Work of the General Register Office, 1836–1952* (Hatfield: Local Population Studies, 2004), chaps. 1–2.

18. On the location of the GRO, see Edward Higgs, *The Information State in England: The Central Collection of Information on Citizens since 1500* (Basingstoke: Palgrave MacMillan, 2004), 80–81.

19. The best account of Farr's life remains John M. Eyler, *Victorian Social Medicine: The Ideas and Methods of William Farr* (Baltimore: Johns Hopkins University Press, 1979).

20. [William Farr], "Vital Statistics, or the Statistics of Health, Sickness, Diseases and Death," in J.R. McCulloch, *A Statistical Account of the British Empire: Exhibiting Its Extent, Physical Capacities, Population, Industry, and Civil and Religious Institutions*, 2 vols. (London: Charles Knight, 1837), 1: 567–601.

21. Higgs, *Life, Death and Statistics*, 46.

22. Quoted in Martin Campbell-Kelly, "Information and Organizational Change in the British Census, 1801–1911," in *Information Technology and Organizational Transformation: History, Rhetoric and Practice,* ed. JoAnne Yates and John Van Maanen (Thousand Oaks, CA: Sage, 2001), 41.

23. Simon Szreter, "The Genesis of the Registrar-General's Social Classification of Occupations," *British Journal of Sociology* 35, no. 4 (1984): 522–46; Edward Higgs, "Disease, Febrile Poisons, and Statistics: The Census as a Medical Survey," *Social History of Medicine*, 4, no. 3 (1991): 465–78.

24. Iwao M. Moriyama, Ruth M. Loy, and Alastair H.T. Robb-Smith, *History of the Statistical Classification of Diseases and Causes of Death*, ed. Harry M. Rosenberg and Donna Hoyert (Washington, DC: National Center for Health Statistics, 2011), chap. 3.

25. *1st ARRG*, No. 187 (1839), 71.

26. For further reflections on this front see esp. K. Codell Carter, "Causes of Disease and Causes of Death," *Continuity and Change* 12, no. 2 (1997): 189–98.

27. Tom Crook, "Suspect Figures: Statistics and Public Trust in Victorian England," in *Statistics and the Public Sphere: Numbers and the People in Modern Britain, c. 1800–2000,* ed. Tom Crook and Glen O'Hara (New York: Routledge, 2011), 165–84.

28. See in particular J.T.S, "The Public Health Bill and the 'Cant about Centralization': To the Editor of the *Morning Chronicle*," in A Citizen, *Centralization or Local Representation: Health of Towns' Bill: The Opinion of the Public Journals*, 3 vols. (London: Thomas Harreld, 1848), 3: 11–16.

29. Henry Wyldbore Rumsey, *Public Health: The Right Use of Records Founded on Local Facts* (London: John W. Parker, 1860), xiii–xiv.

30. *30th ARRG*, No. 4146 (1869), 208.

31. *35th ARRG*, C.1155–I (1875), iii–iv.

32. Simon Szreter, "The GRO and the Public Health Movement in Britain, 1837–1914," *Social History of Medicine* 4, no. 3 (1991): 435–63. See also Simon Szreter, *Fertility, Class and Gender, 1860–1940* (Cambridge: Cambridge University Press, 1996), 85–93.

33. See esp. Margaret Pelling, *Cholera, Fever and English Medicine, 1825–1865* (Oxford: Oxford University Press, 1978), chap. 3.

34. *1st ARRG*, 67. Emphasis in original.

35. At the behest of the first International Statistical Congress of 1853, Farr and a Genevan statistician, Marc d'Espine, had been asked to draw up a uniform nosology of global scope; but owing to disagreements, the plan came to naught. F.M.M. Lewes, "Dr Marc D'Espine's Statistical Nosology," *Medical History* 32, no. 3 (1988): 301–13.

36. [William Farr], *Report on the Nomenclature and Statistical Classification of Diseases for Statistical Returns* (London: HMSO, 1856), 8.

37. *The Nomenclature of Diseases, Drawn Up by a Joint Committee of the Royal College of Physicians* (London: Harrison, 1869). For a fuller discussion see A.H.T. Robb-Smith, "A History of the College's Nomenclature of Diseases: Its Preparation," *Journal of the Royal College of Physicians of London* 3, no. 4 (1969): 341–58.

38. Henry Wyldbore Rumsey, *Essays and Papers on Some Fallacies of Statistics Concerning Life and Death, Health and Disease, with Suggestions towards an Improved Registration System* (London: Smith, Elder, 1875), 115–61.

39. A useful summary of these developments, including those introduced by Tatham in 1903, can be found in the *64th ARRG*, Cd. 1230 (1903), xxx–xlii. Though not mentioned by Tatham, it seems that Ogle's innovations were influenced by the criticisms of Stark, and his own by Bertillon's scheme.

40. Higgs, *Life, Death and Statistics*, 45–46.

41. Quoted in Edward Higgs, "The Determinants of Technological Innovation and Dissemination: The Case of Machine Computation and Data-Processing in the General Register Office, London, 1837–1920," in *Yearbook of European Administrative History*, ed. E.V. Heyer and B. Wunder (Baden-Baden: Nomos Verlagsgesellschaft, 1997), 164.

42. Edward Higgs, "The General Register Office and the Tabulation of Data, 1837–1939," in *The History of Mathematical Tables: From Sumer to Spreadsheets*, ed. Martin Campbell-Kelly, Mary Croarken, Raymond Flood, and Eleanor Robson (Oxford: Oxford University Press, 2003), 214.

43. House of Commons, "First and Second Reports from the Select Committee on Death Certification," *Sessional Papers*, 1893–94 (373 and 402), August 15 and September 1, 1893.

44. Lionel Rose, *The Massacre of the Innocents: Infanticide in Britain, 1800–1939* (London: Routledge and Kegan Paul, 1986), chap. 14.

45. John F.J. Sykes, "Certification and Classification of the Causes of Death, Part II," *Public Health* 2, no. 1 (1889–90): 34.

46. Rumsey, *Public Health*, xiv–xviii; and Rumsey, *Essays and Papers on Some Fallacies of Statistics*, 41–47.

47. *Registration of the Causes of Death: Circulars to Medical Practitioners, and to Registrars* (London: HMSO, 1845), 6. Before the 1858 Medical Act, qualified practitioners were considered to be those possessing the Licentiate of the Society of Apothecaries, and/or membership of the royal colleges of surgeons and physicians.

48. *62nd ARRG*, Cd. 323 (1900), xxxviii.

49. Sykes, "Certification and Classification of the Causes of Death, Part II," 34–38; House of Commons, "First and Second Reports from the Select Committee on Death Certification," 32–34.

50. Anne Hardy, "'Death is the Cure of All Diseases': Using the General Register Office Cause of Death Statistics for 1837–1920," *Social History of Medicine* 7, no. 3 (1994): 475–77.

51. J.R. Kaye, "Certification and Registration of Death: The Urgent Need for Improvement," *Public Health* 14, no. 1 (1901–2): 17.

52. Ian Burney, *Bodies of Evidence: Medicine and the Politics of the English Inquest, 1830–1926* (Baltimore: Johns Hopkins University Press, 2000), chap. 2.

53. House of Commons, "First and Second Reports from the Select Committee on Death Certification," viii.

54. Kaye, "Certification and Registration of Death," 16.

55. *Manual of the International List of Causes of Death, as Adapted for Use in England and Wales* (London: HMSO, 1912), iv, vi.

56. Moriyama, Loy, and Robb-Smith, *History of the Statistical Classification of Diseases*, 13–14.

57. John V. Pickstone, *Ways of Knowing: A New History of Science, Technology and Medicine* (Manchester: Manchester University Press, 2000), chaps. 4–5.

58. Joseph Fletcher, "Moral and Educational Statistics of England and Wales," *JSSL* 10, no. 3 (1847): 194–95.

59. For further discussion see Libby Schweber, *Disciplining Statistics: Demography and Vital Statistics in France and England, 1830–1885* (Durham, NC: Duke University Press, 2006), 113–14.

60. Arthur Ransome and William Royston, *Remarks on Some of the Numerical Tests of the Health of Towns* (Manchester: Powlson, 1863), 4.

61. "Address by W. Farr on Public Health," *TNAPSS: 1866* (London: Longmans, Green, Reader, and Dyer, 1867), 67.

62. *Weekly Return of Births and Deaths in London,* no. 1 (London: HMSO, 1865), 1–3.

63. *Weekly Return of Births and Deaths in London and in Twenty Other Large Towns of the United Kingdom,* no. 1 (London: HMSO, 1875), 3.

64. *Annual Summary of Births, Deaths and Causes of Death in London, and Other Large Cities, 1872* (London: HMSO, 1873), ix.

65. See esp. Dr. Rumsey, "On Certain Fallacies in Local Rates of Mortality," *Transactions of the Manchester Statistical Society* (November 1871): 17–39; and Rumsey, *Essays and Papers on Some Fallacies of Statistics.*

66. Rumsey, *Public Health,* xxiv–xxv.

67. *Public Health: Ninth Report of the Medical Officer of the Privy Council, with Appendix, 1866,* No. 3949 (1867), 13, 18.

68. Henry Letheby, *On the Estimation of the Sanitary Condition of Communities and the Comparative Salubrity of Towns* (London: Charles Knight, 1874). For a fuller discussion see Graham Mooney, "Professionalization in Public Health and the Measurement of Sanitary Progress in Nineteenth-Century England and Wales," *Social History of Medicine* 10, no. 1 (1997): 53–78.

69. "Dr Letheby on Death-Rates," *BMJ,* October 31, 1874, 561–62; and "Dr Letheby's Errors," *Sanitary Record,* October 31, 1874, 310–11.

70. Noel A. Humphreys, "The Value of Death-Rates as a Test of Sanitary Condition," *JSSL* 37, no. 4 (1874): 437.

71. Ibid., 441–63. Humphreys was especially critical of Letheby; but it is evident from a quote included in his paper to the SSL, attributed to a "well known critic of the 'national system,'" that he also had Rumsey in mind.

72. Noel A. Humphreys, "Sanitary Test-Value of the Death-Rate," *TNAPSS: 1884* (London: John W. Parker, 1885), 485.

73. "The Notification of Infectious Diseases," *Sanitary Record*, July 15, 1884, 17.

74. Arthur Newsholme, *Elements of Vital Statistics* (London: Swann Sonnenschein, 1889), chap. 6.

75. *Quarterly Return of Marriages, Births and Deaths Registered in the Divisions, Counties, and Districts of England*, no. 30 (London: HMSO, 1856), 3.

76. *Quarterly Return of Marriages, Births and Deaths Registered in the Divisions, Counties, Districts and Sub-Districts of England and Wales*, no. 235 (London: HMSO, 1907), v.

77. *Report on the Health of Liverpool during the Year 1861* (Liverpool: M'Corquodale, 1862), 3.

78. *Borough of Torquay: Annual Report of the Medical Officer of Health for 1897* (Torquay: Standard, 1897), 4.

79. "Sanitary Inaction in Bristol," *Sanitary Record*, January 18, 1878, 36.

80. "The Death-Rate of Preston," *Sanitary Record*, May 2, 1879, 278.

81. Arthur Ransome, "On the Vital Statistics of Towns," *Transactions of the Manchester Statistical Society* (March 1888): 90.

82. Nikolas Rose, *Powers of Freedom: Reframing Political Thought* (Cambridge: Cambridge University Press, 1999), chap. 6; Ian Hacking, "How Should We Do the History of Statistics?" in *The Foucault Effect: Studies in Governmentality*, ed. Graham Burchell, Colin Gordon, and Peter Miller (Chicago: University of Chicago Press, 1991), 181–96.

83. Quoted in Trevor Fisher, ed., *Prostitution and the Victorians* (Stroud: Sutton, 1997), 70; Robert Giffen, "On International Statistical Comparisons," *Economic Journal* 2, no. 6 (1892): 209.

84. Edward Higgs, "The State and Statistics in Victorian and Edwardian Britain: Promotion of the Public Sphere or Boundary Maintenance?" in Crook and O'Hara, eds., *Statistics and the Public Sphere*, 71–72; Szreter, *Fertility, Class and Gender*, 246–53.

85. William Hoyle, *The Question of the Day; or, Facts and Figures for Electors and Politicians* (London: Simpkin, Marshall, 1874), 14–15.

86. Robert Giffen, "The Progress of the Working Classes in the Last Half Century: Being the Inaugural Address of R. Giffen, President of the Statistical Section, Session, 1883–84," *JSSL* 46, no. 4 (1883): 621–22.

87. B. Seebohm Rowntree, *Poverty: A Study of Town Life* (London: Macmillan, 1901), 304–5.

88. Robert Blatchford, *Merrie England* (London: Clarion Office, 1895), 9.

89. Ibid., 23–27.

90. Ibid., 23. Emphasis in original.

91. Ibid., 53.

92. Crook, "Suspect Figures," 178–79.

93. Alexander Wynter Blyth, "The Desirability of Uniformity in the Reports of Medical Officers of Health," *Public Health* 3, no. 7 (1890–91): 163.

94. W.G. Willoughby, "Mortality Statistics in Annual Reports," *Public Health* 23, no. 5 (1909–10): 165.

95. *Sanitary Reform: Speech of Viscount Morpeth, in the House of Commons, on Tuesday 30th March, 1847* (London: James Ridgway, 1847), 5.

96. Ernest Hart, "Mortality Statistics of Healthy and Unhealthy Districts of London," *Sanitary Record*, August 15, 1884, 57.

97. W.H. Duncan, *On the Physical Causes of the High Rate of Mortality in Liverpool: Read before the Literary and Philosophical Society in February and March, 1843* (Liverpool: Mitchell, Heaton and Mitchell, 1843), 7.

98. Quoted in Gerry Kearns, "Town Hall and Whitehall: Sanitary Intelligence in Liverpool, 1840–63," in *Body and City: Histories of Urban Public Health*, ed. Sally Sheard and Helen Power (Aldershot: Ashgate, 2000), 101.

99. Details of those involved can be found in the *Liverpool Health of Town's Advocate* 1 (September 1845): 1–2. The journal was short-lived, however, and lasted only two years.

100. "Election for St Anne's Ward," *Liverpool Mercury*, December 15, 1866, 5.

101. William Dawbarn, *Letters Addressed to the Mayor, John Grant Morris, on the Sanitary Condition of Liverpool* (Liverpool: James Woollard, 1867), 2–3.

102. Ibid., 4–6.

103. In the course of his reports Shimmin often made specific reference to the work of the city's health committee. See, for instance, Hugh Shimmin, "Sunday in the 'Slums,'" in *Liverpool Sketches, Chiefly Reprinted from the "Porcupine"* (London: W. Tweedie, 1862), 109–17.

104. Brad Beaven, *Visions of Empire: Patriotism, Popular Culture and the City, 1870–1939* (Manchester: Manchester University Press, 2012), chap. 2.

105. "The Birmingham Improvement Scheme: Local Government Enquiry," *Birmingham Daily Post*, March 16, 1876, 6.

106. "Birmingham Municipal Elections: Duddeston Ward Meeting," *Birmingham Daily Post*, October 20, 1877, 5.

107. "St Martin's Ward Conservative Association," *Birmingham Daily Post*, November 28, 1877, 6.

108. "The Birmingham Improvement Scheme," *Birmingham Daily Post*, May 20, 1882, 3.

109. *Progressive Leaflet No. 13: The Housing of the People* (London: London Reform Union, 1898), 1–2.

110. *London County Council Election, 1910: Facts and Arguments for Municipal Reform Speakers and Candidates* (London: London Municipal Society, 1910), 188–90.

111. "Town Council Meetings: Newcastle," *Newcastle Weekly Courant*, December 7, 1889, 4.

112. *Report of the Sanitary Committee on the Memorial Relative to the Death-Rate of Newcastle* (Newcastle: Lambert, 1890), 2–4.

113. Ibid., 8.

114. William Augustus Guy, *Health of Towns' Association: Unhealthiness of Towns, and Its Causes and Remedies, Being a Lecture Delivered at Crosby Hall, Bishopsgate Street* (London: Charles Knight, 1845), 10.

115. Hacking, *Taming of Chance*, 163.

116. Benjamin Ward Richardson, "Address on Health," *TNAPSS: 1875* (London: Longmans, Green, 1876), 119.

117. *Quarterly Return, no. 2, 1843* (London: General Register Office, 1843), 2; *Quarterly Return of the Death and Mortality in 117 Districts of England, for the Quarter Ending March 31st, 1847* [1847–no. 1] (London: HMSO, 1847), 5–7.

118. *16th ARRG* (London: HMSO, 1856), xv–xvi. The first *16th ARRG* had been published shortly before, in 1855, but consisted only of a handful of abstracts. This version, by contrast, was much more elaborate, extending to more than 150 pages.

119. Szreter, "The GRO and the Public Health Movement in Britain, 1837–1914," 439–40.

120. Ewald, "Norms, Discipline and the Law," esp. 151–52, 156–57.

121. Ibid., 152.

122. *Quarterly Return of the Marriages, Births and Deaths Registered in the Divisions, Counties and Districts of England* [1857–no. 36] (London: HMSO, 1858), 5–6.

123. *20th ARRG*, No. 2559 (1859), 174–76.

124. *Annual Summary of Births, Deaths and Causes of Death in London, and Other Large Cities, 1872,* ix.

125. Quoted in Noel A. Humphreys, ed., *Vital Statistics: Memorial Volume of Selections from the Reports and Writings of William Farr* (London: Edward Stanford, 1885), 125.

126. Henry Wyldbore Rumsey, *Essays on State Medicine* (London: John Churchill, 1856), 334–35. See also William Royston, *Variation of the Death Rate in England: Being the Substance of a Paper Read before the Committee of the Manchester and Salford Sanitary Association, November 15th, 1860* (Manchester: Cave and Sever, 1860).

127. John Simon, "Preventibility of Certain Kinds of Premature Death," in *General Board of Health: Papers Relating to the Sanitary State of the People of England,* No. 2415 (1858), iv–x.

128. "Nottingham Town Council," *Nottinghamshire Guardian,* November 23, 1866, 6. Emphasis in original.

129. *Supplement to the 45th ARRG,* C. 4564 (1885), xvi.

130. *Supplement to the 65th ARRG: Part I,* Cd. 2618 (1907), xx.

131. *Supplement to the 55th ARRG: Part II,* C. 8503 (1897), cii–ciii. Emphasis in original.

CHAPTER 4. OFFICIALISM

1. Edward Higgs, *The Information State in England: The Central Collection of Information on Citizens since 1500* (Basingstoke: Palgrave MacMillan, 2004), chap. 3.

2. Jill Pellew, *The Home Office, 1848–1914: From Clerks to Bureaucrats* (London: Heinemann, 1982), 123; Herbert Jones, "Reform of the Public Health Service," *Public Health* 13, no. 4 (1900–1901): 276.

3. Christine Bellamy, *Administering Centre-Local Relations, 1871–1919: The Local Government Board in Its Fiscal and Cultural Context* (Manchester: Manchester University Press, 1988), chap. 4.

4. *Local Government Board Inquiry Committee,* C. 8731 (1898), 4.

5. In 1838, one writer suggested *bureaucracy* was "a term recently borrowed [from France] by English writers," offering "official despotism" as the closest translation. Saxe Bannister, *British Colonization and Coloured Tribes* (London: William Ball, 1838), 161.

6. Hyde Clarke, *A New and Comprehensive Dictionary of the English Language* (London: John Weale, 1855), 53.

7. *Morning Chronicle,* April 4, 1848, 4.

8. On "anonymity" and the corresponding doctrine of "ministerial responsibility," see David Vincent, *The Culture of Secrecy: Britain, 1832–1998* (Oxford: Oxford University Press, 1998), chap. 2.

9. John Stuart Mill, *On Liberty and Other Essays,* ed. John Gray (Oxford: Oxford University Press, 1991), 289–90. On the various meanings of *bureaucracy* during the nineteenth and twentieth centuries see John Greenaway, "British Conservatism and Bureaucracy," *History of Political Thought* 13, no. 1 (1992): 129–60.

10. Ramsay Muir, *Peers and Bureaucrats* (London: Constable, 1910), 8.

11. Sir John Simon, *English Sanitary Institutions, Reviewed in Their Course of Development, and in Some of Their Political and Social Relations* (London: Cassell, 1890), 363, 377, 387–89.

12. Jeanne L. Brand, *Doctors and the State: The British Medical Profession and Government Action in Public Health, 1870–1912* (Baltimore: Johns Hopkins University Press, 1965), 65–72.

13. A useful set of tables—five in total—in relation to numbers of MOsH and sanitary inspectors during the mid-1860s can be found in Alexander P. Stewart and Edward Jenkins, *The Medical and Legal Aspects of Sanitary Reform* (London: R. Hardwick, 1867).

14. *Sanitary Report, by Dr Partridge, Medical Officer of Health* (Stroud: News Office, 1881), 4.

15. "Tenure of Office of Sanitary Inspectors," *Sanitary Record,* October 15, 1889, 199.

16. Milo Roy Maltbie, "English Local Government of To-Day: A Study of the Relations of Central and Local Government," in *Studies in History, Economic and Public Law* 9, no. 1 (1897–98): 102–3.

17. Stewart and Jenkins, *Medical and Legal Aspects of Sanitary Reform,* table 3.

18. James Niven, *Health Officer Report: 1896* (Manchester: Henry Blacklock, 1897), 148–49.

19. W. H. Greg, "The Status and Duties of a Sanitary Inspector in England," *Journal of the Sanitary Institute* 21 (1900): 505.

20. William Blackstone, *Commentaries on the Laws of England, in Four Books,* vol. 3, 16th ed. (London: S. Sweet, 1836), chap. 13. See also Christopher Hamlin, "Public Sphere to Public Health: The Transformation of 'Nuisance,'" in *Medicine, Health and the Public Sphere in Britain, 1600–2000,* ed. Steve Sturdy (London: Routledge, 2002), 189–94; and Joel Franklin Brenner, "Nuisance Law and the Industrial Revolution," *Journal of Legal Studies* 3, no. 2 (1974): 403–8.

21. For a fuller discussion see James G. Hanley, "Parliament, Physicians, and Nuisances: The Demedicalization of Nuisance Law, 1831–1855," *Bulletin of the History of Medicine* 80, no. 4 (2006): 702–32.

22. William Cunningham Glen, *The Law Relating to Public Health and Local Government,* ed. Alexander Glen, 11th ed. (London: Charles Knight, 1895), 160–61.

23. Useful overviews include Derek J. Oddy, "Food Quality in London and the Rise of the Public Analyst, 1870–1939," in *Food and the City in Europe since 1800,* ed. Peter J. Atkins, Peter Lummel, and Derek J. Oddy (Aldershot: Ashgate, 2007), 91–104.

24. Stewart and Jenkins, *Medical and Legal Aspects of Sanitary Reform,* table 3; and Christopher Hamlin, "Nuisances and Community in Mid-Victorian England: The Attractions of Inspection," *Social History* 38, no. 3 (2013): 346–79.

25. "The Sanitary Inspectors' Examination: A Retrospect," *Journal of the Sanitary Institute* 20 (1899): 323.

26. Matthew Chapman, *The Student's Guide to Success in Sanitary Inspectors' Exams* (London: Sanitary Publishing Company, 1901).

27. "The Sanitary Inspectors' Examination," 325.

28. W. R. E. Coles, "The Sanitary Inspectors' Examination Board," *Sanitary Record,* January 5, 1900, 7; H. H. Spears, "The Present System of Examination and Training of Sanitary Inspectors," *Sanitary Record,* August 24, 1905, 161.

29. J. Spottiswoode Cameron, *On Nuisances and Methods of Inspection* (London: Sanitary Publishing Company, 1901), 4.

30. *Public Health: Eleventh Report of the Medical Officer of the Privy Council, 1868,* C. 4127 (1869), 27.

31. Albert Taylor, *The Sanitary Inspector's Handbook,* 2nd ed. (London: H. K. Lewis, 1897), 68–74; Thomas Whiteside Hime, *The Practical Guide to the Public Health Acts: A Vade Mecum for Officers of Health and Inspectors of Nuisances,* 2nd ed. (London: Baillière, Tindall, and Cox, 1901), 71.

32. J. M. Jones, "The Public Health Acts: Difficulties in Administration and Suggestions for Amendment," *Sanitary Inspectors Journal* 1, no. 1 (1895): 250.

33. We still await a detail statistical investigation of the late Victorian and Edwardian periods. Hamlin's study of the mid-1870s, however, suggests that only 1 percent of cases went to court. Christopher Hamlin, "Sanitary Policing and the Local State, 1873–1874: A Statistical Study of English and Welsh Towns," *Social History of Medicine* 18, no. 1 (2005): 55.

34. "Sanitary Inspectors' Reports," *Sanitary Record,* November 15, 1882, 227.

35. Alfred Carpenter, "Remarks on the General Working of the Public Health Administration in Great Britain," *BMJ,* October 16, 1880, 616.

36. Edward Smith, *Handbook for Inspectors of Nuisances* (London: Charles Knight, 1873), 31–32.

37. Edward Smith, *Manual for Medical Officers of Health* (London: Charles Knight, 1873), 323.

38. "Stockton," *York Herald,* January 8, 1880, 7.

39. "New Offices of the Public Health Department at St Helens," *Sanitary Officer* 2 (1910–11): 352–53.

40. "New Health Offices for Blackpool," *Sanitary Officer* 3 (1911–12): 4–5.

41. "The Sanitary Inspection of the City of London," *BMJ,* May 30, 1908, 1322.

42. F. J. Allan, "A House Record," *Public Health* 11, no. 12 (1898–99): 821–22.

43. Albert Palmberg, *A Treatise on Public Health and Its Applications in Different European Countries,* ed. Arthur Newsholme (London: Swan Sonnenschein, 1893), 23.

44. G. Petgrave Johnson, "The Organisation of the Health Department of a Large Town," *Public Health* 27, no. 5 (1913–14): 147.

45. [H. Thomas], "The Opening Meeting," *Sanitary Inspectors Journal* 1, no. 1 (1895): 8.

46. On the duties of MOsH and inspectors see Edward F. Willoughby, *The Health Officer's Pocket-book: A Guide to Sanitary Practice and Law for Medical Officers of Health, Sanitary Inspectors and Members of Sanitary Authorities,* 2nd ed. (London: Crosby Lockwood, 1902), 111–15.

47. Chapman, *Student's Guide to Success in Sanitary Inspectors' Exams,* 43. Emphasis in original.

48. "Powers of Sanitary Inspection," *BMJ,* April 22, 1893, 863.

49. Glen, *Law Relating to Public Health and Local Government,* 164. An excellent discussion of the emergence of this dual status can be found in Hanley, "Parliament, Physicians, and Nuisances."

50. *Noxious Vapours Commission: Report of the Royal Commission on Noxious Vapours,* C. 2159 (1878), 524.

51. Among other instances see "The Distinction between Nuisance at Common Law and Nuisance under the Sanitary Acts," *Public Health* 1, no. 8 (1888–89): 246–47; "Nuisance at Common Law," *Journal of State Medicine* 1, no. 6 (1893): 157–58; "Nuisance of a Burning Pit and Colliery Mound at Wednesbury," *Public Health* 5, no. 4 (1892–93): 186–87.

52. W. A. Holdsworth, *The Public Health (London) Act, 1891* (London: George Routledge, 1891), 36–37.

53. Alexander Wynter Blyth, *Lectures on Sanitary Law* (London: Macmillan, 1893), 16.

54. *Weekly Reports of the Inspector of Nuisances for the District of the Bicester Union, June 1873–September 1873.* PLU2/SN/A1/1, OHC.

55. *Journal of the Inspector of Nuisances for Chipping Norton Urban District, 1879–1883.* BOR1/20/A2/4, OHC.

56. "The Essex Sanitary Inspectors' Association," *Sanitary Record,* November 1, 1878, 280.

57. On various nuisance prosecutions see Glen, *Law Relating to Public Health and Local Government*, 164–79.

58. J. Dixon, "Certain Trade Nuisances," *Public Health* 12, no. 4 (1899–1900): 276–79.

59. *Henley Urban District Council: Annual Report of W. Dyson Wood, Medical Officer of Health for the Year 1896, June 29, 1897*, 5–6. CC3/3/A5, OHC.

60. Thomas Herbert, *The Law on Adulteration, Being the Sale of Food and Drugs Acts, 1875 and 1879, with Notes, Cases and Extracts from Official Reports* (London: Charles Knight, 1884), 35.

61. Maltbie, "English Local Government," 104.

62. A comprehensive discussion of due procedure can be found in H. Mansfield Robinson and Cecil H. Cribb, *The Law and Chemistry of Food and Drugs* (London: F. B. Rebman, 1895), chaps. 4–5.

63. On public analysis laboratories and methods of investigation see Albert E. Leach, *Food Inspection and Analysis* (London: Chapman and Hall, 1904), chaps. 2, 4, and 5.

64. Francis Vacher, "Address: Conference of Sanitary Inspectors," *Journal of the Sanitary Institute* 15 (1894): 410–11.

65. Cameron, *On Nuisances and Methods of Inspection*, 15.

66. On meat inspection more generally see Keir Waddington, *The Bovine Scourge: Meat, Tuberculosis and Public Health, 1850–1914* (Woodbridge: Boydell, 2006), chap. 5.

67. J. Stopford Taylor, *Report of the Health of Liverpool during the Year 1882* (Liverpool: Henry Greenwood, 1883), 57; "Sanitary Inspectors' Reports: Borough of Leicester," *Sanitary Officer* 1 (1909–10): 16.

68. O. W. Andrews, *Hand-Book of Public Health Laboratory Work and Food Inspection* (Portsmouth: Carpenter, 1898), 12.

69. William Robertson, *Meat and Food Inspection* (London: Baillière, Tindall and Cox, 1908), 100.

70. Hugh A. Macewen, *Food Inspection: A Practical Handbook* (London: Blackie, 1909), 48.

71. Francis Vacher, *The Food Inspector's Handbook*, 4th ed. (London: Sanitary Publishing Company, 1905), 6.

72. Chris Otter, *The Victorian Eye: A Political History of Light and Vision in Britain, 1800–1910* (Chicago: University of Chicago Press, 2008), 109–10.

73. T. E. Coleman, *Sanitary House Drainage, Its Principles and Practice* (London: E. and F. N. Spon, 1896), 65–74.

74. Vacher, *Food Inspector's Handbook*, 8–10.

75. Taylor, *Sanitary Inspector's Handbook*, 115–12; and L. C. Parkes, "The Testing of Drains," *Public Health* 15, no. 5 (1902–3): 272–78.

76. Useful overviews of testing include Coleman, *Sanitary House Drainage*, 161–77; and Gerard J. G. Jensen, *Modern Drainage Inspection and Sanitary Surveys* (London: Sanitary Publishing Company, 1899), 76–88.

77. "A Suggestion to Abolish the Term 'Nuisance,'" *Public Health* 23, no. 5 (1909–10): 185.

78. G. H. Anderson, "Address to Conference of Sanitary Inspectors," *Journal of the Royal Sanitary Institute* 29 (1908): 713–14. Emphasis in original.

79. At first the full title was the Association of Public Sanitary Inspectors; the use of "Public" was abandoned in the 1890s.

80. Hugh Alexander, *Inaugural Address Delivered at the Westminster Town Hall, Nov. 5 1887 to the Association of Public Sanitary Inspectors* (London: Potter, 1887), 6; "Sanitary Inspectors' Association: Annual Dinner," *Sanitary Record*, February 11, 1909, 120.

81. "Appointment of Sanitary Inspectors," *Sanitary Inspectors Journal* 3, no. 1 (1897): 21.

82. P.F. Aschrott, *The English Poor Law System, Past and Present*, trans. Herbert Preston-Thomas (London: Charles Knight, 1888), 174.

83. Daniel Duman, "The Creation and Diffusion of a Professional Ideology in Nineteenth-Century England," *Sociological Review* 27, no. 1 (1979): 113–38; and Harold Perkin, *The Rise of Professional Society: England since 1880* (London: Routledge, 1990), chap. 4.

84. Edward S. May, "Tenure of Office of Sanitary Inspectors," in *Association of Public Sanitary Inspectors, First Session, 1883–84* (Manchester: Emmot's Printing Works, 1883), 5.

85. T.M. Legge, "Notes on some Continental Abattoirs," *Public Health* 6, no. 12 (1893–94): 402.

86. E. Petronell Manby, "Meat Inspection and the Abolition of Private Slaughterhouses," *BMJ*, September 2, 1899, 581–84.

87. Macewen, *Food Inspection*, v.

88. "Visit to the Sewage Works," *Sanitary Inspectors Journal* 5, no. 4 (1899): 100–103; "Visit to the Enfield U.D.C. Isolation Hospital," *Sanitary Inspectors Journal* 5, no. 5 (1899): 117–24.

89. "The Association's Visit to the Sanitary Congress in Paris," *Sanitary Inspectors Journal* 1, no. 2. (1895): 93–98.

90. "A Tour in Belgium," *Sanitary Inspectors Journal (Special Belgium Number)* 3 (1897): 1–5.

91. W.H. Grigg, "The Status and Duties of a Sanitary Inspector in England," *Journal of the Sanitary Institute* 21 (1900): 503.

92. Edwin Chadwick, "Sanitation versus Militarianism," in *Edwin Chadwick: Public Health, Sanitation and Its Reform*, ed. David Gladstone (London: Routledge, 1997), 2.

93. Edwin Chadwick, *The Jubilee of Sanitary Science, Being the Annual Address of Edwin Chadwick, C.B., at the Anniversary Dinner of the Association of Public Sanitary Inspectors, February 5, 1887* (London: James Meldrum, 1887), 7.

94. Alexander, *Inaugural Address*, 8.

95. G.B. Jerram, *Association of Public Sanitary Inspectors: The Fourth Inaugural Address, November 6th 1886* (London: Potter, 1886), 5; "North-Western and Midland (North Wales Centre)," *Sanitary Record*, July 1, 1898, 14.

96. "Sanitary Inspectors' Association: Annual Meeting," *Sanitary Record*, October 31, 1907, 388.

97. *Celebration of the Third Anniversary Dinner of the Association of Public Sanitary Inspectors, June 5th, 1886: Report of Speeches* (London: Potter, 1886), 161.

98. Edwin Chadwick, *Sanitary Review of the Session: Read at the Monthly Meeting of the Association of Public Sanitary Inspectors, May 2, 1885* (London: New Otto Works, 1885), 11; "The Opportunity of the General Election," *Sanitary Officer* 1 (1909–10): 151.

99. *Report to the Association of Public Sanitary Inspectors, from a Deputation to the Right Hon. James Stansfeld, M.P., President of the Local Government Board, April 8th, 1886* (London: Potter, 1886).

100. John Highet, "The Need of a State Department of Public Health," *Public Health* 12, no. 12 (1899–1900): 855.

101. *Celebration of the Third Anniversary Dinner, 167.*

102. Taylor, *Sanitary Inspector's Handbook,* 19.

103. "Sanitary Inspection in London," *BMJ,* June 6, 1903, 1333.

104. *Questions for Candidates: Metropolitan Borough Councils, June 1890* (London: Fabian Society, 1900).

105. "Sanitary Inspectors' Association: Annual Dinner, Address by Sir James Crichton-Browne," *Sanitary Record,* February 6, 1908, 114.

106. E. C. Robins, "The Disabilities of Inspectors of Nuisances and Their Remedy," *Transactions of the Sanitary Institute of Great Britain* 5 (1883–84): 121–22. Emphasis in original.

107. John M. Eyler, *Sir Arthur Newsholme and State Medicine, 1885–1935* (Cambridge: Cambridge University Press, 1997), 69–72.

108. Anthony S. Wohl, *Endangered Lives: Public Health in Victorian Britain* (London: Methuen, 1984), chap. 7.

109. May, "Tenure of Office of Sanitary Inspectors," 5–6.

110. Taylor, *Sanitary Inspector's Handbook,* 14–20.

111. C. MacMahon, "Conference of Sanitary Inspectors: Address," *Journal of the Sanitary Institute* 20 (1899): 447–48.

112. Peter Fyfe, "The Sanitary Inspector's Vocation," *Supplement to the Sanitary Record: Sanitary Inspectors' Association Annual Conference,* August 26, 1893, 11–12.

113. "Sanitary Inspection," *BMJ,* January 21, 1899, 172.

114. George Reid, "Address: Conference of Sanitary Inspectors," *Journal of the Sanitary Institute* 17 (1896): 303.

115. Francis Vacher, *Address to the Royal Institute of Public Health: Congress at Blackpool, Conference of Sanitary Inspectors* (London: Baillière, Tindall and Cox, 1899), 12.

116. Dorothy Porter, "Stratification and Its Discontents: Professionalisation and Conflict in the British Public Health Service, 1848–1914," in *A History of Education in Public Health: Health That Mocks the Doctors' Rules,* ed. Elizabeth Fee and Roy M. Acheson (Oxford: Oxford University Press, 1991), 97–98.

117. W. W. West, "Practical Training for Sanitary Inspectors before Certification," *Journal of the Royal Sanitary Institute* 27 (1906): 710–11.

118. Frank Charles Stockman, *A Practical Guide for Sanitary Inspectors,* 2nd ed. (London: Butterworth, 1894), 19–22.

119. H. Mansfield Robinson, "Legal Hints on Sanitary Inspection," *Journal of State Medicine* 1, no. 3 (1893): 119.

120. It was a distinction that became more pronounced and politicized during the late Victorian period, especially in the context of poor law relief. Jane Lewis, "The Boundary between Voluntary and Statutory Social Service in the Late Nineteenth and Early Twentieth Centuries," *Historical Journal* 39, no. 1 (1996): 155–77.

121. Organized domestic visitation dates back to the late eighteenth century, but it underwent an enormous expansion from the 1830s. Frank Prochaska, *Christianity and Social Service in Modern Britain: The Disinherited Spirit* (Oxford: Oxford University Press, 2006), 63–65.

122. David Davies, "The Training, Qualifications and Duties of Nuisance-Inspectors," *BMJ*, November 11, 1871, 554.

123. The name was soon abbreviated to the Ladies' Sanitary Association. See Perry Williams, "The Laws of Health: Women, Medicine and Sanitary Reform, 1850–1900," in *Science and Sensibility: Gender and Scientific Enquiry, 1780–1945*, ed. Marina Benjamin (Oxford: Basil Blackwell, 1991), 60–88.

124. Ladies' Sanitary Association, *Twenty-Fourth Annual Report of the Ladies Sanitary Association: April, 1882* (London: Ladies Sanitary Association, 1882), 6.

125. A. Kidd, *Manchester,* 2nd ed. (Keele: Keele University Press, 1996), 151.

126. A more detailed account of female sanitary inspection and health visiting can be found in Celia Davies, "The Health Visitor as Mother's Friend: A Woman's Place in Public Health, 1900–1914," *Social History of Medicine* 1, no. 1 (1988): 39–59.

127. "Are Women Inspectors Satisfactory?" *Sanitary Record,* October 27, 1904, 408.

128. "Lady Sanitary Inspectors," *Sanitary Record,* October 20, 1899, 346.

129. On the diplomacy of central inspectors see David Roberts, *Victorian Origins of the British Welfare State* (New Haven, CT: Yale University Press, 1960), 287–93.

130. "The Sanitary Inspection of Birmingham," *Birmingham Daily Post,* May 20, 1875, 3.

131. Taylor, *Sanitary Inspector's Handbook,* 29.

132. Alexander Wynter Blyth, "Address: Conference of Sanitary Inspectors," *Public Health* 5, no. 1 (1892–93): 10.

133. Smith, *Handbook for Inspectors of Nuisances,* 29–30.

134. "Inspector of Nuisances," *Sanitary Record,* November 23, 1877, 338.

135. See, for instance, Christopher Dandeker, *Surveillance, Power and Modernity: Bureaucracy and Discipline from 1700 to the Present Day* (Oxford: Polity, 1990).

136. An excellent discussion of the Charity Organization Society along these lines can be found in Lauren M. E. Goodlad, *Victorian Literature and the Victorian State: Character and Governance in a Liberal Society* (Baltimore: Johns Hopkins University Press, 2003), chap. 6.

137. Taylor, *Sanitary Inspector's Handbook,* 29; "Conference of Inspectors of Nuisances," *Sanitary Record,* September 15, 1890, 122; and T. W. Warren, "Office and Duties of a Sanitary Inspector," *Journal of the Royal Sanitary Institute* 29 (1908): 751.

138. Alexander Wynter Blyth, "The Education, Status and Emoluments of Sanitary Inspectors," *Journal of the Sanitary Institute* 18 (1897): 198.

139. "Sanitary Inspectors' Conference at Nottingham," *Sanitary Record,* May 19, 1894, 716.

140. For a broader discussion see G. K. Behlmer, *Friends of the Family: The English Home and Its Guardians, 1850–1940* (Stanford, CA: Stanford University Press, 1998), chap. 1.

141. H. S. Jones, *Victorian Political Thought* (Basingstoke: Macmillan, 2000), 69–73.

142. W. W. West, "Conference of Sanitary Inspectors: Address," *Journal of the Sanitary Institute* 19 (1898): 429, 431.

143. "Death of Burnley Sanitary Inspector," *Blackburn Standard and Weekly Express,* June 10, 1893, 8.

144. William Cunningham Glen, *The Nuisances Removal and Diseases Prevention Acts, 1848 and 1849, with Practical Notes and Appendix,* 3rd ed. (London: Shaw, 1849), 3; Hime, *Practical Guide to the Public Health Acts,* 70.

145. "Sanitary Notice," *Newcastle Courant,* July 30, 1869, 1.

146. Taylor, *Report of the Health of Liverpool during the Year 1882,* 58; *Health of Manchester: Weekly Return of the Medical Officer of Health, Twenty-Fourth Week, Ending 13th June* (Manchester: Henry Blacklock, 1896), 9.

147. Witney Rural Sanitary Authority, *Annual Report of W. Dyson Wood, Medical Officer of Health, for the Year 1892, Oxford, June 24th, 1893,* 4. The printed reports for the years 1890 to 1904 are collected in the Bodleian Library, Oxford.

148. Stockman, *Practical Guide for Sanitary Inspectors,* 22.

149. Smith, *Handbook for Inspectors of Nuisances,* 31.

150. Taylor, *Sanitary Inspector's Handbook,* 26–27.

151. Robinson and Cribb, *Law and Chemistry of Food and Drugs,* 114–15.

152. "Uniforms," *Sanitary Inspectors Journal* 1, no. 6 (1895): 219.

153. "Sanitary Inspector Assaulted at Colchester," *Sanitary Record,* September 14, 1900, 244.

154. "Assaulting a Sanitary Inspector," *Sanitary Inspectors Journal* 4, no. 4 (1898): 72.

155. Vacher, *Food Inspector's Handbook,* 5.

156. "Weekly Report of the Medical Officer of Health for the City of London: Overcrowding of Common Lodging Houses, 14 January, 1860," 7. CLA/006/AD/07/029/05, LMA.

157. "A Day with the County Council Lodging House Inspectors," *London,* October 20, 1898, 671.

158. "The Rights of Sanitary Inspectors," *Sanitary Record,* June 14, 1906, 520.

159. "Refusal to Admit Sanitary Officers," *Public Health* 4, no. 9 (1891–92): 277.

160. The following cases were all resolved in favor of the public. "Important Question as to Entry by an Inspector of Nuisances," *Sanitary Record,* July 10, 1875, 30; "Complaint against a Nuisance Inspector," *Sanitary Record,* April 5, 1878, 219; "Right of Entry," *Public Health* 11, no. 7 (1898–99): 458–59; "A Sanitary Inspector's Appeal," *Sanitary Record,* March 28, 1901, 284.

161. Vacher, *Food Inspector's Handbook*, 4.

162. "Common Lodging Houses and Seamen's Lodging Houses: Register of Police Court Proceedings, 1895–1914." LCC/PH/REG/1/20, LMA.

163. "Law Reports: Lodgson v. Booth," *Public Health* 12, no. 6 (1899–1900): 473–81.

164. London County Council, *Report by the Medical Officer as to the Need for the Extension of the Power of Control over Premises used by Persons of the Common Lodging House Class* (London: London County Council, 1909). LCC/PH/REG/1/24, LMA.

165. David Rutherford, "Conference of Sanitary Inspectors: Presidential Address," *Journal of the Royal Sanitary Institute* 33 (1912): 72.

166. "Sanitary Experts and the Charge of Obstructing Justice," *BMJ*, February 1, 1890, 269–70.

167. "Quite Right To," *Sanitary Inspectors Journal* 1, no. 2 (1896): 20; "Voluntary Evidence by Public Sanitary Officers against Other Sanitary Officers," *Sanitary Inspectors Journal* 1, no. 2 (1896): 1–3.

168. See Robinson, "Legal Hints on Sanitary Inspection," 119–27; and John Lindsay, "The Preparation and Conduct of Cases for Courts of Law," *Journal of State Medicine* 8, no. 6 (1900): 345–54.

169. Quoted in "The Powers of Sanitary Inspectors," *BMJ*, October 9, 1897, 1018.

CHAPTER 5. MATTER IN ITS RIGHT PLACE

1. Bernard Harris, *The Origins of the British Welfare State: Social Welfare in England and Wales, 1800–1945* (Basingstoke: Palgrave Macmillan, 2004), chap. 8; and Derek Fraser, *The Evolution of the British Welfare State: A History of Social Policy since the Industrial Revolution*, 4th ed. (Basingstoke: Palgrave Macmillan, 2009), chap. 3.

2. For an overview of these developments see Robert Millward, "The Political Economy of Urban Utilities," in *The Cambridge Urban History of Britain*, vol. 3, 1840–1950, ed. Martin Daunton (Cambridge: Cambridge University Press, 2000), 315–49.

3. Henry Hartley Fowler, "Municipal Finance and Municipal Enterprise," *Journal of the Royal Statistical Society* 63, no. 3 (1900): 384–86.

4. Although as Ann La Berge has detailed, Chadwick was highly selective in the way he developed their insights. Ann F. La Berge, "Edwin Chadwick and the French Connection," *Bulletin of the History of Medicine* 62, no. 1 (1988): 23–41.

5. See R. A. Buchanan, *The Engineers: A History of the Engineering Profession in Britain, 1750–1914* (London: Jessica Kingsley, 1989), which views this as crucial in terms of establishing a secure organizational base for the profession.

6. On job titles see H. Percy Boulnois, *The Municipal and Sanitary Engineers' Handbook*, 3rd ed. (London: E. and F. N. Spon, 1898), 1–5.

7. Christopher Hamlin, "James Newlands and the Bounds of Public Health," *Transactions of the Historic Society of Lancashire and Cheshire*, no. 143 (1993): 117–39.

8. Lewis Angell, "The Origin, Constitution, and Objects of the Association of Municipal and Sanitary Engineers and Surveyors," *PAMSES, 1884–85: Vol. 9* (1885): 8–17. The association was incorporated in 1890, changing its title slightly. The initial abbreviation, AMSES, is used here.

9. T. de Courcy Meade, "Address of the President," *PAMSES, 1890–91: Vol. 17* (1891): 168–69; E. Purnell Hooley, "The President's Address," *PAMSES, 1908–9: Vol. 35* (1909): 168.

10. For a fuller discussion of this premise see Tom Crook, "Putting Matter in Its Right Place: Dirt, Time and Regeneration in Mid-Victorian Britain," *Journal of Victorian Culture* 13, no. 2 (2008): 200–222.

11. F.S.B.F. de Chaumont, "Modern Sanitary Science," *Sanitary Record,* August 15, 1881, 44.

12. Recent accounts include Ben Marsden and Crosbie Smith, *Engineering Empires: A Cultural History of Technology in Nineteenth-Century Britain* (Basingstoke: Palgrave Macmillan, 2005); and Chris Otter, *The Victorian Eye: A Political History of Light and Vision in Britain, 1800–1910* (Chicago: University of Chicago Press, 2008).

13. A useful summary of an extensive literature can be found in the introduction to William A. Cohen and Ryan Johnson, eds., *Filth: Dirt, Disgust, and Modern Life* (Minneapolis: University of Minnesota Press, 2005).

14. There is now an enormous amount of literature on this subject, and the concern for moral and physical health was hardly new and had first been subject to detailed exploration in the context of prisons by reformers such as John Howard in the 1770s. See H.J. Dyos, "The Slums of Victorian London," *Victorian Studies* 11, no. 1 (1967): 5–40; and Mary Poovey, *Making a Social Body: British Cultural Formation, 1830–1864* (Chicago: University of Chicago Press, 1995), chaps. 2–3.

15. On the Towns Improvement Company see Anthony Brundage, *England's "Prussian Minister": Edwin Chadwick and the Politics of Government Growth, 1832–1854* (University Park: Pennsylvania State University Press, 1988), chap. 6.

16. On Chadwick's "cosmic" ambitions see Paul Dobraszczyk, *Into the Belly of the Beast: Exploring London's Victorian Sewers* (Reading: Spire, 2009), 42–51.

17. The address was subsequently reissued in 1880, along with embellishments by Chadwick and others, as "Circulation or Stagnation; Being the Translation of a Paper by F.O. Ward on the Arterial and Venous System for the Sanitation of Towns," *Transactions of the Sanitary Institute of Great Britain* 2 (1880): 267–71. Emphasis in original. Ward in fact had first outlined the scheme using a similar idiom in his article published in 1851 on "sanitary consolidation," which is discussed in chapter 2.

18. Quoted in S.E. Finer, *The Life and Times of Sir Edwin Chadwick* (London: Methuen, 1952), 222.

19. R.D. Grainger, "Influence of Noxious Effluvia on the Origin and Propagation of Epidemic Diseases," *Association Medical Journal,* March 4, 1853, 184.

20. This is the definition given in *The Laws of Sewers; or, The Office and Authority of Commissioners of Sewers* (London: E. and R. Nutt and R. Gosling, 1726), 25–26.

21. Joseph Hillier, "The Rise of Constant Water in Nineteenth-Century London," *London Journal* 36, no. 1 (2011): 37–53.

22. On the politics of supplying water see, most recently, John Broich, *London: Water and the Making of the Modern City* (Pittsburgh, PA: University of Pittsburgh Press, 2013). On the technical-engineering aspect see Bill Luckin, *Pollution and Control: A Social History of the Thames in the Nineteenth Century* (Bristol: Adam Hilger, 1986), chap. 2.

23. Christopher Hamlin, *Public Health and Social Justice in the Age of Chadwick: Britain, 1800–1854* (Cambridge: Cambridge University Press, 1998), chap. 10.

24. General Board of Health, *Minutes of Information Collected with Reference to Works for the Removal of Soil Water or Drainage of Dwelling Houses and Public Edifices and for the Sewerage and Cleansing of the Sites of Towns,* No. 1535 (1852). The board had earlier circulated similar papers on water supply, and the mapping and surveying of districts.

25. Ibid., 32–36.

26. Robert Rawlinson, "On the Drainage of Towns," *Minutes of Proceedings of the Institution of Civil Engineers,* vol. 12, *Session, 1852–53,* ed. Charles Manby (London: Institution of Civil Engineers, 1853), 36.

27. Ibid., 66–68.

28. Ibid., 105.

29. Baldwin Latham, *Sanitary Engineering: A Guide to the Construction of Works of Sewerage and House Drainage* (London: E. and F. N. Spon, 1873), 48.

30. Robert Rawlinson, "On the Sewering of Towns and Draining of Houses," *Journal of the Society of Arts* 10 (March 1862): 281.

31. Frederick Ashmead, "Report on the Drainage of the City and County of Bristol," *PAMSES, 1877–78: Vol. 4* (1879): 11–12.

32. Edwin Chadwick, "The General History and Principles of Sanitation," *Public Health* 2, no. 7 (1889–90): 200–203.

33. Quoted in Stephen Halliday, *The Great Stink of London: Sir Joseph Bazalgette and the Cleansing of the Victorian Metropolis* (Stroud: Sutton, 1999), 92.

34. Joseph William Bazalgette, "On the Main Drainage of London and the Interception of Sewage from the River Thames," *Minutes of Proceedings of the Institution of Civil Engineers,* vol. 24, *Session, 1864–65,* ed. James Forrest (London: Institution of Civil Engineers, 1865), 291–92.

35. Ibid., 292–93.

36. Ibid., 314.

37. Robert Rawlinson, *Suggestions as to the Preparation of District Maps, and of the Plans for Main Sewerage, Drainage and Water Supply* (London: Charles Knight, 1878), 7–8.

38. E. L. Stephens, "A Concise Description of the Sewerage and Sewage Works of the Borough of Leicester," *PAMSES, 1873–74: Vol. 1* (1875): 208.

39. F. Oscar Kirby, "Notes on Doncaster and Some of Its Municipal Works," *PAMSES, 1908–9: Vol. 35* (1909): 204. Indeed, by the end of the century the "partially separate system" was a recognized variant. See E. C. S. Moore, *Sanitary Engineering: A Practical Treatise on the Collection, Removal and Final Disposal of Sewage,* 2nd ed. (London: B. T. Batsford, 1901), 3.

40. James Lemon, "The Separate System of Drainage," *Sanitary Record,* October 15, 1882, 159.

41. Lewis Angell, "The Separate System of Town Drainage," *PAMSES, 1879–80: Vol. 6* (1880): 32–34; Albert W. Parry, "The Separate System of Sewerage as Carried Out at Reading," *PAMSES, 1882–83: Vol. 9* (1883): 102–11; and Moore, *Sanitary Engineering,* 15.

42. W. H. Corfield and Louis C. Parkes, "The Disposal of Refuse," in *A Treatise on Hygiene and Public Health,* vol. 1, ed. Thomas Stevenson and Shirley F. Murphy (London: J. and A. Churchill, 1892), 836; and Lemon, "The Separate System of Drainage."

43. Herbert L. Sussman, *Victorian Technology: Invention, Innovation, and the Rise of the Machine* (Santa Barbara, CA: Greenwood, 2009), chap. 2.

44. J. Corbett, "A New Sewer Scouring Machine," *Journal of the Sanitary Institute* 23 (1902): 768.

45. Latham, *Sanitary Engineering,* 52–71.

46. David J. Eveleigh, *Bogs, Baths and Basins: The Story of Domestic Sanitation* (Stroud: Sutton, 2006), 38–39.

47. Latham, *Sanitary Engineering,* 179–95.

48. Bazalgette, "On the Main Drainage of London," 315–18, 325–26.

49. See in particular the evidence presented in *First Report of the Commissioners for Inquiring into the State of Large Towns and Populous Districts,* No. 572 (1844), 124–37.

50. Thomas Walker, "Some of the Public Works of Croydon," *PAMSES, 1890–91: Vol. 17* (1891): 10.

51. Ashmead, "Report on the Drainage of the City and County of Bristol," 25.

52. E. G. Mawbey, "The Main Sewerage, Storm Outfall and Sewage Disposal Works of Leicester," *PAMSES, 1893–94: Vol. 20* (1894): 17.

53. Thomas Wicksteed, *An Experimental Inquiry Concerning the Relative Power of, and Useful Effect Produced by, the Cornish and Boulton and Watt Pumping Engines* (London: John Weale, 1841), 1–3.

54. H. P. Boulnois, "The Drainage of Portsmouth," *PAMSES, 1886–87: Vol. 13* (1887): 127.

55. Mawbey, "The Main Sewerage, Storm Outfall and Sewage Disposal Works of Leicester," 25–31.

56. A. S. Jones, "Ten Years' Experience of the Shone System," *PAMSES, 1887–88: Vol. 14* (1888): 312–21; Corfield and Parkes, "The Disposal of Refuse," 847–49; and Moore, *Sanitary Engineering,* 37–42.

57. Charles Tomes, "Shone's Ejector System as Carried Out at Eastbourne," *PAMSES, 1881–82: Vol. 8* (1882): 6–7; and Moore, *Sanitary Engineering,* 41–42.

58. For a fuller discussion on this theme see Christopher Hamlin, "Muddling in Bumbledon: On the Enormity of Large Sanitary Improvements in Four British Towns, 1855–1885," *Victorian Studies* 32, no. 1 (1988): 55–83.

59. House of Commons, "Thames Valley Sewerage: Return of Report of Lieutenant Colonel Cox, R.E., one of the Inspectors of the Local Government Board, to the President of the Board," *Sessional Papers, 1876* (184), April 10, 1876, 1–8.

60. *6th ARLGB,* C.1865 (1877), lxvi, 375–80.

61. Latham, *Sanitary Engineering,* 198.

62. Metropolitan Sanitary Commission, *First Report of the Commissioners Appointed to Inquire Whether Any and What Special Means May Be Requisite for the Improvement of the Health of the Metropolis,* No. 888 (1847), 31.

63. Michelle Allen, *Cleansing the City: Sanitary Geographies in Victorian London* (Athens: Ohio State University Press, 2008), 42–44.

64. S. Sneade Brown, *A Lay Lecture on Sanitary Matters, with a Paper on Sewer Ventilation* (London: Kerby and Endean, 1873), 31.

65. See esp. *Reports by Neil Arnott, Esq., M.D. and Thomas Page, Esq., C.E. on an Inquiry Ordered by the Secretary of State, Relative to the Prevalence of Disease at Croydon, and to the Plan of Sewerage, Together with an Abstract of Evidence Accompanying the Reports,* No. 1648 (1853), 8–10, 33–35.

66. Henry Letheby, *Report to the Honourable Commissioners of Sewers of the City of London, on Sewage and Sewer Gases, and on the Ventilation of Sewers* (London: M. Lownds, 1858).

67. *Times,* December 7, 1871, 9.

68. *Times,* September 22, 1876, 9.

69. Summaries of the debate can be found in H. Alfred Roechling, *Sewer Gas and Its Influence upon Health* (London: Biggs, 1898); and Louis C. Parkes, "Review of Books: 'Is Sewer Air a Source of Disease?'" *Journal of the Sanitary Institute* 16 (1896): 142–52.

70. S. Martin Gaskell, *Building Control: National Legislation and the Introduction of Local Bye-Laws in Victorian England* (London: Bedford Square, 1983), 3–20.

71. [Local Government Board], *Model Bye-Laws for Sanitary Authorities* (London: Eyre and Spottiswoode, 1886), pt. 4, §§ 63–66.

72. Gordon E. Cherry, *Cities and Plans: The Shaping of Urban Britain in the Nineteenth and Twentieth Centuries* (London: Edward Arnold, 1988), 41.

73. Parry, "The Separate System of Sewerage as Carried Out at Reading," 105–6.

74. William Eassie, *Healthy Houses: A Handbook to the History, Defects and Remedies of Drainage, Ventilation, Warming and Kindred Subjects* (London: Simpkin, Marshall, 1872), 31–50.

75. P. Hinckes Bird, *Hints on Drains, Traps, Closets, Sewer Gas, and Sewage Disposal* (Blackpool: Gazette Printing Works, 1877), 33–39.

76. Quoted in Boulnois, *Municipal and Sanitary Engineers' Handbook,* 340.

77. See A. B. Miller, "Cleansing and Ventilating Sewers," *Surveyor,* October 13, 1892, 211–14; and Boulnois, *Municipal and Sanitary Engineers' Handbook,* 340–47.

78. G. F. Deacon, "Notes as to Certain Municipal Works in Liverpool," *PAMSES, 1878–79: Vol. 5* (1879): 29.

79. J. Gordon, "Address of the President," *PAMSES, 1886–87: Vol. 13* (1887): 185.

80. E. B. Ellice-Clark, *Further Remarks on the Ventilation of Sewers* (London: n.p., 1878), 4.

81. Alfred Bostock Hill, "Sewers, in Relation to Medical Officers of Health and Surveyors," *Public Health* 9, no. 9 (1896–97): 164.

82. E. B. Ellice-Clark, "Ventilation of Sewers," *PAMSES, 1873–74: Vol. 1* (1875): 55.

83. H. Gilbert Whyatt, "The Ventilation of Sewers," *Public Health Engineer,* May 14, 1904, 487–88.

84. E. George Mawbey, "Presidential Address on Municipal Engineering and Sewer Ventilation," *Journal of State Medicine* 9, no. 9 (1901): 587.

85. F. B. Smith, *The People's Health, 1830–1910* (London: Croom Helm, 1979), 219.

86. Thomas Cargill, *Sewage and Its General Application to Grass, Cereal and Root Crops, Showing the Results Obtained by Actual Experience* (London: Robertson, Brooman, 1869), 7.

87. Frederick Hahn Danchell, *Concerning Sewage and Its Economical Disposal* (London: Simpkin, Marshall, 1872), 3.

88. On the complexities of setting standards of water purity see Christopher Hamlin, *A Science of Impurity: Water Analysis in Nineteenth Century Britain* (Berkeley: University of California Press, 1990), chaps. 6–8.

89. Quoted in Anthony S. Wohl, *Endangered Lives: Public Health in Victorian Britain* (London: Methuen, 1984), 235.

90. "The 'Cloaca Maxima' of the 'Metropolis Magna,'" *Builder,* December 4, 1875, 1073.

91. *First Report of the Commissioners for Inquiring into the State of Large Towns and Populous Districts,* xiii, 323, and [in appendix] 209–10.

92. For a fuller discussion see Christopher Hamlin, "Providence and Putrefaction: Victorian Sanitarians and the Natural Theology of Health and Disease," *Victorian Studies* 28, no. 3 (1985): 381–411; and Daniel Schneider, *Hybrid Nature: Sewage Treatment and the Contradictions of the Industrial Ecosystem* (Cambridge, MA: MIT Press, 2011), chap. 1.

93. E. D. Girdlestone, *Our Debt and Duty to the Soil; or, The Poetry and Philosophy of Sewage Utilization* (Weston-super-Mare: Robbins, 1878), 41.

94. A. B. Granville, *The Great London Question of the Day; or, Can the Thames Sewage Be Converted into Gold?* (London: Edward Stanford, 1865), 15.

95. *Sewage Disposal: Report of a Committee Appointed by the President of the Local Government Board to Inquire into the Several Modes of Treating Town Sewage,* C. 1410 (1876), 105–15; and Schneider, *Hybrid Nature,* 131.

96. For a fuller discussion of these methods and their many variants, see esp. [Dr. Letheby], *The Sewage Question: Comprising a Series of Reports: Being Investigations into the Condition of the Principal Sewage Farms and Sewage Works of the Kingdom* (London: Bailliere, Tindall and Cox, 1872); and Corfield and Parkes, "The Disposal of Refuse," 850–88.

97. Rawlinson, *Suggestions as to the Preparation of District Maps, and of the Plans for Main Sewerage, Drainage and Water Supply,* 17–18.

98. *Sewage Disposal,* 61–71; [Society of Arts], *Health and Sewage of Towns: Conference, Thursday and Friday, 23rd and 24th May, 1878* (London: W. Trounce, 1878), 61–62.

99. [Letheby], *Sewage Question,* 4, 202–3.

100. Corfield and Parkes, "The Disposal of Refuse," 870.

101. Rawlinson, *Suggestions as to the Preparation of District Maps, and of the Plans for Main Sewerage, Drainage and Water Supply*, 17–19.

102. W. S. Till, "Address of the President," *PAMSES, 1880–81: Vol. 7* (1881): 84–85.

103. The most recent survey is Leslie Rosenthal, *The River Pollution Dilemma in Victorian England: Nuisance Law versus Economic Efficiency* (Farnham: Ashgate, 2014).

104. J. H. Cox, "Municipal Work in Bradford," *PAMSES, 1885–86: Vol. 12* (1886): 90–91.

105. J. B. Reignier Conder, *A Handbook of Sewer and Drain Cases* (London: St. Bride's, 1904).

106. For a fuller discussion see Schneider, *Hybrid Nature*, chap. 4.

107. E. Monson, "The Sewage Difficulty," *PAMSES, 1873–74: Vol. 1* (1875): 64–65.

108. Crawford Barlow, "The London Sewage Question," *PAMSES, 1889–90: Vol. 16* (1890): 154–62.

109. Christopher Hamlin, "William Dibdin and the Idea of Biological Sewage Treatment," *Technology and Culture* 29, no. 2 (1988): 189–218; and Schneider, *Hybrid Nature*, chap. 1.

110. Royal Commission on Sewage Disposal, *Fifth Report of the Commissioners Appointed to Inquire and Report what Methods of Treating and Disposing of Sewage (including any Liquid from any Factory or Manufacturing Process) may Properly be Adopted*, Cd. 4278 (1908), 9.

111. Useful overviews include Samuel Rideal, *Sewage and the Bacterial Purification of Sewage*, 3rd ed. (London: Sanitary Publishing Company, 1906), chaps. 9–11.

112. Moore, *Sanitary Engineering*, 596–97.

113. Ibid., 596.

114. William Ackroyd, *The Scientific Aspects of the Sewage Question* (London: Wrightman, 1897), 1.

115. Hamlin, "Providence and Putrefaction."

116. M. J. Daunton, *House and Home in the Victorian City: Working-Class Housing, 1850–1914* (London: Edward Arnold, 1983), chaps. 2–3.

117. *Report of a Committee of the Manchester Statistical Society, on the Condition of the Working Classes, in an Extensive Manufacturing District, in 1834, 1835, and 1836* (London: James Ridgway, 1838), 14–15.

118. "Report on the Condition of the Town of Leeds and of its Inhabitants," *JSSL* 2, no. 6 (1840): 401–2.

119. The best overview is Richard Rodger, *Housing in Urban Britain, 1780–1914* (Cambridge: Cambridge University Press, 1995), chaps. 3–7.

120. House of Commons, "Report from Select Committee on Buildings Regulation and Improvement of Boroughs," *Sessional Papers, 1842* (372), June 27, 1842, 51.

121. Manchester Corporation, *Health Committee Minutes*, vol. 1 (April 6, 1868–April 22, 1872), 91. M595/1/1/1, MALSC.

122. Daunton, *House and Home in the Victorian City*, chaps. 2–3.

123. [Local Government Board], *Model Bye-Laws*, pt. 4, §§ 67–69.

124. T.R. Marr, *Housing Conditions in Manchester and Salford* (London: Sherratt and Hughes, 1904), 45–46.

125. Latham, *Sanitary Engineering*, 328.

126. Figures cited in William Morley Egglestone, *House Drainage and Sanitary Catalogue* (Stanhope: Egglestone, 1889), 18.

127. Thomas Hewson, "Town Sewers," *PAMSES, 1879–80: Vol. 6* (1880): 157.

128. J.J. Rowley, *The Difficult and Vexed Question of the Age. Sewage of Towns: How to Dispose of It, by Making None* (Sheffield: Leader, 1884), 4.

129. *Sewage Disposal: Report of a Committee Appointed by the President of the Local Government Board to Inquire into the Several Modes of Treating Town Sewage*, xxv.

130. Frederick Charles Krepp, *The Sewage Question: Being a General Review of all the Systems and Methods Hitherto Employed in Various Countries for Draining Cities and Utilizing Sewage* (London: Longmans, Green, 1867); and "Health Committee," *Liverpool Mercury*, October 9, 1874, 8.

131. "Pneumatic Drainage," *York Herald*, June 26, 1874, 2.

132. For a summary see Eveleigh, *Bogs, Baths and Basins*, 45–51.

133. [Letheby], *Sewage Question*, 112–15.

134. See, for example, George Vivian Poore, *Essays on Rural Hygiene* (London: Longmans, Green, 1893).

135. Krepp, *Sewage Question*, chap. 10; and Henry Moule, *Town Refuse: The Remedy for Local Taxation* (London: William Ridgway, 1872).

136. *Twelfth Report of the Medical Officer of the Privy Council: 1869*, C. 208 (1870), 111–15, 127–28; and Daunton, *House and Home in the Victorian City*, 249–51.

137. General Board of Health, *Report on the Supply of Water to the Metropolis (Appendix No. 4: The Cesspool System in Paris)*, No. 1284 (1850).

138. *Reports of the Medical Officer of the Privy Council and Local Government Board (New Series, No. II): Supplementary Report to the Local Government Board on Some Recent Inquiries under the Public Health Act, 1858*, C. 1066 (1874), 171–78, 185–88.

139. "Birmingham Sewage Works: Discussion," *PAMSES, 1880–81: Vol. 7* (1881): 89.

140. [W.A. Power], *Filth Removal: Progress at Liverpool and Birmingham* (Dublin: Alexander Thom, 1877), 9.

141. [W.A. Power], *Filth Removal: Progress at Manchester* (Dublin: Alexander Thom, 1877), 1; and Charles J. Lomax, *Collection, Treatment and Disposal of Town Refuse* (Bolton: R. Whewell, 1892), 21.

142. George J.C. Broom, "Water-Closets *v.* Privies and Pails," *Journal of State Medicine* 3, no. 6 (1895): 429.

143. "Report by Dr Buchanan and Mr J. Netten Radcliffe on the Systems in Use in Various Northern Towns," in *Twelfth Report of the Medical Officer of the Privy Council: 1869*, 111–40.

144. Thomas Hewson, "On the Manufacture of Manure from Town Refuse," *PAMSES, 1878–79: Vol. 5* (1879): 110, 114.

145. See also the discussion in Harold L. Platt, *Shock Cities: The Environmental Transformation and Reform of Manchester and Chicago* (Chicago: University of Chicago Press, 2005), chap. 5.

146. *First Report of the Royal Sanitary Commission, with the Minutes of Evidence up to 5th August 1869*, No. 4218 (1870), 136.

147. [Dr Syson], *The Great Sanitary Question of the Day: How to Dispose of our Refuse* (Manchester: James F. Wilkinson, 1869), 5.

148. J. Conyers Morrell, *The High Death Rate: An Answer to the Question, What Is to Be Done?* (Manchester: Powlson, 1869), 6–8.

149. Hewson, "On the Manufacture of Manure from Town Refuse," 111.

150. Eveleigh, *Bogs, Baths and Basins*, chap. 2.

151. By 1900, a sixth edition was in press. S. Stevens Hellyer, *The Plumber and Sanitary Houses: A Practical Treatise on the Principles of Internal Plumbing Work, or the Best Means for Effectually Excluding Noxious Gases from Our Houses*, 4th ed. (London: B.T. Batsford, 1887), 192.

152. Eveleigh, *Bogs, Baths and Basins*, appendix 1.

153. "Drainage and Plumbing Work: Past, Present and Future," *Sanitary Record*, April 3, 1896, 773.

154. George Wilson, *Handbook of Sanitary Science*, 3rd ed. (London: J. and A. Churchill, 1877), 288–89.

155. General Board of Health, *Minutes of Information*, 163–65.

156. *Twelfth Report of the Medical Officer of the Privy Council: 1869*, 139.

157. *20th ARLGB: Supplement Containing the Report of the Medical Officer for 1890*, C. 6461 (1891), 159–88.

158. See esp. Philip Boobbyer, "Ten Years' Experience of Enteric Fever in a Midland Town, and Its Lessons," *Transactions of the Epidemiological Society of London*, vol. 18, *Session 1898–99* (1899), 88–110; and Roechling, *Sewer Gas and Its Influence upon Health*, 20–25.

159. William H. Maxwell, *The Removal and Disposal of Town Refuse* (London: Sanitary Publishing Company, 1898), 51.

160. Ibid., 63. Emphasis in original.

161. "Property Owners and Manchester Sanitation," *Manchester Guardian*, December 1, 1892, 7; "Compensation for Sanitary Improvements," *Manchester Guardian*, March 16, 1906, 5; and "Manchester Rates: Deputations to the Lord Mayor," *Manchester Guardian*, May 20, 1908, 10.

162. T.H. Yabbicom, "A Description of the Corporation Depot at Albert Road, St. Philip's, Bristol," *PAMSES, 1896–97: Vol. 23* (1897): 8–9.

163. Arthur A. Salmon, "The Disposal of House Refuse," *Sanitary Record*, April 15, 1889, 471; D. Richards, "The Removal and Disposal of House-Refuse in London," *Sanitary Record*, March 15, 1890, 423.

164. Thomas Codrington, *Report on the Destruction of Town Refuse* (London: HMSO, 1888), 4–6.

165. H. Percy Boulnois, *Dirty Dustbins and Sloppy Streets: A Practical Treatise on the Scavenging and Cleansing of Cities and Towns* (London: E. and F.N. Spon, 1881), chap. 4.

166. [Local Government Board], *Model Bye-Laws*, pt. 4, § 83.

167. Charles Mason, "Scavenging and Disposal of Refuse," *Sanitary Record,* April 21, 1894, 640.

168. W. H. Hamblett, "The Disposal of Towns' Refuse," *Journal of the Sanitary Institute* 23 (1902): 777.

169. Codrington, *Report on the Destruction of Town Refuse,* 5.

170. Lomax, *Collection, Treatment and Disposal of Town Refuse,* 71–74.

171. Henry Whiley, "Work and Cost of the Manchester Corporation Health Department," *Transactions of the Manchester Statistical Society* (January 1886): 51.

172. W. Francis Goodrich, "Twenty-five Years' Progress in Final and Sanitary Refuse Disposal," *Sanitary Record,* September 24, 1903, 315.

173. W. Francis Goodrich, *The Economic Disposal of Towns' Refuse* (London: P. S. King, 1901), 19.

174. Maxwell, *Removal and Disposal of Town Refuse,* chap. 5

175. "Dust Destructors," *BMJ,* July 8, 1893, 85.

176. J. Spottiswoode Cameron, "Destruction of Town Refuse by Heat," *Public Health* 8, no. 2 (1895–96): 49.

177. Charles Jones, "Disposal of House and Town Refuse," *Transactions of the Sanitary Institute* 13 (1892): 49.

178. "Saltley and Refuse Destructors," *Birmingham Daily Post,* March 29, 1894, 4.

179. "Refuse Destructors at Birkenhead," *Liverpool Mercury,* January 8, 1892, 7; and "Birkenhead Town Council," *Liverpool Mercury,* April 2, 1896, 7.

180. Codrington, *Report on the Destruction of Town Refuse,* 29–31.

181. "Electric Light from House Refuse: A London Vestry's Enterprise," *Sanitary Record,* July 2, 1897, 412.

182. Timothy Cooper, "Burying the 'Refuse Revolution': The Rise of Controlled Tipping in Britain, 1920–1960," *Environment and Planning (A)* 42 (2010): 1033–48.

183. Goodrich, *Economic Disposal of Towns' Refuse,* chaps. 17–24.

184. Maxwell, *Removal and Disposal of Town Refuse,* 114.

185. Hamblett, "The Disposal of Towns' Refuse," 780.

CHAPTER 6. STAMPING OUT

1. See esp. Dorothy Porter, *Health, Civilization and the State: A History of Public Health from Ancient to Modern Times* (London: Routledge, 1999), chap. 8; and Peter Baldwin, *Contagion and the State in Europe, 1830–1930* (Cambridge: Cambridge University Press, 1999). Recent accounts include Nadja Durbach, *Bodily Matters: The Anti-Vaccination Movement in England, 1853–1907* (Durham, NC: Duke University Press, 2005); Deborah Brunton, *The Politics of Vaccination: Practice and Policy in England, Wales, Ireland, and Scotland, 1800–1874* (Rochester, NY: University of Rochester Press, 2008); and Catherine Lee, *Policing Prostitution, 1856–1886: Deviance, Surveillance and Morality* (London: Pickering and Chatto, 2012).

2. We continue to conflate the two today, and the distinction is not an absolute one. See Bob Heyman, "The Concept of Risk," in *Risk, Safety and Clinical*

Practice: Health Care through the Lens of Risk, ed. Bob Heyman, Andy Alaszewski, Monica Shaw and Mike Titterton (Oxford: Oxford University Press, 2010), 25–31.

3. On complexities of organization and process see esp. Graham Mooney, "'A Tissue of the Most Flagrant Anomalies': Smallpox and the Centralisation of Sanitary Administration in Late Nineteenth-Century London," *Medical History* 41, no. 3 (1997): 261–90; and Miles Ogborn, "Law and Discipline in Nineteenth-Century English State Formation: The Contagious Diseases Acts, 1864, 1866 and 1869," *Historical Sociology* 6, no. 1 (1993): 28–54.

4. [John Simon], *General Board of Health: Papers Relating to the History and Practice of Vaccination,* No. 2239 (1857), 180.

5. William Budd, "Can the Government, Further, Beneficially Interfere in the Prevention of Infectious Diseases?" *TNAPSS: 1869* (London: Longmans, Green, Reader and Dyer, 1870), 392.

6. Ibid., 400–401.

7. *Report of the Board of Education, 1899–1900,* vol. 3, *Appendix to Report,* Cd. 330 (1900), 67.

8. On the use of these terms, which was often confused, see Christopher Hamlin, *Cholera: The Biography* (Oxford: Oxford University Press, 2009), chap. 1.

9. Boyd Hilton, *The Age of Atonement: The Influence of Evangelicalism on Social and Economic Thought, 1795–1865* (Oxford: Clarendon, 1988). See also Pamela K. Gilbert, *Cholera and Nation: Doctoring the Social Body in Victorian England* (Albany: State University of New York Press, 2008), chaps. 1–3.

10. "The Cholera Morbus and the Sanitary Movement," *Times,* September 12, 1849, 3; "The Cholera Morbus and the Sanitary Movement," pt. 2, *Times,* September 13, 1849, 7.

11. John Liddle, *Board of Works, Whitechapel District: Report on the Epidemic of Cholera in 1866* (London: T. Penny, 1867), 27–30.

12. The coining of the term *international* is attributed to Jeremy Bentham in 1789 in the context of legal reform. Georgios Varouxakis, *Liberty Abroad: J. S. Mill on International Relations* (Cambridge: Cambridge University Press, 2013), 19–20.

13. House of Commons, "Correspondence Respecting the Quarantine Laws, Since the Correspondence Last Presented to Parliament," *Sessional Papers, 1846* (718), May 19, 1846, 1–6, 10–13.

14. David P. Fidler, *International Law and Infectious Diseases* (Oxford: Clarendon, 1999), chap. 2.

15. Fraser Brockington, "Public Health at the Privy Council, 1805–6," *Medical History* 7, no. 1 (1963): 13–31. Contrary to Brockington's suggestion, however, the term "Central Board of Health" was never used in 1805. The five handwritten reports of the board, for instance, were signed off by the "Board of Health." PC 1/3637, and PC1/3666, TNA. The quote is from C. C. Greville to Local Boards, November 11, 1831, PC1/102, TNA.

16. D. Barry, "On the Statistics of Epidemic Cholera," *Transactions of the Statistical Society of London, Volume I–Part I* (London: Charles Knight, 1837), 83–91.

17. Tom Koch, "1831: The Map That Launched the Idea of Global Health," *International Journal of Epidemiology* 43, no. 4 (2014): 1014–20.

18. John Booker, *Maritime Quarantine: The British Experience, c. 1650–1900* (Aldershot: Ashgate, 2007), 461–74.

19. Figure derived from House of Commons, "Quarantine: Return, in Detail, of All Vessels Which Have Been Detained in Quarantine during the Five Years Ending the 1st day of July 1853, in Great Britain," *Sessional Papers, 1852–53* (993), July 7, 1853; and House of Commons, "Quarantine: Return of the Number, Name, Tonnage, Port from Whence Last Arrived of Each Vessel, Distinguishing Whether English or Foreign," *Sessional Papers, 1867* (423), June 3, 1867.

20. Mark Harrison, *Contagion: How Commerce Has Spread Disease* (Padstow: Yale University Press, 2012), chap. 4; and Krista Maglen, *The English System: Quarantine, Immigration, and the Making of a Port Sanitary Zone* (Manchester: Manchester University Press, 2014), chap. 1.

21. General Board of Health, *Report on Quarantine*, No. 1070 (1849), 123–28, 157–59.

22. *Report by the General Board of Health, on the Measures Adopted for the Execution of the Nuisances Removal and Diseases Prevention Act, and the Public Health Act, up to July 1849*, No. 1115 (1849), 5–7, 116–22.

23. Michael Durey, *The Return of the Plague: British Society and the Cholera, 1831–2* (Dublin: Gill and Macmillan, 1979), 90–91.

24. David McLean, *Public Health and Politics in the Age of Reform: Cholera, the State and the Royal Navy in Victorian Britain* (London: I.B. Tauris, 2006), 81.

25. James G. Hanley, "Parliament, Physicians, and Nuisances: The Demedicalization of Nuisance Law, 1831–1855," *Bulletin of the History of Medicine* 80, no. 4 (2006): 720–32.

26. Paul Slack, *The Impact of Plague in Tudor and Stuart England* (Oxford: Clarendon, 1990), chap. 8; and Kira L.S. Newman, "Shutt Up: Bubonic Plague and Quarantine in Early Modern England," *Journal of Social History* 45, no. 3 (2012): 809–34.

27. "The Cholera," *Morning Post*, December 8, 1831, 3.

28. *Report of the General Board of Health on the Epidemic Cholera of 1848 and 1849*, No. 1273 (1850), 101–3 (appendix A).

29. S.E. Finer, *The Life and Times of Sir Edwin Chadwick* (London: Methuen, 1952), 350–51; and R.A. Lewis, *Edwin Chadwick and the Public Health Movement* (London: Longmans and Green, 1952), 204–5.

30. The records have now been published as Alan Kidd and Terry Wyke, eds., *The Challenge of Cholera: Proceedings of the Manchester Special Board of Health, 1831–1833* (Bristol: The Record Society of Lancashire and Cheshire, 2010).

31. "The Public Health," *Morning Post*, November 2, 1866, 3; Liddle, *Board of Works, Whitechapel District*, 18.

32. Henry Wentworth Acland, *Memoir on the Cholera at Oxford, in the Year 1854, with Considerations Suggested by the Epidemic* (London: John Churchill, 1856), pt. 2, chap 1.

33. House of Commons, "Quarantine: Return of the Number of Vessels Placed in Quarantine in the British Colonies in Each of the Ten Years Ending 31 December 1854," *Sessional Papers, 1857–58* (103), February 17, 1858, 10.

34. House of Commons, "Quarantine: Copy of the Papers Relating to Quarantine, Communicated to the Board of Trade on the 30th Day of July 1861," *Sessional Papers, 1861* (544), August 5, 1861, 36–38.

35. *Public Health: Ninth Report of the Medical Officer of the Privy Council, with Appendix: 1866*, No. 3949 (1867), 25–26.

36. *Public Health: Eighth Report of the Medical Officer of the Privy Council, with Appendix: 1865*, No. 3645 (1866), 41.

37. Ibid., 44.

38. J. Lane Notter, "International Sanitary Conferences of the Victorian Era: Inaugural Address of Session 1897–98," *Transactions of the Epidemiological Society of London*, vol. 17, *Session 1897–98* (1898), 3.

39. Similar arrangements became common throughout the capital after 1855, when MOsH were appointed to all districts. Royston Lambert, *Sir John Simon, 1816–1904, and English Sanitary Administration* (London: Macgibbon and Kee, 1963), 114–15, 139–40; and Edward Ballard, "The Work of the Metropolitan Medical Officers of Health: Their Success and Their Difficulties," *TNAPSS: 1862* (London: John W. Parker and Bourne, 1863), 657–59.

40. *5th ARLGB*, C. 1585 (1876), xllvii; *13th ARLGB*, Cd. 746 (1901), xxv.

41. Alfred Ashby, "The Medical Officer of Health," in *A Treatise on Hygiene and Public Health*, vol. 2, ed. Thomas Stevenson and Shirley F. Murphy (London: J. and A. Churchill, 1893), 743.

42. House of Commons, "Report from the Select Committee on Medical Poor Relief," *Sessional Papers, 1844* (531), July 29, 1844, 554–55, 560–61; and Henry Wyldbore Rumsey, *Essays on State Medicine* (London: John Churchill, 1856), 105–9, 278–79.

43. [Benjamin Ward Richardson], "The Registration of Disease in England," *Journal of Public Health and Sanitary Review* 3 (January 1858): 317–26.

44. Arthur Ransome, *Statistical Review of Ten Years of Disease in Manchester and Salford, Being an Analysis of the Weekly Returns of Health and Meteorology Issued by the Manchester and Salford Sanitary Association, 1861–1870* (Manchester: Heywood, 1870), 3–6.

45. A useful overview is Arthur Newsholme, "A National System of Notification and Registration of Sickness," *Journal of the Royal Statistical Society* 59, no. 1 (1896): 3–9.

46. J. M. Walker, *History of the Meteorological Office* (Cambridge: Cambridge University Press, 2012), 34–45.

47. Lyon Playfair, "Address on Health," *TNAPSS: 1874* (London: Longmans, Green, 1875), 101.

48. Newsholme, "A National System of Notification and Registration of Sickness," 14–21.

49. J. Y. Simpson, *Proposal to Stamp Out Small-Pox and Other Contagious Diseases* (Edinburgh: Edmonston and Douglas, 1868), 11, 18–19.

50. William Hardwicke, "On the Same," *TNAPSS: 1869* (London: Longmans, Green, Reader, and Dyer, 1870), 404–5.

51. Alfred Carpenter, "The Right of the State to Enforce Notification of Infectious Disease, and the Best Method of Doing It," in *International Health Exhibition, London, 1884: Transactions of the Conference in Domestic Sanitation in Urban and Rural Districts* (London: William Clowes, 1884), 204, 206.

52. Ernest Hart, "Report on Local Legislation as to Infectious Diseases," *BMJ*, March 12, 1881, 375–81; and House of Commons, "Report from the Select Committee on Police and Sanitary Regulations," *Sessional Papers, 1882* (226), June 9, 1882.

53. F. T. Bond, "Spread of Infectious Fevers," *TNAPSS: 1876* (London: Longmans, Green, 1877), 479.

54. For a full reconstruction see Graham Mooney, "Public Health versus Private Practice: The Contested Development of Compulsory Infectious Disease Notification in Late Nineteenth-Century Britain," *Bulletin of the History of Medicine* 73, no. 2 (1999): 238–67.

55. Edward Sergeant, "On the Compulsory Registration of Infectious Diseases with Special Reference to Its Workings at Bolton," *Sanitary Record,* October 25, 1878, 266–67; "The Registration of Infectious Disease," *Sanitary Record,* April 4, 1879, 212; and "The Leicester Improvement Bill," *Leicester Chronicle and the Leicestershire Mercury,* May 24, 1879, 8.

56. Mooney, "Public Health versus Private Practice," 247–51; "The Compulsory Notification of Infectious Diseases," *Sanitary Record,* April 15, 1883, 455–56; and Robert Hamilton, *Compulsory Notification of Infectious Diseases Considered* (London: J. and A. Churchill, 1883).

57. F. H. Moger, "Notification of Infectious Diseases," *BMJ*, June 16, 1883, 1187–88.

58. William Carter, "Is the Compulsory Notification of Infectious Diseases by Medical Men Practically Useful?" *BMJ*, September 16, 1882, 509.

59. J. W. Moore, "The Notification of Infectious Diseases," *BMJ*, November 5, 1881, 736.

60. Carpenter, "The Right of the State to Enforce Notification of Infectious Disease, and the Best Method of Doing It," 210–12.

61. W. H. Michael, "Is It (a) Desirable That There Should Be a System of Compulsory Notification of Infectious Diseases; and, If So, (b) What Is the Best Method of Carrying Such a System into Effect; and (c) What Is the Best Mode of Enforcing the Isolation of Cases of Infectious Disease?" *TNAPSS: 1881* (London: Longmans, Green, 1882), 538.

62. House of Commons, "Notification of Infectious Diseases: Return Showing the Districts wherein Local Acts for the Notification of Infectious Diseases Are in Force in England and Wales and Scotland Respectively," *Sessional Papers, 1889* (150), March 11, 1889.

63. House of Commons, "Returns: Infectious Disease (Notification) Act, 1889; Infectious Disease (Prevention) Act, 1890; and Public Health Acts Amendment Act, 1890," *Sessional Papers, 1892* (194), March 7, 1892.

64. *Morning Post,* November 30, 1889, 4.

65. T. Orme Dudfield, "Address: Conference of Medical Officers of Health," *Journal of the Sanitary Institute* 20 (1899): 410–14.

66. "Discussion," in *International Health Exhibition, London, 1884,* 236–37.

67. J. Spottiswoode Cameron, *Hints as to the Working of the Infectious Disease (Notification) Act, 1889* (Huddersfield: Alfred Jubb, 1889), 17–19.

68. "Compulsory Notification of Infectious Diseases," *BMJ,* November 5, 1887, 1021; Arthur Newsholme, "The Notification of Infectious Disease," *Public Health* 10, no. 7 (1897–98): 228.

69. "Proceedings of the Home Counties Branch of the Incorporated Society of Medical Officers of Health," *Public Health* 10, no. 2 (1897–98): 44.

70. W. G. Woodforde, "The Working of the Infectious Disease (Notification) Act," *Public Health* 4, no. 9 (1891–92): 258–59; T. A. Green, "Some Difficulties Met with in the Isolation of Infectious Diseases," *Public Health* 13, no. 6 (1900–1901): 428–29.

71. Jeremy Taylor, *Hospital and Asylum Architecture in England, 1840–1914: Building for Health Care* (London: Mansell, 1991), 105–9.

72. *44th ARLGB, Part III–(a) Public Health and Local Administration,* Cd. 8197 (1916), 26–27.

73. A useful overview of these provisions is Louis C. Parkes, *Infectious Diseases: Notification and Prevention* (London: H. K. Lewis, 1894), pt. 1.

74. "The New Despotism," *Pall Mall Gazette,* October 21, 1882, 1.

75. Charles Bell Taylor, *For Liberty: A Speech* (Nottingham: Stevenson, Bailey and Smith, 1885), 6. The Vigilance Association was established in 1871.

76. John Livy, "The Notification of Infectious Diseases," *BMJ,* August 12, 1882, 291–92.

77. "Discussion," *International Health Exhibition, London, 1884,* 243.

78. Anthony King, "Hospital Planning: Revised Thoughts on the Origin of the Pavilion Principle in England," *Medical History* 10, no. 4 (1966): 360–73.

79. *10th ARLGB: Supplement Containing Report and Papers Submitted by the Board's Medical Officer on the Use and Influence of Hospitals for Infectious Diseases,* C. 3290 (1882), esp. 6–27 for an overview.

80. *1st ARLGB,* C. 516 (1872), 321–24.

81. *17th ARLGB: Supplement Containing the Report of the Medical Officer for 1887,* C. 5526–I (1888), 199–201; and *40th ARLGB: Supplement in Continuation of the Report of the Medical Officer of the Board for 1910–11, Containing a Report on Isolation Hospitals by H. Franklin Parsons, M.D.,* Cd. 6342 (1912), appendix A.

82. R. S. Rounthwaite, "Sunderland Hospital Accommodation," *PAMSES, 1888–89: Vol. 15* (1889): 28–31.

83. The most thorough account remains Gwendoline M. Ayers, *England's First State Hospitals and the Metropolitan Asylums Board, 1867–1930* (London: Wellcome Institute, 1971).

84. Dudfield, "Address: Conference of Medical Officers of Health," 424.

85. "Leicester's New Isolation Hospital," *Leicester Chronicle and the Leicestershire Mercury,* April 1, 1899, 3.

86. R. Forsyth, "Difficulties in the Provision of Isolation Hospitals," *Public Health* 15, no. 4 (1902–3): 193–95. See also John V. Pickstone, *Medicine and Industrial Society: A History of Hospital Development in Manchester and Its Region, 1752–1946* (Manchester: Manchester University Press, 1985), 173–77.

87. See, for instance, "Discussion on Charges for Maintenance in Hospitals for Infectious Disease," *Public Health* 3, no. 1 (1890–91): 2–9; and "Isolation Hospital Charges," *Journal of State Medicine* 6, no. 2 (1898): 66–67.

88. Meredith Young, "Practical Hints on Isolation Hospital Construction," *Public Health* 15, no. 4 (1902–3): 182.

89. Whooping cough was also discussed alongside measles, even if the focus was generally on the latter. Calls were also made to add influenza and chickenpox to the list of notifiable diseases.

90. *24th ARLGB,* C. 7867 (1895), clx; and J. Howard Jones, "The Control of Measles: A Plea for United Action," *Public Health* 16, no. 9 (1903–4): 532.

91. Ayers, *England's First State Hospitals,* 72–74.

92. Dudfield, "Address: Conference of Medical Officers of Health," 425.

93. "Law Reports: High Court of Justice; Chancery Division—before Mr Justice Chitty—*Does the Establishment of a Small-Pox Hospital Constitute an Offensive Trade?*—Withington Local Board v. Corporation of Manchester," *Public Health* 5, no. 5 (1892–93): 185–86.

94. *40th ARLGB: Supplement in Continuation of the Report of the Medical Officer of the Board for 1910–11, Containing a Report on Isolation Hospitals by H. Franklin Parsons, M.D.,* 47.

95. *Hospitals Commission: Report of the Commissioners Appointed to Inquire Respecting Small-pox and Fever Hospitals,* C. 3314 (1882).

96. John M. Eyler, "Scarlet Fever and Confinement: The Edwardian Debate over Isolation Hospitals," *Bulletin of the History of Medicine* 61, no. 1 (1987): 1–24.

97. Michael Worboys, *Spreading Germs: Disease Theories and Medical Practice in Britain, 1865–1900* (Cambridge: Cambridge University Press, 2000), 254–65.

98. *40th ARLGB: Supplement in Continuation of the Report of the Medical Officer of the Board for 1910–11, Containing a Report on Isolation Hospitals by H. Franklin Parsons, M.D.,* 23–25.

99. W. Noble Twelvetrees, "Disinfection: Physical, Chemical and Mechanical," *Sanitary Inspectors Journal* 3, no. 1 (1897): 22, 28; and B. Arthur Whitelegge and George Newman, *Hygiene and Public Health* (London: Cassell, 1905), 312.

100. See Henry Bollmann Condy, *Disinfection and the Prevention of Disease* (London: John W. Davis, 1862), 2–4; and "Dr Baxter's Report on an Experimental Study of Certain Disinfectants," in *Public Health: Reports of the Medical Officer of the Privy Council and Local Government Board,* C.1371 (1875), 216–56.

101. John Dougall seems to have been the first to promote it as such in an address to the NAPSS in 1874. See "The Science of Disinfection," *BMJ,* October 24, 1874, 530–31.

102. *14th ARLGB: Supplement Containing the Report of the Medical Officer for 1884,* C. 4516 (1885), 183–303.

103. Overviews include John Gay, *Disinfection and Disinfectants* (London: Allman, 1895), 6–10; and George Newman, *Bacteriology and the Public Health,* 3rd ed. (London: John Murray, 1904), 439–44.

104. For a fuller discussion on the merits and applications of steam see Albert Taylor, *The Sanitary Inspector's Handbook,* 2nd ed. (London: H.K. Lewis, 1897), 196–204; and Twelvetrees, "Disinfection," 24–27.

105. Arthur Newsholme, *The Role of "Missed" Cases in the Spread of Infectious Diseases (a Lecture at the Victoria University of Manchester)* (London: Sherratt and Hughes, 1904), 7–8.

106. Worboys, *Spreading Germs,* chap. 7.

107. See esp. Ashby, "The Medical Officer of Health," 797–802.

108. Parkes, *Infectious Diseases,* 12–14.

109. Dudfield, "Address: Conference of Medical Officers of Health," 425.

110. By definition, however, the codes only applied to public elementary schools, exclusive of voluntary ones. Ashby, "The Medical Officer of Health," 803.

111. "Infectious Disease Prevention and the London School Board," *Public Health* 3, no. 10 (1890–91): 309–10.

112. *20th ARLGB: Supplement Containing the Report of the Medical Officer for 1890,* C. 6461 (1891), 213–17.

113. M.A. Adams, "School Closure for Infectious Diseases in Towns," *Public Health* 6, no. 9 (1893–94): 312.

114. William R. Smith, "Inaugural Address to the London Congress of the British Institute of Public Health," *Journal of State Medicine* 2, no. 4 (1894): 153.

115. G.S. Graham-Smith, "The Measures Taken to Check the Diphtheria Outbreak of 1901 at Colchester," *Journal of Hygiene* 2, no. 2 (1902): 180.

116. Conflict was not entirely absent, however. See "The Right of Entry of the Officials of a Sanitary Authority in Schools," *Journal of State Medicine* 7, no. 3 (1899): 168–70; and John J. Boyd, "School Notification of Infectious Disease," *Public Health* 16, no. 2 (1903–4): 94–98.

117. "Prosecution as to the Exposure of an Infectious Person under the Public Health (London) Act," *Public Health* 4, no. 10 (1891–92): 307–8; and "Removal by Force of Two Cases of Scarlet Fever," *Public Health* 3, no. 3 (1890–91): 147.

118. A. Wellesley Harris, "Some Difficulties Connected with Sanitary Legislation," *Journal of State Medicine* 3, no. 3 (1895): 182–83.

119. Alderman T. Windley, "Leicester and Small-pox: Thirty years' Experience," *Journal of State Medicine* 11, no. 1 (1903): 21–30.

120. Matthew L. Newsom Kerr, "'Perambulating Fever Nests of Our London Streets': Cabs, Omnibuses, Ambulances and Other 'Pest-Vehicles' in the Victorian Metropolis," *Journal of British Studies* 49, no. 2 (2010): 283–310. See also *Hospitals Commission,* xx–xxi.

121. Parkes, *Infectious Diseases,* 16–19, 61–65.

122. G.J.H. Evatt, *Ambulance Organization, Equipment and Transport* (London: William Clowes, 1884), 2.

123. Alexander Wynter Blyth, *A Dictionary of Hygiène and Public Health* (London: Charles Griffin, 1876), 51.

124. *10th ARLGB: Supplement Containing Report and Papers Submitted by the Board's Medical Officer on the Use and Influence of Hospitals for Infectious Diseases,* 72, 103, 190, 203.

125. Roger Cooter, "The Moment of the Accident: Culture, Militarism and Modernity in Late-Victorian Britain," in *Accidents in History: Injuries, Fatalities and Social Relations,* ed. Roger Cooter and Bill Luckin (Amsterdam: Rodopi, 1997), 107–46.

126. George A. Hutton, "First Aid and Transport of Sick and Wounded in Civil Life in Large Towns," *BMJ,* September 8, 1900, 623.

127. Ayers, *England's First State Hospitals,* 84, 100, and chap. 16.

128. T. Duncombe Mann, "The Metropolitan Asylums Board," *Public Health (Supplement to the International Congress of Hygiene and Demography)* (1891): 9.

129. John F. J. Sykes, *Public Health Problems* (London: Walter Scott, 1892), 219.

130. Metropolitan Asylums Board, *Annual Report of the Metropolitan Asylums Board: 1898* (London: McCorquodale, 1899), 13–14.

131. Judith Flanders, *The Victorian House: Domestic Life from Childbirth to Deathbed* (London: Harper Perennial, 2003), chap. 10.

132. Graham Mooney, "Infection and Citizenship: (Not) Visiting Isolation Hospitals in Mid-Victorian Britain," in *Permeable Walls: Historical Perspectives on Hospital and Asylum Visiting,* ed. Graham Mooney and Jonathan Reinarz (Amsterdam: Rodopi, 2009), 147–73.

133. C. Killick Millard, "The Hospital Isolation of Scarlet Fever: Some Points of Uncertainty," *Public Health* 14, no. 5 (1901–2): 292.

134. On the Parisian and English variants of the cubicle or barrier system see *40th ARLGB: Supplement in Continuation of the Report of the Medical Officer of the Board for 1910–11, containing a Report on Isolation Hospitals by H. Franklin Parsons, M.D.,* 30–38, 129–33.

135. H. G. Howse, "Hospital Hygiene," in *Treatise on Hygiene and Public Health,* vol. 1, ed. Stevenson and Murphy, 785.

136. *10th ARLGB: Supplement Containing Report and Papers Submitted by the Board's Medical Officer on the Use and Influence of Hospitals for Infectious Diseases,* 27–28. See also Mooney, "Infection and Citizenship," 159–65.

137. Roger McNeill, *The Prevention of Epidemics and the Construction and Management of Isolation Hospitals* (London: J. and A. Churchill, 1894), 182–83.

138. Ibid., 143.

139. T. W. Aldwinckle, "The Planning of Fever Hospitals," *Journal of State Medicine* 3, no. 6 (1895): 405–6.

140. *Hospitals Commission,* xx.

141. J. Lane Notter and W. H. Horrocks, *The Theory and Practice of Hygiene,* 2nd ed. (London: J. and A. Churchill, 1900), 736–38.

142. "The Corporation Disinfecting Station," *Birmingham Daily Post,* October 7, 1876, 5; "A Public Disinfecting Station for Ipswich," *Ipswich Journal,* October 28, 1876, 6.

143. "The Work of Disinfection in London," *BMJ,* June 24, 1893, 1336–37.

144. Gay, *Disinfection and Disinfectants,* 11.

145. Worboys, *Spreading Germs,* chap. 5; and Graham A. J. Ayliffe and Mary P. English, *Hospital Infection: From Miasmas to MRSA* (Cambridge: Cambridge University Press, 2003), chap. 8.

146. C. Killick Millard, "The Etiology of 'Return Cases' of Scarlet Fever," *BMJ*, September 3, 1898, 616.

147. *10th ARLGB: Supplement Containing Report and Papers Submitted by the Board's Medical Officer on the Use and Influence of Hospitals for Infectious Diseases*, 77.

148. Howse, "Hospital Hygiene," 795–96.

149. A. Knyvett Gordon, "Some Practical Points in the Management of an Isolation Hospital," *Public Health* 17, no. 6 (1904–5): 384–87.

150. R. Thorne Thorne, "On Sea-Borne Cholera: British Measures of Prevention v. European Measures of Restriction," *BMJ*, August 13, 1887, 339.

151. Harry Leach, "The Duties and Responsibilities of Port Sanitary Authorities, Particularly with Reference to Epidemic Diseases and Quarantine," *TNAPSS: 1875* (London: Longmans, Green, 1876), 570.

152. W. Collingridge, "The Milroy Lectures on Quarantine," *BMJ*, March 20, 1897, 713.

153. *Public Health: Reports of the Medical Officer of the Privy Council and Local Government Board: Papers, Concerning the European Relations of Asiatic Cholera, Submitted to the Local Government Board in Supplement to the Annual Report of the Present Year*, C.1370 (1875), 212–16.

154. Baldwin, *Contagion and the State in Europe*, chap. 2; Maglen, *English System*.

155. "The International Sanitary Conference, Paris, 1903," *BMJ*, December 12, 1903, 1549–50; "Disappearing Quarantine," *BMJ*, January 2, 1904, 34–35.

156. *10th ARLGB*, C. 2982 (1881), lxxv; *33rd ARLGB*, Cd. 2214 (1904), 657–68.

157. Booker, *Maritime Quarantine*, 537–51; Maglen, *English System*, chap. 1.

158. *15th ARLGB: Supplement Containing Reports and Papers on Cholera Submitted by the Board's Medical Officer*, C. 4873 (1886), 129–200; and Local Government Board, *Reports and Papers on the Port and Riparian Sanitary Survey of England and Wales, 1893–94*, C. 7812 (1895).

159. "Quarantine and our Port Authorities," *Public Health* 5, no. 2 (1892–93): 44–45.

160. "Association of Port Sanitary Authorities," *BMJ*, September 30, 1899, 862.

161. *Port of London Sanitary Committee, with the Half-Yearly Report of the Medical Officer for the Port of London, to 30th June, 1890* (London: Charles Skipper and East, 1890), 27.

162. John W. Mason, "Port Sanitary Administration," *Public Health* 4, no. 1 (1891–92): 5.

163. Henry E. Armstrong, "Port Sanitary Administration on the Tyne: A Seven Years' Retrospect (1881–87)," *Public Health* 1, no. 2 (1888–89): 37.

164. Anne Hardy, "Cholera, Quarantine and the English Preventive System, 1850–1895," *Medical History* 37, no. 3 (1993): 261–67.

165. "General Memorandum on the Proceedings Which Are Advisable in Places Attacked or Threatened by Epidemic Disease." MH19/244, 232, TNA.

166. A detailed overview of the preventive methods employed can be found in Local Government Board, *Reports and Papers on Bubonic Plague, by Dr R. Bruce Low,* Cd. 748 (1901), 34–55.

167. "Discussion on Cholera," *BMJ,* August 12, 1893, 365–66.

168. E. W. Hope, "Plague," *Public Health* 14, no. 6 (1901–2): 346–48.

169. *16th ARLGB,* C. 5131 (1887), 2–3, 12–13, 45–46.

170. Armstrong, "Port Sanitary Administration on the Tyne," 38–41.

171. Local Government Board, *Reports and Papers on Bubonic Plague,* 54–55.

172. "The Health of the Port of London," *BMJ,* May 14, 1904, 1144.

173. D. S. Davies, "Plague: Its Exclusion and Control," *Public Health* 14, no. 6 (1901–2): 332–34.

174. Shane Ewen, *Fighting Fires: Creating the British Fire Service, 1800–1978* (Basingstoke: Palgrave Macmillan, 2010); Cooter, "The Moment of the Accident"; and John Calder, *The Prevention of Factory Accidents* (London: Longmans, Green, 1899), chap. 3.

CHAPTER 7. PERSONAL HYGIENE

1. Annmarie Adams, *Architecture in the Family Way: Doctors, Houses and Women, 1870–1900* (Montreal: McGill-Queen's University Press, 1996); Victoria Kelley, *Soap and Water: Cleanliness, Dirt and the Working Classes in Victorian and Edwardian Britain* (London: I. B. Tauris, 2010).

2. Earl of Shaftesbury, "Address on Public Health," *TNAPSS: 1858* (London: Savill and Edwards, 1859), 84–85.

3. Benjamin Ward Richardson, "Lecture: Woman as Sanitary Reformer," *Transactions of the Sanitary Institute of Great Britain* 2 (1880): 188.

4. L. J. Rather, "The 'Six Things Non-Natural': A Note on the Origins and Fate of a Doctrine and a Phrase," *Clio Medica* 3 (1968): 337–47; and Virginia Smith, *Clean: A History of Personal Hygiene and Purity* (Oxford: Oxford University Press, 2007), chaps. 7–8.

5. The distinction might be traced back further. William Buchan's best-selling handbook on household regimen, *Domestic Medicine* (1769), noted how it steered clear of those "public means" of preserving health, such as street cleansing and the provision of water. The point here is that it became an established one during the Victorian period.

6. Andrew Wear, "The History of Personal Hygiene," in *Companion Encyclopedia of the History of Medicine,* ed. W. F. Bynum and Roy Porter, 2 vols. (London: Routledge, 1997), 2: 1283–308.

7. Alexander Kilgour, *Lectures on the Ordinary Agents of Life as Applicable to Therapeutics and Hygiene* (London: Longman, Rees, Orme, Brown, Green, Longman, 1834), xi.

8. E. A. Parkes, *Manuals of Health: On Personal Care of Health* (London: Society for Promoting Christian Knowledge, 1876), 4–5.

9. Alexander Wynter Blyth, *A Dictionary of Hygiène and Public Health* (London: Charles Griffin, 1876), 293–94.

10. *Reports of the Medical Officer of the Privy Council and Local Government Board*, C. 1066 (1874), 7.

11. George Crabb, *English Synonymes Explained, in Alphabetical Order* (London: Simpkin, Marshall, 1846), 265.

12. Samuel Smiles, *Self-Help: With Illustrations of Character and Conduct* (London: John Murray, 1859), 2.

13. Martin J. Wiener, *Reconstructing the Criminal: Culture, Law and Policy in England, 1830–1914* (Cambridge: Cambridge University Press, 1990), chap. 4; and James C. Livingston, *Religious Thought in the Victorian Age: Challenges and Reconceptions* (London: Continuum, 2006), chap. 6.

14. Francis Vacher, "Public Baths," *Sanitary Record*, March 6, 1876, 225. Emphasis and translations in the original.

15. It seems the phrase was first used by Edward Bulwer-Lytton in the opening "Dedicatory Epistle" of his 1830 novel *Paul Clifford*, where it referred to critics of an earlier work.

16. Edwin Chadwick, "Skin Cleanliness: Head to Foot Washing; Public Measures Proposed for Its Promotion," *Journal of the Society of Arts* 25 (August 1877): 885.

17. Lyon Playfair, "An Address on the Progress of Sanitary Reform," *BMJ*, October 10, 1874, 457.

18. Richard Metcalfe, *Sanitas Sanitatum et Omnia Sanitas* (London: Co-operative Printing Company, 1877), 41, 91–94; and Agnes Campbell, *The Carnegie United Kingdom Trust: Report on Public Baths and Wash-Houses in the United Kingdom* (Edinburgh: Constable, 1918), 6–7.

19. Thomas Webster, *An Encyclopaedia of Domestic Economy* (London: Longman, Brown, Green and Longmans, 1844), 1216–26.

20. W. Hale White, "Baths," in *A Treatise on Hygiene and Public Health*, vol. 1, ed. Thomas Stevenson and Shirley F. Murphy (London: J. and A. Churchill, 1892), 645.

21. On the founding of the London Committee, see Baths and Wash-houses for the Labouring Classes, *Statement of the Preliminary Measures Adopted for the Purpose of Promoting the Establishment of Baths and Wash-houses for the Labouring Classes* (London: Blades and East, 1845).

22. Herbert G. Coales, "Public Baths for a Small Town," *PAMSES, 1896–97: Vol. 23* (1897): 160.

23. W. Hawes, "Baths and Washhouses," *TNAPSS: 1857* (London: John W. Parker, 1858), 595.

24. "Public Baths and Washhouses," *Manchester Weekly Times*, September 30, 1876, 5.

25. London County Council, *Comparative Municipal Statistics, 1912–13* (London: Odham, 1915), 46.

26. Baths and Wash-houses for the Labouring Classes, *Statement of the Preliminary Measures*, 13; and Campbell, *Carnegie United Kingdom Trust*, 28.

27. A. Hessell Tiltman, "Public Baths and Washhouses," *Journal of the Royal Institute of British Architects* 6, no. 7 (1899): 178.

28. For a detailed discussion see Sally Sheard, "Profit Is a Dirty Word: The Development of Public Baths and Wash-houses in Britain, 1847–1915," *Social History of Medicine* 13, no. 1 (2000): 62–85.

29. "Baths and Wash-houses in Manchester and Salford," *Builder*, August 14, 1858, 654; "New Public Baths in Hulme, Manchester," *Builder*, June 30, 1860, 414–45.

30. "Establishment of the Baths and Wash-houses at St Mary's," *Morning Post*, September 22, 1853, 6.

31. "Opening of New Corporation Baths at Birkenhead," *Liverpool Mercury*, March 2, 1883, 7.

32. Vacher, "Public Baths," 226.

33. "The Rusholme Public Baths: Local Government Inquiry," *Manchester Guardian*, September 12, 1901, 9; "Preston's Public Baths: Ratepayers Oppose New Scheme," *Manchester Guardian*, February 19, 1908, 4.

34. "Gorton Public Baths," *Manchester Guardian*, July 1, 1890, 9.

35. House of Commons, "Report from the Joint Select Committee of the House of Lords and the House of Commons on Municipal Trading," *Sessional Papers, 1900* (305), July 27, 1900, 180.

36. Charles Clement Walker, "Baths for the People," *Transactions of the Sanitary Institute of Great Britain* 10 (1888–89): 230–31.

37. The most notable champion was the leading public baths architect A. Hessell Tiltman, who had visited establishments in Germany and Austria as part of five years of research. See esp. Tiltman, "Public Baths and Washhouses."

38. Walter W. Thomas, "People's Baths," *Public Health Engineer*, July 12, 1902, 53–54.

39. M. J. Daunton, *House and Home in the Victorian City: Working-Class Housing, 1850–1914* (London: Edward Arnold, 1983), 246–47.

40. Arthur Ransome, "Cleanliness," in *Health Lectures for the People Delivered in Manchester, Fourth and Fifth Series: 1880–81–82* (Manchester: John Heywood, 1883), 5; and H. G. Brooke, "Washing and Bathing," in *Health Lectures for the People Delivered in Manchester, 1883 and 1884*, vol. 7 (Manchester: John Heywood, 1884), 25–26.

41. Benjamin Ward Richardson, "Addresses to the Wage Classes: On Health at Home," *Transactions of the Sanitary Institute of Great Britain* 1 (1879): 287.

42. R. Sydney Marsden, "Sanitary Difficulties in Connection with the Personal Cleanliness of the Lower Working-Classes and of the Submerged Tenth," *Public Health* 8, no. 3 (1895–96): 83.

43. *4th ARLGB*, C. 1328 (1875), 127.

44. *16th ARLGB*, C. 5131 (1887), 1–2.

45. Recent accounts of the politics of municipal water provision include Harriet Ritvo, *The Dawn of Green: Manchester, Thirlmere, and Modern Environmentalism* (Chicago: University of Chicago Press, 2009); and John Broich, *London: Water and the Making of the Modern City* (Pittsburgh, PA: University of Pittsburgh Press, 2013).

46. *First Report of the Commissioners for Inquiring into the State of Large Towns and Populous Districts*, No. 572 (1844), 195–98 (appendix).

47. General Board of Health, *Report on the Supply of Water to the Metropolis: Appendix No. III. Reports and Evidence–Medical, Chemical, Geological and Miscellaneous*, No. 1283 (1850), 222–25.

48. House of Commons, "Special Report from the Select Committee on the Metropolis Water (No. 2) Bill," *Sessional Papers, 1871* (381), July 25, 1871, 14–16.

49. Anne Hardy, "Parish Pump to Private Pipes: London's Water Supply in the Nineteenth Century," *Medical History* 35, supplement no. 11 (1991): 88.

50. W. George Laws and H. E. Armstrong, *Report on the Water Supply of Newcastle-upon-Tyne and District* (Newcastle: Health Department, 1884), 41–42.

51. P. P. Baly, *A Statement of the Proceedings of the Committee Appointed to Promote the Establishment of Baths and Washhouses for the Labouring Classes; and a Report Upon the Buildings, Erected and Erecting; with Plans and Estimates* (London: Effingham Wilson, 1852).

52. [Jane Dukinfield], *A Memoir of the Rev. Sir Henry Robert Dukinfield* (London: W. H. Dalton, 1861), 60–64; and Hawes, "Baths and Washhouses," 595.

53. A. Ashpitel and J. Whichcord, *Observations on Baths and Wash-houses, with an Account of their History; an Abstract of the Acts of Parliament Relating Thereto; Their Applicability and Advantage to Provincial Towns; and a Description of the Principles Adopted*, 3rd ed. (London: John Weale, 1852).

54. [Local Government Board], *Model Bye-Laws for Sanitary Authorities* (London: Eyre and Spottiswoode, 1886), pt. 9.

55. "Construction of Baths," *Builder*, February 20, 1847, 84.

56. Robert Owen Allsop, *Public Baths and Washhouses* (London: E. and F. N. Spon, 1894), 26–28.

57. S. Stevens Hellyer, *The Plumber and Sanitary Houses: A Practical Treatise on the Principles of Internal Plumbing Work, or the Best Means for Effectually Excluding Noxious Gases from Our Houses*, 4th ed. (London: B. T. Batsford, 1887), 239.

58. Daniel J. Eveleigh, *Bogs, Baths and Basins: The Story of Domestic Sanitation* (Stroud: Sutton, 2006), 99.

59. W. J. Wells, "Modern Sanitary Appliances for Interior of Dwelling-Houses," *Sanitary Record*, March 26, 1897, 266.

60. Eveleigh, *Bogs, Baths and Basins*, 74–80.

61. Allsop, *Public Baths and Washhouses*, chap. 8; and Alfred W. S. Cross, *Public Baths and Wash-houses: A Treatise on Their Planning, Design, Arrangement and Fitting* (London: B. T. Batsford, 1906), chap. 9.

62. Overviews include William R. Maguire, *Domestic Sanitary Drainage and Plumbing* (London: Kegan Paul, Trench and Trübner, 1890), chap. 9; and F. W. Raynes, *Domestic Sanitary Engineering and Plumbing* (London: Longmans, Green, 1909), chaps. 13–14.

63. W. Eassie, "The Systems of Heating Water in Basements of Houses for Supply of Hot Water There, and also Hot Water for Upstairs Purposes," *Sanitary Record*, January 15, 1885, 295–97.

64. Anne Hardy, *The Epidemic Streets: Infectious Disease and the Rise of Preventive Medicine, 1856–1900* (Oxford: Clarendon, 1993), 169–72.

65. Manchester Corporation, *Letter Books of the Baths and Washhouses Committee,* vol. 1 (October 4, 1876–January 27, 1881), 118–20. M9/73/1/1, MALSC.

66. Vanessa Taylor and Frank Trentmann, "Liquid Politics: Water and the Politics of Everyday Life in the Modern City," *Past and Present,* no. 211 (2011): 199–241.

67. Ibid., 212–15.

68. "The Bradford Water Famine," *Sheffield and Rotherham Independent,* October 28, 1884, 3; *Liverpool Mercury,* July 28, 1885, 5; and "Leicester Water Supply," *Leicester Chronicle and the Leicestershire Mercury,* October 7, 1893, 6.

69. Taylor and Trentmann, "Liquid Politics," 220–28.

70. This was but one of a number of regulations. The bylaws of Manchester Corporation's Bath and Washhouses Committee, for instance, contained twenty-three rules in total, prohibiting, among other things, loitering in corridors and the use of foul language. Manchester Corporation, *Proceedings of the Manchester Baths and Washhouses Committee,* vol. 1 (August 17, 1876–February 17, 1881), 252–54. M9/73/2/1, MALSC.

71. Alfred Ebsworth, *Facts and Inferences Drawn from an Inspection of the Public Baths and Washhouses in This Metropolis* (London: William Brickhill, 1853), 6.

72. Dawson W. Turner, *Dirt and Drink* (London: Longmans, 1884), 7.

73. Baths and Wash-houses for the Labouring Classes, *Statement of the Preliminary Measures,* 11–12.

74. Erasmus Wilson, *Healthy Skin: A Popular Treatise on the Skin and Hair, Their Preservation and Management,* 5th ed. (London: John Churchill, 1855), xiii.

75. Henry Rumsey, "Address on Health," *TNAPSS: 1868* (London: Longmans, Green, Reader and Dyer, 1869), 81.

76. "Lord Derby on Sanitary Legislation and Sanitary Duties," *Manchester Guardian,* April 11, 1872, 6.

77. *Hints on District Visiting Societies: A Plan for Their Formation and Suggestions to Visitors* (London: Longman, Rees, Orme, Brown, Green and Longman, 1836), 30.

78. Hugh Stowell Brown, *Cleanliness Is Next to Godliness* (Liverpool: Gabriel Thomson, 1858), 4.

79. Major Lamorock Flower, "Cleanliness: An Address to the Working Classes," *Transactions of the Sanitary Institute of Great Britain* 9 (1887–88): 449.

80. *Education Department: New Code of Regulations,* C.1170 (1875), 6; and *New Code of 1882: Instructions to H.M. Inspectors, England and Wales,* C.3335 (1882), 8.

81. See, for instance, W.F. Richards, *Manual of Method: For the Use of Teachers in Elementary Schools* (London: National Society's Depository, 1854); John Gill, *Introductory Text-book to School Education, Method and School Management,* 9th ed. (London: Longmans, Green, 1863); and John Richard Blakiston, *The Teacher: Hints on School Management* (London: Macmillan, 1879).

82. See Harry Hendrick, *Child Welfare: England, 1872–1989* (London: Routledge, 1994), chaps. 2–3; and, most recently, Ina Zweiniger-Bargielowska, *Managing the Body: Beauty, Health and Fitness in Britain, 1880–1939* (Oxford: Oxford University Press, 2010), chaps. 1–3.

83. Christopher Love, *A Social History of Swimming in England, 1800–1918: Splashing in the Serpentine* (Abingdon: Routledge, 2008), chap. 7.

84. "School Hygiene in Manchester," *Public Health* 21, no. 4 (1907–8): 163.

85. See esp. Georges Vigarello, *Concepts of Cleanliness: Changing Attitudes in France since the Middle Ages,* trans. Jean Birrel (Cambridge: Cambridge University Press, 1988), 39–84.

86. Michael Curtin, *Propriety and Position: A Study of Victorian Manners* (London: Garland, 1987), chaps. 1–2.

87. William Hardwicke, *On the Moral and Physical Advantages of Baths and Washhouses* (London: Robert Hardwicke, 1874), 13.

88. G. Dickson, *On Cleanliness* (Edinburgh: J.D. Lowe, 1855), 1, 6–7. Emphasis in original.

89. Alfred Carpenter, "Education by Proverb in Sanitary Work," *Transactions of the Sanitary Institute of Great Britain* 6 (1884–85): 397–419.

90. Brooke, "Washing and Bathing," 29.

91. On the soap industry see Brian Lewis, *"So Clean": Lord Leverhulme, Soap and Civilization* (Manchester: Manchester University Press, 2008), chap. 2.

92. Eveleigh, *Bogs, Baths and Basins,* 164; and W. Lawrence Gadd, *Soap Manufacture: A Practical Treatise on the Fabrication of Hard and Soft Soaps and Analytical Methods for the Determination of Their Chemical Composition* (London: George Bell, 1893), 3.

93. For further discussion see Anne McClintock, *Imperial Leather: Race, Gender and Sexuality in the Colonial Contest* (London: Routledge, 1995), chap. 5.

94. "Pears' Soap Has Passed into a Proverb," *Penny Illustrated Paper and Illustrated Times,* April 4, 1896, 221.

95. H.R. Jennings, *Our Homes, and How to Beautify Them,* 3rd ed. (London: Harrison, 1902), 236–37.

96. Samuel Smiles, *Thrift* (London: John Murray, 1875), 382–83.

97. A Journeyman Engineer [Thomas Wright], "Working Men's Saturdays," in *Some Habits and Customs of the Working Classes* (London: Tinsley, 1867), 188.

98. Kelley, *Soap and Water.*

99. Vigarello, *Concepts of Cleanliness;* Keith Thomas, "Cleanliness and Godliness in Early Modern England," in *Religion, Culture and Society in Early Modern Britain: Essays in Honour of Patrick Collinson,* ed. Anthony Fletcher and Peter Roberts (Cambridge: Cambridge University Press, 1994), 56–83.

100. John Harrison Curtis, *Observations on the Preservation of Health in Infancy, Youth, Manhood and Age,* 4th ed. (London: John Churchill, 1842), 225. Emphasis in original.

101. This was linked to the gradual eclipse of a broadly humoral model of bodily health by one that was anatomical and physiological; which is to say, based around the integrity of the body's structures (e.g., bones, tissues, and

cells) and systems (e.g., digestive and respiratory). A useful discussion of this shift can be found in Virginia Smith, "Physical Puritanism and Sanitary Science: Material and Immaterial Beliefs in Physiology, 1650–1840," in *Medical Fringe and Medical Orthodoxy,* ed. W. F. Bynum and Roy Porter (London: Croom Helm, 1987), 174–97.

102. Brooke, "Washing and Bathing," 23.

103. A contemporary overview of the science from an international perspective is Malcolm Morris, "An Address Delivered at the Opening of the Section of Dermatology: The Rise and Progress of Dermatology," *BMJ,* September 18, 1897, 697–702.

104. Benjamin Ward Richardson, "The Next to Godliness: An Address to the Working Classes," *Transactions of the Sanitary Institute of Great Britain* 9 (1887–88): 256.

105. Wilson, *Healthy Skin,* 42–43.

106. *How to Behave: A Pocket Manual of Etiquette, and Guide to Correct Personal Habits* (London: Houlston and Wright, 1865), 17.

107. Wilson, *Healthy Skin,* 163.

108. See, for example, Metropolitan Working Classes' Association for Improving the Public Health, *Bathing and Personal Cleanliness* (London: John Churchill, 1847), 9–10.

109. Wilson, *Healthy Skin,* xv.

110. James Black, *Observations and Instructions on Cold and Warm Bathing* (Manchester: Simms and Dinham, 1846), 3–4.

111. Hardwicke, *On the Moral and Physical Advantages of Baths and Washhouses,* 9–10.

112. James Baird, *The Management of Health: A Manual of Home and Personal Hygiene* (London: Virtue, 1867), 73.

113. M. Loane, *An Englishman's Castle* (London: Edward Arnold, 1909), 164–68; Mrs Pember Reeves, *Round About a Pound a Week* (London: George Bell, 1913), 54–57.

114. [Wright], "Working Men's Saturdays," 188.

115. Mrs Caddy, *Household Organization* (London: Chapman and Hall, 1877), 165–69.

116. Eveleigh, *Bogs, Baths and Basins,* chap. 5.

117. Walker, "Baths for the People," 233–35.

118. Hugh Shimmin, "Cornwallis Street Baths," in *Low Life and Moral Improvement in Mid-Victorian Britain: Liverpool through the Journalism of Hugh Shimmin,* ed. John K. Walton and Alastair Wilcox (Leicester: Leicester University Press, 1991), 216–17.

119. Malcolm Morris, *Ethics of the Skin: A Lecture, Delivered in the Lecture Room of the Exhibition, June 19th, 1884* (London: William Clowes, 1884), 1, 5.

120. "In Praise of the Tub," *Sanitary Record,* May 15, 1893, 551.

121. White, "Baths," 618–19.

122. Recent accounts of the birth of hydropathy include James Bradley, "Medicine on the Margins? Hydropathy and Orthodoxy in Britain, 1840–1860," in *Plural Medicine, Tradition and Modernity, 1800–2000,* ed. Waltraud Ernst (London: Routledge, 2002), 19–39; and Hilary Marland and Jane Adams,

"Hydropathy at Home: The Water Cure and Domestic Healing in Mid-Nineteenth-Century Britain," *Bulletin of the History of Medicine* 83, no. 3 (2009): 499–529.

123. David Blackbourn, "'Taking the Waters': Meeting Places of the Fashionable World," in *The Mechanics of Internationalism: Culture, Society and Politics, from the 1840s to the First World War*, ed. Martin H. Geyer and Johannes Paulmann (Oxford: Oxford University Press, 2001), 435–57.

124. David Urquhart, *The Pillars of Hercules; or, A Narrative of Travels in Spain and Morocco in 1848*, 2 vols. (London: Richard Bentley, 1850), 2: 14–19, 36.

125. Ibid., 75–78.

126. Metcalfe, *Sanitas Sanitatum et Omnia Sanitas*, 101–105.

127. Edward Haughton, *The Facts and Fallacies of the Turkish Bath Question; or, What Kind of Bath Shall We Have?* (Dublin: William Robertson, 1860).

128. "The Turkish-Roman Bath: What Are Its right uses?" *BMJ*, March 2, 1861, 231–32.

129. See, for instance, the various works of the entrepreneur Charles Bartholomew, including *Lecture on Turkish Baths, Delivered before the Balloon Society of Great Britain, at Westminster Hall, London, March 26th, 1886* (London: Marshall, 1886), and *Illustrated Guide to the Turkish Baths, Medicated and Other Baths* (London: Marshall, 1887).

130. Frederic C. Coley, *The Turkish Bath: Its History and Uses* (London: Walter Scott, 1887), 30–41.

131. Francis Drake, *The Anglo-Roman, or Turkish Bath: Its History, Proper Construction, Present Status and Various Uses* (London: Ward and Lock, 1862), 12–17.

132. Robert Owen Allsop, *The Turkish Bath: Its Design and Construction* (London: E. and F. N. Spon, 1890), 64–69.

133. See the diagram which features in Edward Haughton, *On the Remains of Ancient Roman Baths in England* (London: Simpkin, Marshall, 1861).

134. "New Public Baths in Hulme, Manchester," *Builder*, June 30, 1860, 414–15; Metcalfe, *Sanitas Sanitatum et Omnia Sanitas*, 167–70.

135. "Manchester Corporation Baths: Proposed Additions to the Public Baths," *Manchester Guardian*, September 21, 1899, 9; I. Brooke-Adler, "London's Washhouses and Baths," in *Living London*, ed. George R. Sims, 3 vols. (London: Cassell, 1906), 2: 369.

136. Erasmus Wilson, *The Eastern or Turkish Bath: Its History, Revival in Britain and Application to the Purposes of Health* (London: John Churchill, 1861), 50, 70–72.

137. Baird, *Management of Health*, 73.

138. [Alfred Mellett Peirson], *Turkish Baths: Their Relation to Health and the Senses* (Yeovil: Western Chronicle Office, 1898), 19.

139. Daniel Noble, "Causes Reducing the Effects of Sanitary Reform," in *Health Lectures for the People: Health Lectures Delivered in Manchester, 1875–76, 1876–77, 1877–78* (Manchester: John Heywood, 1878), 12–13.

140. Stephen Reynolds, *A Poor Man's House* (London: John Lane, 1909), 88–89.

CHAPTER 8. CONCLUSION

1. *An Outline of the Practice of Preventive Medicine: A Memorandum Addressed to the Minister of Health,* by Sir George Newman, Cmd. 363 (1919), 46–100.

2. The precise role that public health initiatives played in the epidemiological transition toward more chronic conditions as the principal cause of death has been much debated; but surely these initiatives played some role, and even a significant one. See esp. Simon Szreter, "The Importance of Social Intervention in Britain's Mortality Decline, c. 1850–1914: A Re-interpretation of the Role of Public Health," *Social History of Medicine* 1, no. 1 (1988): 1–37; and Anne Hardy, *The Epidemic Streets: Infectious Disease and the Rise of Preventive Medicine, 1856–1900* (Oxford: Clarendon, 1993).

3. Recent accounts include Bernard Harris, *The Origins of the British Welfare State: Social Welfare in England and Wales, 1800–1945* (Basingstoke: Palgrave Macmillan, 2004), chaps. 15–16; Martin Gorsky, "Local Government Health Services in Interwar England: Problems of Quantification and Interpretation," *Bulletin of the History of Medicine* 85, no. 3 (2011): 384–412; and Barry M. Doyle, *The Politics of Hospital Provision in Early Twentieth-Century Britain* (London: Pickering and Chatto, 2014).

4. Dorothy Porter and Roy Porter, "What Was Social Medicine? An Historiographical Essay," *Historical Sociology* 1, no. 1 (1988): 90–109; Ben Pimlott, "The Myth of Consensus," in *The Making of Britain: Echoes of Greatness,* ed. Lesley M. Smith (Basingstoke: Palgrave Macmillan, 1988), 129–42; and Charles Webster, "Conflict and Consensus: Explaining the British Health Service," *Twentieth Century British History* 1, no. 2 (1990): 115–51.

5. Ann F. La Berge, *Mission and Method: The Early Nineteenth-Century French Public Health Movement* (Cambridge: Cambridge University Press, 1992), chap. 8. On struggles regarding the institutionalization of "public health" in France see also William Coleman, *Death Is a Social Disease: Public Health and Political Economy in Early Industrial France* (Madison: University of Wisconsin Press, 1982); and Martha Lee Hildreth, *Doctors, Bureaucrats and Public Health in France, 1888–1902* (New York: Garland Publishing, 1987).

6. Dorothy Porter, *Health, Civilization and the State: A History of Public Health from Ancient to Modern Times* (London: Routledge, 1999), 104.

7. One should also mention, however, a federal Marine Hospital Service, which dates back to 1798; a National Board of Health had also been briefly established during the period 1879–83. There is, of course, no shortage of complexities in the American case. See Manfred Waserman, "The Quest for a National Health Department in the Progressive Era," *Bulletin of the History of Medicine* 49, no. 3 (1975): 353–80; and John Duffy, *The Sanitarians: A History of American Public Health* (Urbana: University of Illinois Press, 1990).

8. See esp. David Arnold, *Colonizing the Body: State Medicine and Epidemic Disease in Nineteenth-Century India* (Berkeley: University of California Press, 1993); Alison Bashford, *Imperial Hygiene: A Critical History of Colonialism, Nationalism and Public Health* (Basingstoke: Palgrave Macmillan, 2004); and Ryan Johnson and Amna Khalid, eds., *Public Health in the British Empire:*

Intermediaries, Subordinates and the Practice of Public Health, 1850–1960 (New York: Routledge, 2012).

9. Peter Baldwin, "Beyond Weak and Strong: Rethinking the State in Comparative Policy History," *Journal of Policy History* 17, no. 1 (2005): 19.

10. Philip Harling, "The Centrality of the Locality: The Local State, Local Democracy and Local Consciousness in Late-Victorian and Edwardian Britain," *Journal of Victorian Culture* 9, no. 2 (2004): 216–34; and James Vernon, *Distant Strangers: How Britain Became Modern* (Berkeley: University of California Press, 2014), 69–72.

11. See esp. James F. Stark, *The Making of Modern Anthrax, 1875–1920: Uniting Local, National and Global Histories of Disease* (London: Pickering and Chatto, 2013); and Shane Ewen and Pierre-Yves Saunier, eds., *Another Global City: Historical Explorations into the Transnational Municipal Moment, 1850–2000* (New York: Palgrave, 2008).

12. These are among only the most striking developments, of course. A recent survey of the multiple agents involved is Paul Weindling, "International Health between Public and Private in the Twentieth Century," in *Healthcare in Private and Public from the Early Modern Period to 2000,* ed. Paul Weindling (London: Routledge, 2015), 194–214.

13. Alan Petersen and Deborah Lupton, *The New Public Health: Health and Self in the Age of Risk* (London: Sage, 1996), chap. 3; and Virginia Berridge, *Health and Society in Britain since 1939* (Cambridge: Cambridge University Press, 1999), 48–54.

14. Porter, *Health, Civilization and the State,* 147, 219, 239, 264; La Berge, *Mission and Method,* chaps. 8–9.

15. See esp. Philippa Levine, *Prostitution, Race, and Politics: Policing Venereal Disease in the British Empire* (New York: Routledge, 2003), chap. 3.

16. See, for instance, John M. Eyler, *Sir Arthur Newsholme and State Medicine, 1885–1935* (Cambridge: Cambridge University Press, 1997), 354–74; and Glen O'Hara, *Governing Post-war Britain: The Paradoxes of Progress, 1951–1973* (Basingstoke: Palgrave Macmillan, 2012), chap. 3.

17. C.A. Bayly, *The Birth of the Modern World, 1780–1914: Global Connections and Comparisons* (Oxford: Blackwell, 2004); Pierre-Yves Saunier, *Transnational History* (Basingstoke: Palgrave Macmillan, 2013); and Diego Olstein, *Thinking History Globally* (Basingstoke: Palgrave Macmillan, 2015).

18. See, for instance, Martin V. Melosi, *The Sanitary City: Urban Infrastructure in America from Colonial Times to the Present* (Baltimore: Johns Hopkins University Press, 2000), chaps. 3, 5, and 8; Andrew R. Aisenberg, *Contagion: Disease, Government, and the "Social Question" in Nineteenth-Century France* (Stanford, CA: Stanford University Press, 1999), 105–12; Ian F. McNeely, *"Medicine on a Grand Scale": Rudolf Virchow, Liberalism and the Public Health* (London: Wellcome Trust, 2002), chap. 3; and Mark Harrison, *Public Health in British India: Anglo-Indian Preventive Medicine, 1859–1914* (Cambridge: Cambridge University Press, 1994), chap. 8.

19. See, for instance, *Report on a General Scheme for Extramural Sepulture,* No. 1158 (1850); and G.F. McCleary, "The Infants' Milk Depot: Its History and Function," *Journal of Hygiene* 4, no. 3 (1904): 329–68; and Helen Jones,

Health and Society in Twentieth-Century Britain (London: Longman, 1994), 23–24.

20. Peter Baldwin, *Contagion and the State in Europe, 1830–1930* (Cambridge: Cambridge University Press, 1999), chap. 5; and Levine, *Prostitution, Race, and Politics,* chap. 4.

21. Ann F. La Berge, "Edwin Chadwick and the French Connection," *Bulletin of the History of Medicine* 62, no. 1 (1988): 23–41.

22. Henry Wyldbore Rumsey, *Essays on State Medicine* (London: John Churchill, 1856), 61.

23. For a recent review of this literature, most of which has been pioneered in the political sciences, see Eugene McCann and Kevin Ward, "Policy Assemblages, Mobilities and Mutations: Toward a Multidisciplinary Conversation," *Political Studies Review* 10, no. 3 (2012): 325–32.

24. Constance A. Nathanson, *Disease Prevention as Social Change: The State, Society, and Public Health in the United States, France, Great Britain, and Canada* (New York: Russell Sage Foundation, 2007), 4.

25. See esp. Lauren M. E. Goodlad, *Victorian Literature and the Victorian State: Character and Governance in a Liberal Society* (Baltimore: Johns Hopkins University Press, 2003); Patrick Joyce, *The Rule of Freedom: Liberalism and the Modern City* (London: Verso, 2003); Chris Otter, *The Victorian Eye: A Political History of Light and Vision in Britain, 1800–1910* (Chicago: University of Chicago Press, 2008); Simon Gunn and James Vernon, eds., *The Peculiarities of Liberal Modernity in Imperial Britain* (Berkeley: University of California Press, 2011); and Joyce, *Rule of Freedom.*

26. Alfred Carpenter, "Education by Proverb in Sanitary Work," *Transactions of the Sanitary Institute of Great Britain* 6 (1884–85): 413–14.

27. "Sanitary Inspectors' Association: Annual Dinner," *Sanitary Record,* February 6, 1908, 115.

28. Joyce, *Rule of Freedom.*

Selected Bibliography

This bibliography is not exhaustive. It lists only those primary and secondary sources that have been most relevant to the construction of the argument. For more details on sources, readers are directed to the notes.

PRIMARY SOURCES

Manuscript Sources

CLA/006/AD, papers relating to the City of London's sanitary functions (1848–88); and LCC/PH/REG/1, papers relating to the inspection and regulation of common lodging houses under the London County Council (1895–1910). London Metropolitan Archives.

H7, papers of the Banbury board of health (1844–89); BOR1/20, papers of the Chipping Norton urban sanitary authority (1872–1910); PLU2/SN, papers of the Bicester rural sanitary authority (1873–97); and CC3/3/A5, papers of the urban and rural sanitary authorities of Banbury, Bicester, Chipping Norton, Henley, and Woodstock (1889–1910). Oxfordshire History Centre, Oxford.

M595/1/1, minutes of the health committee, Manchester Corporation (1868–90); M9/73/1, the letter books of the baths and washhouses committee, Manchester Corporation (1876–91); and M9/73/2, proceedings of the baths and washhouses committee, Manchester Corporation (1876–1911). Manchester Archives and Local Studies Centre.

PC1, papers of the Board of Health (1805–6) and Central Board of Health (1831–32); and MH19, papers of the Local Government Board (1871–1919) in relation to specific diseases. The National Archives, London.

Newspapers, Journals, and Annual Proceedings

Birmingham Daily Post.
British Medical Journal.
Builder.
Edinburgh Review.
Journal of Hygiene.
Journal of Public Health and Sanitary Review.
Journal of the Royal Institute of British Architects.
Journal of the Royal Sanitary Institute.
Journal of the Royal Statistical Society.
Journal of the Sanitary Institute.
Journal of the Society of Arts.
Journal of State Medicine.
Journal of the Statistical Society of London.
Lancet.
Liverpool Mercury.
Manchester Guardian.
Minutes of Proceedings of the Institution of Civil Engineers.
Proceedings of the Association of Municipal and Sanitary Engineers and Surveyors.
Public Health.
Public Health Engineer.
Sanitary Inspectors Journal.
Sanitary Officer.
Sanitary Record.
Times.
Transactions of the Epidemiological Society of London.
Transactions of the Manchester Statistical Society.
Transactions of the National Association for the Promotion of Social Science.
Transactions of the Sanitary Institute of Great Britain.

Official and Parliamentary Sources

Annual Reports of the Local Government Board.
Annual Reports of the Medical Officer of the Privy Council.
Annual Reports of the Registrar-General.
Annual Summaries of Births, Deaths and Causes of Death in London and Other Large Cities (titles varied).
Hansard Parliamentary Debates, 3rd and 4th series.
House of Commons Sessional Papers.
Quarterly Returns of Marriages, Births and Deaths Registered in the Divisions, Counties, and Districts of England (titles varied).
Reports and Minutes of Evidence of Royal Commissions of Inquiry.
Reports, Papers and Minutes of Information of the General Board of Health.
Supplements to the Annual Reports of the Local Government Board.
Supplements to the Annual Reports of the Registrar-General.

Weekly Returns of Births and Deaths in London and Other Towns of the United Kingdom (titles varied).

Books, Pamphlets, and Articles

Ackroyd, William. *The Scientific Aspects of the Sewage Question.* London: Wrightman, 1897.

Acland, Henry Wentworth. *Memoir on the Cholera at Oxford, in the Year 1854, with Considerations Suggested by the Epidemic.* London: John Churchill, 1856.

[Addison, Christopher]. *The Health of the People, and How It May Be Improved, From a Speech Delivered by Dr Christopher Addison, MP, at the Whitehall Rooms, February, 6th, 1914.* London: University of London Press, 1914.

Alexander, Hugh. *Inaugural Address Delivered at the Westminster Town Hall, Nov. 5. 1887 to the Association of Public Sanitary Inspectors.* London: Potter, 1887.

Allsop, Robert Owen. *Public Baths and Washhouses.* London: E. and F. N. Spon, 1894.

Andrews, O. W. *Hand-Book of Public Health Laboratory Work and Food Inspection.* Portsmouth: Carpenter, 1898.

Ashpitel, A., and J. Whichcord. *Observations on Baths and Wash-houses, with an Account of their History; an Abstract of the Acts of Parliament Relating Thereto; Their Applicability and Advantage to Provincial Towns; and a Description of the Principles Adopted.* 3rd ed. London: John Weale, 1852.

Baird, James. *The Management of Health: A Manual of Home and Personal Hygiene.* London: Virtue, 1867.

Baly, P. P. *A Statement of the Proceedings of the Committee Appointed to Promote the Establishment of Baths and Washhouses for the Labouring Classes; and a Report Upon the Buildings, Erected and Erecting; with Plans and Estimates.* London: Effingham Wilson, 1852.

Baths and Wash-houses for the Labouring Classes. *Statement of the Preliminary Measures Adopted for the Purpose of Promoting the Establishment of Baths and Wash-houses for the Labouring Classes.* London: Blades and East, 1845.

Blackstone, William. *Commentaries on the Laws of England, Book the Fourth.* Oxford: Clarendon, 1769.

Blatchford, Robert. *Merrie England.* London: Clarion Office, 1895.

Blyth, Alexander Wynter. *A Dictionary of Hygiène and Public Health.* London: Charles Griffin, 1876.

Boulnois, H. Percy. *Dirty Dustbins and Sloppy Streets: A Practical Treatise on the Scavenging and Cleansing of Cities and Towns.* London: E. and F. N. Spon, 1881.

———. *The Municipal and Sanitary Engineers' Handbook.* 3rd ed. London: E. and F. N. Spon, 1898.

Brooke, H. G. "Washing and Bathing." In *Health Lectures for the People Delivered in Manchester, 1883 and 1884,* vol. 7, 13–32. Manchester: John Heywood, 1884.

Brown, Hugh Stowell. *Cleanliness Is Next to Godliness.* Liverpool: Gabriel Thomson, 1858.

Brown, S. Sneade. *A Lay Lecture on Sanitary Matters, with a Paper on Sewer Ventilation.* London: Kerby and Endean, 1873.

Bulwer, Henry Lytton. *The Monarchy of the Middle Classes: France, Social, Literary, Political.* 2 vols. London: Richard Bentley, 1836.

Cameron, J. Spottiswoode. *Hints as to the Working of the Infectious Disease (Notification) Act, 1889.* Huddersfield: Alfred Jubb, 1889.

———. *On Nuisances and Methods of Inspection.* London: Sanitary Publishing Company, 1901.

Cargill, Thomas. *Sewage and Its General Application to Grass, Cereal and Root Crops, Showing the Results Obtained by Actual Experience.* London: Robertson, Brooman, 1869.

[Chadwick, Edwin]. *An Article on the Principles and Progress of the Poor Law Amendment Act; and Also on the Nature of the Central Control and Improved Local Administration Introduced by That Statute.* London: Charles Knight, 1837.

———. "Centralization: Public Charities in France." *London Review* 1, no. 2 (1829): 536–65.

———. *The Comparative Results of the Chief Principles of the Poor-Law Administration in England and Ireland, as Compared with That of Scotland.* London: E. Faithfull, 1864.

———. *The Jubilee of Sanitary Science, Being the Annual Address of Edwin Chadwick, C.B., at the Anniversary Dinner of the Association of Public Sanitary Inspectors, February 5, 1887.* London: James Meldrum, 1887.

———. *On the Evils of Disunity in Central and Local Administration, Especially with Reference to the Metropolis and Also on the New Centralisation for the People.* London: Longmans, Green, 1885.

———. *A Paper on the Chief Methods of Preparation for Legislation, Especially as Applicable to the Reform of Parliament.* London: Charles Knight, 1859.

———. *Report on the Sanitary Condition of the Labouring Population of Great Britain.* Ed. M.W. Flinn. Edinburgh: Edinburgh University Press, 1965.

Chalmers, M.D. *Local Government.* London: Macmillan, 1883.

A Citizen. *Centralization or Local Representation: Health of Towns' Bill; The Opinion of the Public Journals.* 3 vols. London: Thomas Harreld, 1848.

Codrington, Thomas. *Report on the Destruction of Town Refuse.* London: Her Majesty's Stationery Office, 1888.

Coleman, T.E. *Sanitary House Drainage, Its Principles and Practice.* London: E. and F.N. Spon, 1896.

Conder, J.B. Reignier. *A Handbook of Sewer and Drain Cases.* London: St. Bride's, 1904.

Condy, Henry Bollmann. *Disinfection and the Prevention of Disease.* London: John W. Davis, 1862.

Cross, Alfred W.S. *Public Baths and Wash-houses: A Treatise on Their Planning, Design, Arrangement and Fitting.* London: B.T. Batsford, 1906.

Curtis, John Harrison. *Observations on the Preservation of Health in Infancy, Youth, Manhood and Age.* 4th ed. London: John Churchill, 1842.

Danchell, Frederick Hahn. *Concerning Sewage and Its Economical Disposal.* London: Simpkin, Marshall, 1872.

Dickson, G. *On Cleanliness.* Edinburgh: J.D. Lowe, 1855.

Disraeli, Benjamin. *The Chancellor of the Exchequer in Scotland, Being Two Speeches Delivered by Him in the City of Edinburgh on 29th and 30th October 1867.* Edinburgh: William Blackwood, 1867.

Drake, Francis. *The Anglo-Roman, or Turkish Bath: Its History, Proper Construction, Present Status and Various Uses.* London: Ward and Lock, 1862.

Duncan, W.H. *On the Physical Causes of the High Rate of Mortality in Liverpool: Read before the Literary and Philosophical Society in February and March, 1843.* Liverpool: Mitchell, Heaton and Mitchell, 1843.

Eassie, William. *Healthy Houses: A Handbook to the History, Defects and Remedies of Drainage, Ventilation, Warming and Kindred Subjects.* London: Simpkin, Marshall, 1872.

Ebsworth, Alfred. *Facts and Inferences Drawn from an Inspection of the Public Baths and Washhouses in This Metropolis.* London: William Brickhill, 1853.

Engineers and Officials: An Historical Sketch of the Progress of 'Health of Towns Works' in London and the Provinces. London: Edward Stanford, 1856.

Evatt, G.J.H. *Ambulance Organization, Equipment and Transport.* London: William Clowes, 1884.

[Farr, William]. *Report on the Nomenclature and Statistical Classification of Diseases for Statistical Returns.* London: Her Majesty's Stationery Office, 1856.

———. "Vital Statistics, or the Statistics of Health, Sickness, Diseases and Death." In *A Statistical Account of the British Empire: Exhibiting Its Extent, Physical Capacities, Population, Industry, and Civil and Religious Institutions,* 2 vols., ed. J.R. McCulloch, 1: 567–601. London: Charles Knight, 1837.

Gadd, W. Lawrence. *Soap Manufacture: A Practical Treatise on the Fabrication of Hard and Soft Soaps and Analytical Methods for the Determination of Their Chemical Composition.* London: George Bell, 1893.

Gay, John. *Disinfection and Disinfectants.* London: Allman, 1895.

Glen, William Cunningham. *The Law Relating to Public Health and Local Government.* Ed. Alexander Glen. 11th ed. London: Charles Knight, 1895.

Goodrich, W. Francis. *The Economic Disposal of Towns' Refuse.* London: P.S. King, 1901.

Granville, A.B. *The Great London Question of the Day; or, Can the Thames Sewage Be Converted into Gold?* London: Edward Stanford, 1865.

Guy, William Augustus. *Health of Towns' Association: Unhealthiness of Towns, and Its Causes and Remedies, Being a Lecture Delivered at Crosby Hall, Bishopsgate Street.* London: Charles Knight, 1845.

Hamilton, Robert. *Compulsory Notification of Infectious Diseases Considered.* London: J. and A. Churchill, 1883.

Hardwicke, William. *On the Moral and Physical Advantages of Baths and Washhouses*. London: Robert Hardwicke, 1874.

Haughton, Edward. *The Facts and Fallacies of the Turkish Bath Question; or, What Kind of Bath Shall We Have?* Dublin: William Robertson, 1860.

Hellyer, S. Stevens. *The Plumber and Sanitary Houses: A Practical Treatise on the Principles of Internal Plumbing Work, or the Best Means for Effectually Excluding Noxious Gases from Our Houses*. 4th ed. London: B. T. Batsford, 1887.

Herbert, Thomas. *The Law on Adulteration, Being the Sale of Food and Drugs Acts, 1875 and 1879, with Notes, Cases and Extracts from Official Reports*. London: Charles Knight, 1884.

Hime, Thomas Whiteside. *The Practical Guide to the Public Health Acts: A Vade Mecum for Officers of Health and Inspectors of Nuisances*. 2nd ed. London: Baillière, Tindall, and Cox, 1901.

Hoyle, William. *The Question of the Day; or, Facts and Figures for Electors and Politicians*. London: Simpkin, Marshall, 1874.

Hyndman, H. M. *A Commune for London*. London: Justice Printery, 1887.

Jenks, Edward. *An Outline of English Local Government*. London: Methuen, 1894.

Jennings, H. R. *Our Homes, and How to Beautify Them*. 3rd ed. London: Harrison, 1902.

Jensen, Gerard J. G. *Modern Drainage Inspection and Sanitary Surveys*. London: Sanitary Publishing Company, 1899.

Jerram, G. B. *Association of Public Sanitary Inspection: The Fourth Inaugural Address, November 6th 1886*. London: Potter, 1886.

Kilgour, Alexander. *Lectures on the Ordinary Agents of Life as Applicable to Therapeutics and Hygiene*. London: Longman, Rees, Orme, Brown, Green, Longman, 1834.

Krepp, Frederick Charles. *The Sewage Question: Being a General Review of all the Systems and Methods Hitherto Employed in Various Countries for Draining Cities and Utilizing Sewage*. London: Longmans, Green, 1867.

Latham, Baldwin. *Sanitary Engineering: A Guide to the Construction of Works of Sewerage and House Drainage*. London: E. and F. N. Spon, 1873.

Leach, Albert E. *Food Inspection and Analysis*. London: Chapman and Hall, 1904.

Letheby, Henry. *On the Estimation of the Sanitary Condition of Communities and the Comparative Salubrity of Towns*. London: Charles Knight, 1874.

———. *Report to the Honourable Commissioners of Sewers of the City of London, on Sewage and Sewer Gases, and on the Ventilation of Sewers*. London: M. Lownds, 1858.

———. *The Sewage Question: Comprising a Series of Reports: Being Investigations into the Condition of the Principal Sewage Farms and Sewage Works of the Kingdom*. London: Baillière, Tindall and Cox, 1872.

Lomax, Charles J. *Collection, Treatment and Disposal of Town Refuse*. Bolton: R. Whewell, 1892.

Maguire, William R. *Domestic Sanitary Drainage and Plumbing*. London: Kegan Paul, Trench and Trübner, 1890.

Maxwell, William H. *The Removal and Disposal of Town Refuse*. London: Sanitary Publishing Company, 1898.

McNeill, Roger. *The Prevention of Epidemics and the Construction and Management of Isolation Hospitals*. London: J. and A. Churchill, 1894.

Metcalfe, Richard. *Sanitas Sanitatum et Omnia Sanitas*. London: Co-operative Printing Company, 1877.

Metropolitan Working Classes' Association for Improving the Public Health. *Bathing and Personal Cleanliness*. London: John Churchill, 1847.

Mill, John Stuart. *On Liberty and Other Essays*. Ed. John Gray. Oxford: Oxford University Press, 1991.

Moore, E. C. S. *Sanitary Engineering: A Practical Treatise on the Collection, Removal and Final Disposal of Sewage*. 2nd ed. London: B. T. Batsford, 1901.

Morrell, J. Conyers. *The High Death Rate: An Answer to the Question, What Is to Be Done?* Manchester: Powlson, 1869.

Moule, Henry. *Town Refuse: The Remedy for Local Taxation*. London: William Ridgway, 1872.

Muir, Ramsay. *Peers and Bureaucrats*. London: Constable, 1910.

Newman, George. *Bacteriology and the Public Health*. 3rd ed. London: John Murray, 1904.

Newsholme, Arthur. *Elements of Vital Statistics*. London: Swann Sonnenschein, 1889.

———. *The Role of "Missed" Cases in the Spread of Infectious Diseases (a Lecture at the Victoria University of Manchester)*. London: Sherratt and Hughes, 1904.

Parkes, E. A. *Manuals of Health: On Personal Care of Health*. London: Society for Promoting Christian Knowledge, 1876.

Poore, George Vivian. *Essays on Rural Hygiene*. London: Longmans, Green, 1893.

Ransome, Arthur. *Statistical Review of Ten Years of Disease in Manchester and Salford, Being an Analysis of the Weekly Returns of Health and Meteorology Issued by the Manchester and Salford Sanitary Association, 1861–1870*. Manchester: Heywood, 1870.

Ransome, Arthur, and William Royston. *Remarks on Some of the Numerical Tests of the Health of Towns*. Manchester: Powlson, 1863.

Rawlinson, Robert. *Suggestions as to the Preparation of District Maps, and of the Plans for Main Sewerage, Drainage and Water Supply*. London: Charles Knight, 1878.

Raynes, F. W. *Domestic Sanitary Engineering and Plumbing*. London: Longmans, Green, 1909.

Reeves, Mrs. Pember. *Round About a Pound a Week*. London: George Bell, 1913.

Reynolds, Stephen. *A Poor Man's House*. London: John Lane, 1909.

Richardson, Benjamin Ward. *A Ministry of Health and Other Essays*. London: Chatto and Windus, 1879.

Rideal, Samuel. *Sewage and the Bacterial Purification of Sewage*. 3rd ed. London: Sanitary Publishing Company, 1906.

Robertson, William. *Meat and Food Inspection*. London: Baillière, Tindall and Cox, 1908.

Robinson, H. Mansfield, and Cecil H. Cribb. *The Law and Chemistry of Food and Drugs*. London: F. B. Rebman, 1895.

Roechling, H. Alfred. *Sewer Gas and Its Influence upon Health*. London: Biggs, 1898.

Rowley, J. J. *The Difficult and Vexed Question of the Age: Sewage of Towns: How to Dispose of It, by Making None*. Sheffield: Leader, 1884.

Rumsey, Henry Wyldbore. *Essays and Papers on Some Fallacies of Statistics Concerning Life and Death, Health and Disease, with Suggestions towards an Improved Registration System*. London: Smith, Elder, 1875.

———. *Essays on State Medicine*. London: John Churchill, 1856.

———. "The Health and Sickness of Town Populations." *New Quarterly Review; or Home, Foreign and Colonial Journal* 13 (April 1846): 1–42.

———. *On Sanitary Legislation and Administration in England: An Address*. London: John Churchill, 1857.

———. *On State Medicine in Great Britain and Ireland*. London: William Ridgway, 1867.

———. *Public Health: The Right Use of Records Founded on Local Facts*. London: John W. Parker, 1860.

Shimmin, Hugh. *Liverpool Sketches, Chiefly Reprinted from the "Porcupine."* London: W. Tweedie, 1862.

Simon, John. *English Sanitary Institutions, Reviewed in Their Course of Development, and in Some of Their Political and Social Relations*. London: Cassell, 1890.

Simpson, J. Y. *Proposal to Stamp Out Small-Pox and Other Contagious Diseases*. Edinburgh: Edmonston and Douglas, 1868.

Smiles, Samuel *Self-Help: With Illustrations of Character and Conduct*. London: John Murray, 1859.

———. *Thrift*. London: John Murray, 1875.

Smith, Edward. *Handbook for Inspectors of Nuisances*. London: Charles Knight, 1873.

———. *Manual for Medical Officers of Health*. London: Charles Knight, 1873.

Smith, J. Toulmin. *Government by Commissions Illegal and Pernicious: The Nature and Effects of All Commissions of Inquiry and Other Crown-Appointed Commissions*. London: S. Sweet, 1849.

———. *The Laws of England Relating to Public Health*. London: S. Sweet, 1848.

———. *Local Self-Government and Centralization: The Characteristics of Each; and Its Practical Tendencies, as Affecting Social, Moral and Political Welfare and Progress*. London: John Chapman, 1851.

———. *Local Self-Government Un-Mystified: A Vindication of Common Sense, Human Nature and Practical Improvement, against the Manifesto of Centralism Put Forth at the Social Science Association, 1857*. London: Edward Stanford, 1857.

———. *The Parish: Its Power and Obligations*. London: S. Sweet, 1854.

———. *Practical Proceedings for the Removal of Nuisances and Execution of Drainage Works in Every Parish, Town and Place in England and Wales, under the Nuisances Removal Act, 1855.* London: Henry Sweet, 1855.

Stevenson, Thomas, and Shirley F. Murphy, ed. *A Treatise on Hygiene and Public Health.* 3 vols. London: J. and A. Churchill, 1892–94.

Stewart, Alexander P., and Edward Jenkins, *The Medical and Legal Aspects of Sanitary Reform.* London: R. Hardwick, 1867.

Stockman, Frank Charles. *A Practical Guide for Sanitary Inspectors.* 2nd ed. London: Butterworth, 1894.

Sykes, John F. J. *Public Health Problems.* London: Walter Scott, 1892.

Taylor, Albert. *The Sanitary Inspector's Handbook.* 2nd ed. London: H. K. Lewis, 1897.

Taylor, Charles Bell. *For Liberty: A Speech.* Nottingham: Stevenson, Bailey and Smith, 1885.

Turner, Dawson W. *Dirt and Drink.* London: Longmans, 1884.

Urquhart, David. *The Pillars of Hercules; or, A Narrative of Travels in Spain and Morocco in 1848.* Vol. 2. London: Richard Bentley, 1850.

Vacher, Francis. *Address to the Royal Institute of Public Health: Congress at Blackpool, Conference of Sanitary Inspectors.* London: Baillière, Tindall and Cox, 1899.

———. *The Food Inspector's Handbook.* 4th ed. London: Sanitary Publishing Company, 1905.

[Ward, F. O.] "Sanitary Consolidation." *Quarterly Review* 88 (March 1851): 435–92.

Webb, Sidney. *The Reform of London.* London: Eighty Club, 1894.

Whitelegge, B. Arthur, and George Newman. *Hygiene and Public Health.* London: Cassell, 1905.

Willoughby, Edward F. *The Health Officer's Pocket-book: A Guide to Sanitary Practice and Law for Medical Officers of Health, Sanitary Inspectors and Members of Sanitary Authorities.* 2nd ed. London: Crosby Lockwood, 1902.

Wilson, Erasmus. *The Eastern or Turkish Bath: Its History, Revival in Britain and Application to the Purposes of Health.* London: John Churchill, 1861.

———. *Healthy Skin: A Popular Treatise on the Skin and Hair, Their Preservation and Management.* 5th ed. London: John Churchill, 1855.

Wilson, George. *Handbook of Sanitary Science.* 3rd ed. London: J. and A. Churchill, 1877.

[Wright, Thomas]. *Some Habits and Customs of the Working Classes.* London: Tinsley, 1867.

SECONDARY SOURCES

Ackerknecht, Erwin H. "Anticontagionism between 1821 and 1867." *Bulletin of the History of Medicine* 22, no. 5 (1948): 562–93.

Adams, Annmarie. *Architecture in the Family Way: Doctors, Houses and Women, 1870–1900.* Montreal: McGill-Queen's University Press, 1996.

Allen, Michelle. *Cleansing the City: Sanitary Geographies in Victorian London.* Athens: Ohio State University Press, 2008.

Arnold, David. *Colonizing the Body: State Medicine and Epidemic Disease in Nineteenth-Century India.* Berkeley: University of California Press, 1993.

Ayers, Gwendoline M. *England's First State Hospitals and the Metropolitan Asylums Board, 1867–1930.* London: Wellcome Institute, 1971.

Baldwin, Peter. "Beyond Weak and Strong: Rethinking the State in Comparative Policy History." *Journal of Policy History* 17, no. 1 (2005): 12–33.

———. *Contagion and the State in Europe, 1830–1930.* Cambridge: Cambridge University Press, 1999.

Bashford, Alison. *Imperial Hygiene: A Critical History of Colonialism, Nationalism and Public Health.* Basingstoke: Palgrave Macmillan, 2004.

Bellamy, Christine. *Administering Centre-Local Relations, 1871–1919: The Local Government Board in Its Fiscal and Cultural Context.* Manchester: Manchester University Press, 1988.

Bennett, Tony, and Patrick Joyce, eds. *Material Powers: Cultural Studies, History and the Material Turn.* London: Routledge, 2010.

Bentley, Michael. "'Boundaries' in Theoretical Language about the British State." In *The Boundaries of the State in Modern Britain*, ed. S. J. D. Green and R. C. Whiting, 29–56. Cambridge: Cambridge University Press, 1996.

Bevir, Mark. *Governance: A Very Short Introduction.* Oxford: Oxford University Press, 2012.

Booker, John. *Maritime Quarantine: The British Experience, c. 1650–1900.* Aldershot: Ashgate, 2007.

Braddick, Michael J. *State Formation in Early Modern England, c. 1550–1700.* Cambridge: Cambridge University Press, 2000.

Brand, Jeanne L. *Doctors and the State: The British Medical Profession and Government Action in Public Health, 1870–1912.* Baltimore: Johns Hopkins University Press, 1965.

Brenner, Joel Franklin. "Nuisance Law and the Industrial Revolution." *Journal of Legal Studies* 3, no. 2 (1974): 403–33.

Broich, John. *London: Water and the Making of the Modern City.* Pittsburgh, PA: University of Pittsburgh Press, 2013.

Brundage, Anthony. *England's "Prussian Minister": Edwin Chadwick and the Politics of Government Growth, 1832–1854.* University Park: Pennsylvania State University Press, 1988.

Brunton, Deborah. *The Politics of Vaccination: Practice and Policy in England, Wales, Ireland, and Scotland, 1800–1874.* Rochester, NY: University of Rochester Press, 2008.

Buchanan, R. A. *The Engineers: A History of the Engineering Profession in Britain, 1750–1914.* London: Jessica Kingsley, 1989.

Burney, Ian. *Bodies of Evidence: Medicine and the Politics of the English Inquest, 1830–1926.* Baltimore: Johns Hopkins University Press, 2000.

Burrow, J. W. *A Liberal Descent: Victorian Historians and the English Past.* Cambridge: Cambridge University Press, 1981.

Carroll, Patrick E. "Medical Police and the History of Public Health." *Medical History* 46, no. 4 (2002): 461–94.

Carter, K. Codell. "Causes of Disease and Causes of Death." *Continuity and Change* 12, no. 2 (1997): 189–98.

Clark, J. C. D. *English Society, 1660–1832: Religion, Ideology and Politics during the Ancien Regime.* 2nd ed. Cambridge: Cambridge University Press, 2000.

Crook, Tom. "Suspect Figures: Statistics and Public Trust in Victorian England." In *Statistics and the Public Sphere: Numbers and the People in Modern Britain, c. 1800–2000,* ed. Tom Crook and Glen O'Hara, 165–84. New York: Routledge, 2011.

Dandeker, Christopher. *Surveillance, Power and Modernity: Bureaucracy and Discipline from 1700 to the Present Day.* Oxford: Polity, 1990.

Daunton, M. J. *House and Home in the Victorian City: Working-Class Housing, 1850–1914.* London: Edward Arnold, 1983.

Davies, Celia. "The Health Visitor as Mother's Friend: A Woman's Place in Public Health, 1900–1914." *Social History of Medicine* 1, no. 1 (1988): 39–59.

Dobraszczyk, Paul. *Into the Belly of the Beast: Exploring London's Victorian Sewers.* Reading: Spire, 2009.

Doyle, Barry M. "The Changing Functions of Urban Governance: Councillors, Officials and Pressure Groups." In *The Cambridge Urban History of Britain,* vol. 3, 1840–1950, ed. Martin Daunton, 287–314. Cambridge: Cambridge University Press, 2000.

Duman, Daniel. "The Creation and Diffusion of a Professional Ideology in Nineteenth-Century England." *Sociological Review* 27, no. 1 (1979): 113–38.

Durbach, Nadja. *Bodily Matters: The Anti-Vaccination Movement in England, 1853–1907.* Durham, NC: Duke University Press, 2005.

Eastwood, David. "'Amplifying the Province of the Legislature': The Flow of Information and the English State in the Early Nineteenth Century." *Historical Research* 62, no. 149 (1989): 276–94.

———. *Government and Community in the English Provinces, 1700–1870.* Basingstoke: Palgrave Macmillan, 1997.

Ewald, François. "Norms, Discipline and the Law." *Representations* 30, no. 1 (1990): 138–61.

Eyler, John M. *Sir Arthur Newsholme and State Medicine, 1885–1935.* Cambridge: Cambridge University Press, 1997.

———. *Victorian Social Medicine: The Ideas and Methods of William Farr.* Baltimore: Johns Hopkins University Press, 1979.

Fabian, Johannes. *Time and the Other: How Anthropology Makes Its Object.* New York: Columbia University Press, 1983.

Fidler, David P. *International Law and Infectious Diseases.* Oxford: Clarendon, 1999.

Finer, S. E. *The Life and Times of Sir Edwin Chadwick.* London: Methuen, 1952.

Foucault, Michel. *"Society Must Be Defended": Lectures at the Collège de France, 1975–76.* Ed. Mauro Bertani and Alessandro Fontana. Trans. David Macey. London: Allen Lane, 2003.

Fraser, Derek. *The Evolution of the British Welfare State: A History of Social Policy since the Industrial Revolution.* 4th ed. Basingstoke: Palgrave Macmillan, 2009.

———. *Power and Authority in the Victorian City.* Oxford: Basil Blackwell, 1979.

Fritzsche, Peter. *Stranded in the Present: Modern Time and the Melancholy of History.* Cambridge, MA: Harvard University Press, 2004.

Gauchet, Marcel. *The Disenchantment of the World: A Political History of Religion.* Trans. Oscar Burge. Princeton, NJ: Princeton University Press, 1999.

Giddens, Anthony. *The Consequences of Modernity.* Oxford: Polity, 2004.

Gilbert, Pamela K. *Cholera and Nation: Doctoring the Social Body in Victorian England.* Albany: State University of New York Press, 2008.

———. *The Citizen's Body: Desire, Health, and the Social in Victorian England.* Athens: Ohio State University Press, 2007.

Goldman, Lawrence. *Science, Reform and Politics in Victorian Britain: The Social Science Association, 1857–1886.* Cambridge: Cambridge University Press, 2002.

Goodlad, Lauren M. E. *Victorian Literature and the Victorian State: Character and Governance in a Liberal Society.* Baltimore: Johns Hopkins University Press, 2003.

Greenaway, John. "British Conservatism and Bureaucracy." *History of Political Thought* 13, no. 1 (1992): 129–60.

Gunn, Simon, and James Vernon, eds. *The Peculiarities of Liberal Modernity in Imperial Britain.* Berkeley: University of California Press, 2011.

Hacking, Ian. *The Taming of Chance.* Cambridge: Cambridge University Press, 1990.

Halliday, Stephen. *The Great Stink of London: Sir Joseph Bazalgette and the Cleansing of the Victorian Metropolis.* Stroud: Sutton, 1999.

Hamlin, Christopher. *Cholera: The Biography.* Oxford: Oxford University Press, 2009.

———. "Muddling in Bumbledon: On the Enormity of Large Sanitary Improvements in Four British Towns, 1855–1885." *Victorian Studies* 32, no. 1 (1988): 55–83.

———. "Nuisances and Community in Mid-Victorian England: The Attractions of Inspection." *Social History* 38, no. 3 (2013): 346–79.

———. "Providence and Putrefaction: Victorian Sanitarians and the Natural Theology of Health and Disease." *Victorian Studies* 28, no. 3 (1985): 381–411.

———. "Public Health." In *The Oxford Handbook of the History of Medicine,* ed. Mark Jackson, 411–28. Oxford: Oxford University Press, 2011.

———. "Public Sphere to Public Health: The Transformation of 'Nuisance.'" In *Medicine, Health and the Public Sphere in Britain, 1600–2000,* ed. Steve Sturdy, 189–204. London: Routledge, 2002.

———. "Sanitary Policing and the Local State, 1873–1874: A Statistical Study of English and Welsh Towns." *Social History of Medicine* 18, no. 1 (2005): 39–61.

———. *A Science of Impurity: Water Analysis in Nineteenth Century Britain.* Berkeley: University of California Press, 1990.

Hanley, James G. "Parliament, Physicians, and Nuisances: The Demedicalization of Nuisance Law, 1831–1855." *Bulletin of the History of Medicine* 80, no. 4 (2006): 702–32.

Hardy, Anne. "'Death is the Cure of All Diseases': Using the General Register Office Cause of Death Statistics for 1837–1920," *Social History of Medicine* 7, no. 3 (1994): 472–92.

———. *The Epidemic Streets: Infectious Disease and the Rise of Preventive Medicine, 1856–1900.* Oxford: Clarendon, 1993.

———. "The Public in Public Health." In *Beyond Habermas: Democracy, Knowledge and the Public Sphere,* ed. Christian J. Emden and David Midgley, 87–98. New York: Berghahn Books, 2013.

Harling, Philip. "The Centrality of the Locality: The Local State, Local Democracy and Local Consciousness in Late-Victorian and Edwardian Britain." *Journal of Victorian Culture* 9, no. 2 (2004): 216–34.

Harris, Bernard. *The Origins of the British Welfare State: Social Welfare in England and Wales, 1800–1945.* Basingstoke: Palgrave Macmillan, 2004.

Harrison, Mark. *Contagion: How Commerce Has Spread Disease.* Padstow: Yale University Press, 2012.

———. *Public Health in British India: Anglo-Indian Preventive Medicine, 1859–1914.* Cambridge: Cambridge University Press, 1994.

Harvey, David. *The Condition of Postmodernity: An Enquiry into the Origin of Cultural Change.* Oxford: Basil Blackwell, 1989.

Hennock, E. P. *Fit and Proper Persons: Ideal and Reality in Nineteenth-Century Urban Government.* London: Edward Arnold, 1973.

Hewitt, Martin. "Why the Notion of Victorian Britain *Does* Make Sense." *Victorian Studies* 48, no. 3 (2006): 395–438.

Higgs, Edward. "The General Register Office and the Tabulation of Data, 1837–1939." In *The History of Mathematical Tables: From Sumer to Spreadsheets,* ed. Martin Campbell-Kelly, Mary Croarken, Raymond Flood, and Eleanor Robson, 209–34. Oxford: Oxford University Press, 2003.

———. *The Information State in England: The Central Collection of Information on Citizens since 1500.* Basingstoke: Palgrave MacMillan, 2004.

———. *Life, Death and Statistics: Civil Registration, Censuses and the Work of the General Register Office, 1836–1952.* Hatfield: Local Population Studies, 2004.

Hillier, Joseph. "The Rise of Constant Water in Nineteenth-Century London." *London Journal* 36, no. 1 (2011): 37–53.

Hilton, Boyd. *The Age of Atonement: The Influence of Evangelicalism on Social and Economic Thought, 1795–1865.* Oxford: Clarendon, 1988.

Hobsbawm, Eric. "Introduction: Inventing Traditions." In *The Invention of Tradition,* ed. Eric Hobsbawm and Terence Ranger, 1–14. Cambridge: Cambridge University Press, 1984.

Howlett, Peter, and Mary S. Morgan, eds. *How Well Do Facts Travel? The Dissemination of Reliable Knowledge.* Cambridge: Cambridge University Press, 2011.

Huber, Valeska. "The Unification of the Globe by Disease? The International Sanitary Conferences on Cholera, 1851–1894." *Historical Journal* 49, no. 2 (2006): 453–76.

Hugill, Peter J. "The Shrinking Victorian World." In *The Victorian World,* ed. Martin Hewitt, 73–89. Abingdon: Routledge, 2012.

Innes, Joanna, "Central Government 'Interference': Changing Conceptions, Practices, and Concerns, *c.* 1700–1850." In *Civil Society in British History: Ideas, Identities, Institutions,* ed. Jose Harris, 39–60. Oxford: Oxford University Press, 2003.

———. "Forms of 'Government Growth,' 1780–1830." In *Structures and Transformations in Modern British History,* ed. David Feldman and Jon Lawrence, 74–99. Cambridge: Cambridge University Press, 2011.

———. *Inferior Politics: Social Problems and Social Policies in Eighteenth-Century Britain.* Oxford: Oxford University Press, 2009.

Jessop, Bob. *State Power.* Cambridge: Polity, 2007.

Jones, H. S. *Victorian Political Thought.* Basingstoke: Macmillan, 2000.

Joyce, Patrick. *The Rule of Freedom: Liberalism and the Modern City.* London: Verso, 2003.

———. *The State of Freedom: A Social History of the British State since 1800.* Cambridge: Cambridge University Press, 2013.

Kelley, Victoria. *Soap and Water: Cleanliness, Dirt and the Working Classes in Victorian and Edwardian Britain.* London: I. B. Tauris, 2010.

Kidd, Alan, and Terry Wyke, eds. *The Challenge of Cholera: Proceedings of the Manchester Special Board of Health, 1831–1833.* Bristol: The Record Society of Lancashire and Cheshire, 2010.

King, Anthony. "Hospital Planning: Revised Thoughts on the Origin of the Pavilion Principle in England." *Medical History* 10, no. 4 (1966): 360–73.

Koch, Tom. "1831: The Map That Launched the Idea of Global Health." *International Journal of Epidemiology* 43, no. 4 (2014): 1014–20.

Koselleck, Reinhart. *Futures Past: On the Semantics of Historical Time.* Trans. Keith Tribe. New York: Columbia University Press, 2004.

———. *The Practice of Conceptual History: Timing History, Spacing Concepts.* Trans. Todd Samuel Presner. Stanford, CA: Stanford University Press, 2002.

La Berge, Ann F. "Edwin Chadwick and the French Connection." *Bulletin of the History of Medicine* 62, no. 1 (1988): 23–41.

———. *Mission and Method: The Early Nineteenth-Century French Public Health Movement.* Cambridge: Cambridge University Press, 1992.

Lambert, Royston. *Sir John Simon, 1816–1904, and English Sanitary Administration.* London: Macgibbon and Kee, 1963.

Laxton, Paul, and Richard Rodger, *Insanitary City: Henry Littlejohn and the Condition of Edinburgh.* Lancaster: Carnegie, 2014.

Lewis, Brian. *"So Clean": Lord Leverhulme, Soap and Civilization.* Manchester: Manchester University Press, 2008.

Lewis, Jane. "The Boundary between Voluntary and Statutory Social Service in the Late Nineteenth and Early Twentieth Centuries." *Historical Journal* 39, no. 1 (1996): 155–77.

Lewis, R. A. *Edwin Chadwick and the Public Health Movement.* London: Longmans and Green, 1952.

Levine, Philippa. *Prostitution, Race, and Politics: Policing Venereal Disease in the British Empire.* New York: Routledge, 2003.

Lucey, Donnacha Seán, and Virginia Crossman, eds. *Healthcare in Ireland and Britain from 1850: Voluntary, Regional and Comparative Perspectives*. London: Institute of Historical Research, 2014.

Luckin, Bill. *Pollution and Control: A Social History of the Thames in the Nineteenth Century*. Bristol: Adam Hilger, 1986.

MacDonagh, Oliver. "The Nineteenth-Century Revolution in Government: A Reappraisal." *Historical Journal* 1, no. 1 (1958): 52–67.

MacLeod, Roy, ed. *Government and Expertise: Specialists, Administrators and Professionals, 1860–1919*. Cambridge: Cambridge University Press, 1988.

Maglen, Krista. *The English System: Quarantine, Immigration and the Making of a Port Sanitary Zone*. Manchester: Manchester University Press, 2014.

Magnello, Eileen. "The Introduction of Mathematical Statistics into Medical Research: The Roles of Karl Pearson, Major Greenwood, and Austin Bradford Hill." In *The Road to Medical Statistics*, ed. Eileen Magnello and Anne Hardy, 95–123. Amsterdam: Rodopi, 2002.

Mandler, Peter. *Aristocratic Government in the Age of Reform: Whigs and Liberals, 1830–1852*. Oxford: Clarendon, 1990.

———. "Introduction: State and Society in Victorian Britain." In *Liberty and Authority in Victorian Britain*, ed. Peter Mandler, 1–21. Oxford: Oxford University Press, 2006.

Manent, Pierre. *A World beyond Politics? A Defense of the Nation-State*. Trans. Marc LePain. Princeton, NJ: Princeton University Press, 2006.

Marsden, Ben, and Crosbie Smith. *Engineering Empires: A Cultural History of Technology in Nineteenth-Century Britain*. Basingstoke: Palgrave Macmillan, 2005.

McClintock, Anne. *Imperial Leather: Race, Gender and Sexuality in the Colonial Contest*. London: Routledge, 1995.

McLean, David. *Public Health and Politics in the Age of Reform: Cholera, the State and the Royal Navy in Victorian Britain*. London: I. B. Tauris, 2006.

Meadowcroft, James. *Conceptualizing the State: Innovation and Dispute in British Political Thought, 1880–1914*. Oxford: Clarendon, 1995.

Mitchell, Timothy. *Rule of Experts: Egypt, Techno-Politics, Modernity*. Berkeley: University of California Press, 2002.

Mooney, Graham. "Infection and Citizenship: (Not) Visiting Isolation Hospitals in Mid-Victorian Britain." In *Permeable Walls: Historical Perspectives on Hospital and Asylum Visiting*, ed. Graham Mooney and Jonathan Reinarz, 147–73. Amsterdam: Rodopi, 2009.

———. "Professionalization in Public Health and the Measurement of Sanitary Progress in Nineteenth-Century England and Wales." *Social History of Medicine* 10, no. 1 (1997): 53–78.

———. "Public Health versus Private Practice: The Contested Development of Compulsory Infectious Disease Notification in Late Nineteenth-Century Britain." *Bulletin of the History of Medicine* 73, no. 2 (1999): 238–67.

———. "'A Tissue of the Most Flagrant Anomalies': Smallpox and the Centralisation of Sanitary Administration in Late Nineteenth-Century London." *Medical History* 41, no. 3 (1997): 261–90.

Nathanson, Constance A. *Disease Prevention as Social Change: The State, Society, and Public Health in the United States, France, Great Britain, and Canada.* New York: Russell Sage Foundation, 2007.

Newman, Kira L. S. "Shutt Up: Bubonic Plague and Quarantine in Early Modern England." *Journal of Social History* 45, no. 3 (2012): 809–34.

Olstein, Diego. *Thinking History Globally.* Basingstoke: Palgrave Macmillan, 2015.

Osborne, Peter. *The Politics of Time: Modernity and Avant-Garde.* London: Verso, 1995.

Otter, Chris. *The Victorian Eye: A Political History of Light and Vision in Britain, 1800–1910.* Chicago: University of Chicago Press, 2008.

Parry, Jonathan. *The Politics of Patriotism: English Liberalism, National Identity and Europe, 1830–1886.* Cambridge: Cambridge University Press, 2006.

———. *The Rise and Fall of Liberal Government in Victorian Britain.* New Haven, CT: Yale University Press, 1993.

Pelling, Margaret. *Cholera, Fever and English Medicine, 1825–1865.* Oxford: Oxford University Press, 1978.

Perkin, Harold. *The Rise of Professional Society: England since 1880.* London: Routledge, 1990.

Pickstone, John V. "Dearth, Dirt and Fever Epidemics: Rewriting the History of British 'Public Health,' 1780–1850." In *Epidemics and Ideas: Essays on the Historical Perception of Pestilence,* ed. Terence Ranger and Paul Slack, 125–48. Cambridge: Cambridge University Press, 1992.

———. *Ways of Knowing: A New History of Science, Technology and Medicine.* Manchester: Manchester University Press, 2000.

Poovey, Mary. *A History of the Modern Fact: Problems of Knowledge in the Sciences of Wealth and Society.* Chicago: University of Chicago Press, 1998.

———. *Making a Social Body: British Cultural Formation, 1830–1864.* Chicago: University of Chicago Press, 1995.

Porter, Bernard. "'Bureau and Barrack': Early Victorian Attitudes towards the Continent." *Victorian Studies* 27, no. 4 (1984): 407–33.

Porter, Dorothy. *Health, Civilization and the State: A History of Public Health from Ancient to Modern Times.* London: Routledge, 1999.

———, ed. *The History of Public Health and the Modern State.* Amsterdam: Rodopi, 1994.

Porter, Dorothy, and Roy Porter. "What Was Social Medicine? An Historiographical Essay." *Historical Sociology* 1, no. 1 (1988): 90–109.

Porter, Theodore M. *The Rise of Statistical Thinking, 1820–1900.* Princeton, NJ: Princeton University Press, 1986.

———. *Trust in Numbers: The Pursuit of Objectivity in Science and Public Life.* Princeton, NJ: Princeton University Press, 1996.

Prest, John. *Liberty and Locality: Parliament, Permissive Legislation and Ratepayers' Democracies in the Nineteenth Century.* Oxford: Clarendon, 1990.

Price, Richard. *British Society, 1680–1880: Dynamism, Containment and Change.* Cambridge: Cambridge University Press, 1999.

Prochaska, Frank. *Christianity and Social Service in Modern Britain: The Disinherited Spirit.* Oxford: Oxford University Press, 2006.

Pugh, Martin. *The Making of Modern British Politics, 1867–1939.* 2nd ed. Oxford: Basil Blackwell, 1996.

Randeraad, Nico. *States and Statistics in the Nineteenth Century: Europe by Numbers.* Trans. Debra Molnar. Manchester: Manchester University Press, 2010.

Rawcliffe, Carole. *Urban Bodies: Communal Health in Late Medieval English Towns and Cities.* Woodbridge: Boydell, 2013.

Riley, James C. *The Eighteenth-Century Campaign to Avoid Disease.* Basingstoke: Macmillan, 1987.

Ritvo, Harriet. *The Dawn of Green: Manchester, Thirlmere, and Modern Environmentalism.* Chicago: University of Chicago Press, 2009.

Rose, Nikolas. *Powers of Freedom: Reframing Political Thought.* Cambridge: Cambridge University Press, 1999.

Rosenthal, Leslie. *The River Pollution Dilemma in Victorian England: Nuisance Law versus Economic Efficiency.* Farnham: Ashgate, 2014.

Rusnock, Andrea A. *Vital Accounts: Quantifying Health and Population in Eighteenth-Century England and France.* Cambridge: Cambridge University Press, 2002.

Saunier, Pierre-Yves. *Transnational History.* Basingstoke: Palgrave Macmillan, 2013.

Saunier, Pierre-Yves, and Shane Ewen, eds. *Another Global City: Historical Explorations into the Transnational Municipal Moment, 1850–2000.* New York: Palgrave, 2008.

Schneider, Daniel. *Hybrid Nature: Sewage Treatment and the Contradictions of the Industrial Ecosystem.* Cambridge, MA: MIT Press, 2011.

Schweber, Libby. *Disciplining Statistics: Demography and Vital Statistics in France and England, 1830–1885.* Durham, NC: Duke University Press, 2006.

Scott, James C. *Seeing Like a State: How Certain Schemes to Improve the Human Condition Have Failed.* New Haven, CT: Yale University Press, 1998.

Searle, G.R. *The Quest for National Efficiency: A Study in British Politics and Political Thought, 1899–1914.* London: Ashfield, 1990.

Sheard, Sally. "Profit Is a Dirty Word: The Development of Public Baths and Wash-houses in Britain, 1847–1915." *Social History of Medicine* 13, no. 1 (2000): 62–85.

Skinner, Quentin. "The State." In *Political Innovation and Conceptual Change,* ed. Terence Ball, James Farr, and Russell L. Hanson, 90–126. Cambridge: Cambridge University Press, 1989.

Slack, Paul. *From Reformation to Improvement: Public Welfare in Early Modern England.* Oxford: Clarendon, 1999.

———. *The Impact of Plague in Tudor and Stuart England.* Oxford: Clarendon, 1990.

Smith, Virginia. *Clean: A History of Personal Hygiene and Purity.* Oxford: Oxford University Press, 2007.

Stark, James F. *The Making of Modern Anthrax, 1875–1920: Uniting Local, National and Global Histories of Disease.* London: Pickering and Chatto, 2013.

Steinmetz, George. *State/Culture: State-Formation after the Cultural Turn.* Ithaca, NY: Cornell University Press, 1999.

Szreter, Simon. *Fertility, Class and Gender, 1860–1940.* Cambridge: Cambridge University Press, 1996.

———. "The GRO and the Public Health Movement in Britain, 1837–1914." *Social History of Medicine* 4, no. 3 (1991): 435–63.

Taylor, Jeremy. *Hospital and Asylum Architecture in England, 1840–1914: Building for Health Care.* London: Mansell, 1991.

Taylor, Vanessa, and Frank Trentmann. "Liquid Politics: Water and the Politics of Everyday Life in the Modern City." *Past and Present*, no. 211 (2011): 199–241.

Trentmann, Frank. "Materiality in the Future of History: Things, Practices and Politics." *Journal of British Studies* 48, no. 2 (2009): 283–307.

Vernon, James. *Distant Strangers: How Britain Became Modern.* Berkeley: University of California Press, 2014.

Vigarello, Georges. *Concepts of Cleanliness: Changing Attitudes in France since the Middle Ages.* Trans. Jean Birrel. Cambridge: Cambridge University Press, 1988.

Vincent, David. *The Culture of Secrecy: Britain, 1832–1998.* Oxford: Oxford University Press, 1998.

Waddington, Keir. *The Bovine Scourge: Meat, Tuberculosis and Public Health, 1850–1914.* Woodbridge: Boydell, 2006.

Wagner, Peter. *Modernity as Experience and Interpretation: A New Sociology of Modernity.* Cambridge: Polity, 2008.

Waller, P.J. *Town, City and Nation: England, 1850–1914.* Oxford: Oxford University Press, 1983.

Wear, Andrew. "The History of Personal Hygiene." In *Companion Encyclopaedia of the History of Medicine,* ed. W.F. Bynum and Roy Porter, 2: 1283–308. London: Routledge, 1997.

Weinstein, Ben. *Liberalism and Local Government in Early Victorian London.* Woodbridge: Boydell and Brewer, 2011.

———. "'Local Self-Government Is True Socialism': Joshua Toulmin Smith, the State and Character Formation." *English Historical Review* 123, no. 504 (2008): 1193–228.

Williams, Perry. "The Laws of Health: Women, Medicine and Sanitary Reform, 1850–1900." In *Science and Sensibility: Gender and Scientific Enquiry, 1780–1945,* ed. Marina Benjamin, 60–88. Oxford: Basil Blackwell, 1991.

Wohl, Anthony S. *Endangered Lives: Public Health in Victorian Britain.* London: Methuen, 1984.

Worboys, Michael. *Spreading Germs: Disease Theories and Medical Practice in Britain, 1865–1900.* Cambridge: Cambridge University Press, 2000.

———. "Was There a Bacteriological Revolution in Late Nineteenth-Century Medicine?" *Studies in History and Philosophy of Biological and Biomedical Sciences* 38, no. 1 (2007): 20–42.

Zürn, Michael. "Global Governance as Multi-Level Governance." In *The Oxford Handbook of Governance*, ed. David Levi-Faur, 730–44. Oxford: Oxford University Press, 2012.

Zweiniger-Bargielowska, Ina. *Managing the Body: Beauty, Health and Fitness in Britain, 1880–1939*. Oxford: Oxford University Press, 2010.

Index